Embodied Rhe...

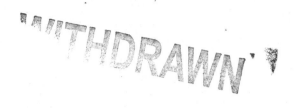

D1565380

Embodied Rhetorics

Disability in Language and Culture

Edited by
James C. Wilson and
Cynthia Lewiecki-Wilson

Southern Illinois University Press
Carbondale and Edwardsville

Library of Congress Cataloging-in-Publication Data

Embodied rhetorics : disability in language and culture / edited by
James C. Wilson and Cynthia Lewiecki-Wilson.
   p. cm.
   Includes bibliographical references and index.
   1. Handicapped—Social conditions. 2. Handicapped—Education. 3.
Handicapped in literature. 4. Handicapped in mass media. 5.
Rhetoric. 6. Language and culture. 7. Language and education. I.
Wilson, James C., 1948– II. Lewiecki-Wilson, Cynthia.

HV1568 .E45 2001
305.9'0816—dc21
ISBN 0-8093-2393-1 (pbk. : alk. paper)   00-050473

The paper used in this publication meets the minimum requirements of American National Standard for Information Sciences—Permanence of Paper for
Printed Library Materials, ANSI Z39.48-1992. ⊗

Contents

Part Three: Cultural and Spatial Rhetorics of Disability

Figures and Tables

Preface

Many streams, flowing together, have contributed to the creation of *Embodied Rhetorics*. This book emerges from the confluence of our personal and professional lives and is fed by the tributaries of several academic disciplines. As parents of a disabled child, as teachers of college writing, and as active members of the disability community, we have come to understand the interconnection of rhetoric and disability. In the nearly twenty years since our son was born, a wide array of scholarship on the social construction of knowledge and postmodern discourse in rhetoric/composition, feminism, postcolonial studies, and later in disability studies provided us with theories and modes of analysis that helped us make sense of our experiences and generalize beyond our own situation to critically analyze social constructions of disability.

When the field of disability studies emerged in the 1990s, we began to bring the private and public streams of our lives together. Because of our experiences parenting our son—grappling with school systems, co-constructing individual education plans, and brainstorming alternative ways of learning—we felt better enabled to meet the needs of the growing number of disabled students appearing in our classes. According to the American Council on Education, 154,520, or 9.4 percent of college freshmen identified themselves in 1998 as having some kind of disability, and of that number 41 percent reported having a learning disability. In light of these facts, merging the two streams of our lives not only made sense but seemed imperative. There is a need for those in higher education to learn more about disability studies. After all, one powerful reason why college professors, and especially compositionists who teach first-year students, should be interested in becoming more theoretically informed about disability is that they will have increasing numbers of disabled students in their classrooms. We also feel that the new field of disability studies has much to learn from rhetoric/composition, which has always paid attention to the learning processes of students in the classroom even as it has developed a body of scholarly work on the social construction of knowledge, histories of rhetoric, and literacy practices. All these currents joined together to form *Embodied Rhetorics*.

Our title refers to the body, by which the disabled have historically been defined, and to rhetoric in the plural to indicate that there are many kinds of rhetoric that have been and can be deployed about disability. The title further signifies that rhetoric is closely aligned with the body and that rhetorical arguments appear in embodied forms. Arguments about disability or the place of the disabled are embodied in social spaces and cultural practices (e.g., curb cuts, wheelchair ramps and lifts, or the lack thereof), embodied in pedagogies, expressed through bodies and adaptive technologies (ASL, voice synthesizers, adapted computer keyboards), as well as in a variety of discourses both within and beyond those traditionally classified as rhetoric.

The essays collected here are arranged in categories—Identity and Rhetoricity, Rhetorics of Literacy, and Cultural and Spatial Rhetorics—meant to evoke both familiar *topoi* and to complicate commonplace assumptions about subjectivity, education, and culture. The essays touch on a number of disabilities—various physical disabilities, mental illness, diseases such as multiple sclerosis and AIDS, deafness, learning disabilities, and blindness. However, they are not meant to represent (or limit) types of disability; rather, they suggest the range of interests and diverse methods of analysis employed by disability studies scholars working at the intersection of several disciplines. Each of the authors is positioned differently in relation to disability as well as to language theory. Several are themselves disabled, or have family members who are disabled, as we do. While all the authors collected here regard their analytic approaches and epistemology as evidencing a disability studies perspective, each essay establishes its own critical relationship to definitions of disability and postmodern theories of language. The authors also come from various academic fields—English studies, education, history, and sociology—and thus consider the relations between discourse and disability from different critical positions and epistemologies. The collected essays present a range of views and employ differing methodologies: historical excavation and interpretation, rhetorical analysis, redeployment of theory, reflective narrative, literary analysis, Marxist analysis, historical study of rhetoric, and interpretation of cultural codes, practices, and images. Comprising conversation and contestation, the collection, as a whole, is thus rhetorical.

Chapter 1, "Disability, Rhetoric, and the Body," contests everyday thinking about disability as a bodily defect. We argue for its social and political constitution in culture, and we lay out our theoretical reasons for aligning rhetoric/composition and disability studies: disability studies contributes to an understanding of postmodern rhetoric as an embodied rhetoric of difference. In arguing for a postmodern view of rhetoric as the art of critique, refutation, position, and action, we are entering into debate with the contributors who follow rather than laying down foundational principles to which all adhere.

The five essays in part one explore subjectivity and identity. Holmes and Couser examine the rhetorical strategies in autobiographical narratives from Victorian England and contemporary memoirs, respectively, whereby the disabled use, elude, resist, or rewrite the culturally authorized scripts of disability identity. Krummel recounts her struggles to construct her own identity after being diagnosed with MS, a struggle that enriches her understanding that the self is composed of diverse subjectivities, and this, in turn, influences her teaching. Taken together, the very different essays of Prendergast and Erevelles show how disability provides a critical perspective from which to rethink the construction of subjectivity, out of which concepts of individual "rights" flow. Prendergast examines the loss of rhetorical agency in the case of schizophrenia and criticizes a "rhetoric of rights" that regards the mentally disabled as needing not treatment but "social empowerment and liberation"; she also notes the lack of "a corresponding rhetoric of public responsibility" that leaves the mentally disabled wandering the streets or in jail. Approaching the disabled subject through a Marxist analysis, Erevelles criticizes postmodern readings of the material body and contests a merely rhetorical theory of the disabled body. She uses disability as a critical theoretical category with which to analyze labor and subjectivity under capitalism. Actively excluded from a productive role in the economy, the disabled are thus excluded in capitalism from anything but a "debilitating" subjectivity as dependent, even "parasitical."

The three essays in part two expose the conflicts between dominant literacy education and the particular needs and interests of the disabled, conflicts that may lead to clashes, resistance, or withdrawal. Brueggemann argues that deaf students are "contained" and "restrained" by a literacy education that severs the two parts of Quintilian's concept of the "good man speaking well" and emphasizes pragmatic communication over language used for expressive interaction, social growth, and civic life. The effect on deaf students has been a "violence of literacy." From her standpoint as both a disabled student and a disabled teacher (of disabled and nondisabled students), Lott analyzes classroom identity and authority and explores teacher and student strategies for confronting cultural assumptions about disability and challenging limiting conceptions of normalcy. Joyner, working with primary materials from the Brashear-Lawrence Family Papers at the University of North Carolina, explores the conflict in one Louisiana family created by the cultural shift in Deaf education from manualism to oralism.

The authors in part three read the meanings of disability in cultural images and social spaces. Barton documents the representations of disability in the United Way campaigns in the Detroit area in the 1940s and 1950s. She concludes that these charity campaigns erased the complexity of the experiences of the disabled, replacing them with stereotypes of pity and fear, with images emphasizing success, and with a focus "extolling the United Way as a model American business"—all of which maintained the segregation of the disabled. Michalko and Titchkosky examine the spatial rhetoric of public places, which are oriented to the nondisabled. After discussing the "intentionality" of this inhospitable environment, they critique the common response of "pragmatically justified exclusion." Nye examines the rhetoric of AIDS as a recent example of the social construction of disability and documents the language and metaphors commonly used to describe AIDS. These include military metaphors, end-of-the-world metaphors, plague metaphors, and contamination or pollution metaphors. Against these, she proposes a new taxonomy of AIDS discourse. In the final essay, Franks analyzes the presence and meaning of disability in the first one hundred Grimms' fairy tales. Her findings are not what most readers would expect: 75 percent of disabled characters play "positive" roles (as heroes, heroines, helpers, donors, and dispatchers). Her conclusion is that "fairy tales do *not* convey an overwhelmingly negative picture of the function of disability." However, the positive picture of disability presented in Grimms' fairy tales contrasts with negative messages about disability that Franks's students later remembered.

Transforming disability includes transforming its negative legacy, as well as promoting active social change and more opportunities for the disabled, but it also entails more than just including the disabled. True transformation would permeate the entire social order and generate changes in economic organization, ethical thought, educational practices, the organization and design of social space, and the interactions and habits of people in all aspects of daily living. We hope the essays collected here contribute to this larger transformation.

We wish to acknowledge our debt to the Society for Disability Studies and to the disability community. We would particularly like to thank Brenda Jo Brueggemann for her friendship, collegiality, and support as well as for her brilliance in convening "Enabling the Humanities: A Colloquium on Disability Studies in Higher Education" in April 1998 at The Ohio State University, where so many of us working in disability studies exchanged ideas and were enriched by our mutual endeavors and experiences. We also want to thank Martha Stoddard Holmes for her diplomacy in moderating the boisterous, sometimes contentious DS-HUM listserv.

At Southern Illinois University Press, we would like to thank editor Karl Kageff for his support and guidance and reviewers of this manuscript, Gary Olson and Patricia A. Dunn, for their enthusiasm and helpful suggestions. In gratitude, we dedicate this book to all the members, families, and friends of the disability community and, of course, especially to our son Sam Wilson.

Embodied Rhetorics

1

Disability, Rhetoric, and the Body
James C. Wilson and Cynthia Lewiecki-Wilson

[T]he body provides a point of mediation between what is perceived as purely internal and accessible only to the subject and what is external and publicly observable, a point from which to rethink the opposition between the inside and the outside, the private and the public, the self and other, and all the other binary pairs associated with the mind/body opposition.
— Elizabeth Grosz, *Volatile Bodies: Toward a Corporeal Feminism*

Language sustains the body not by bringing it into being or feeding it in a literal way; rather, it is by being interpellated within the terms of language that a certain social existence of the body first becomes possible. To understand this, one must imagine an impossible scene, that of a body that has not yet been given social definition, a body that is, strictly speaking, not accessible to us, that nevertheless becomes accessible on the occasion of an address, a call, an interpellation that does not 'discover' this body, but constitutes it fundamentally.
— Judith Butler, *Excitable Speech: A Politics of the Performative*

[L]et there be a law that no deformed child shall be reared.
— Aristotle, *The Politics*

A project of disability studies scholars and the disability rights movement has been to bring into sharp relief the processes by which disability has been imbued with the meaning(s) it has and to reassign a meaning that is consistent with a sociopolitical analysis of disability.
— Simi Linton, *Claiming Disability: Knowledge and Identity*

Disability in Language and Culture

At first glance, Simi Linton's call to "reassign" a sociopolitical meaning to disability might seem to be an example of postmodernist social (re)construction at its most excessive, identity politics carried to an extreme, language presuming to alter fact. After all, when Americans think, talk, and write about disability, they usually consider it as a tragedy, illness, or defect that an individual body "has"—that is, as personal and accidental, before or without sociopolitical significance. Although this commonplace view of disability may feel as right as common sense, we cite Judith Butler to point out that this version of disability is actually "an impossible scene." As the citation from Aristotle makes clear, disability has had a political definition—of exclusion—for well over two thousand years. Why is disability still strongly "imbued" with a meaning that not only points to the personal but actually restricts thinking about disability in any other way? We argue that this "natural" view of disability is tied to the dominant views of language and the body, and we turn to Judith Butler, in part, for an explanation. Language functions performatively, in Butler's term, as an address interpellating the body, not "discovering" but calling this naturalized meaning of disability into circulation, where it accords with and reinforces a host of other dualities such as "the inside and the outside, the private and the public, the self and other, and all the other binary pairs associated with the mind/ body opposition," in the words of Elizabeth Grosz. This view of disability persists, then, as a component of the old and familiar dualist tradition.

One of the most familiar and powerful of these binaries casts language in opposition to the world. Such a construction assumes "the *mental*" rather than "the *material* character" of discourse (Laclau and Mouffe 108), and a reflective rather than a productive relation between language and material reality (Williams 38). In arguing against the dualist tradition, we cite cultural studies and new left theory, corporeal feminism, and postmodern rhetoric, not to elide their different approaches to materiality and discourse but to suggest some possible openings for rethinking the relations of disability to rhetoric and the material world and to suggest possible alignments that could help in the project of transforming the social order.

Postmodern rhetoricians argue that rhetoric is not a neutral "instrument" to reflect or describe the world, not the art of "rational" debate, but the art of critique, refutation, position, and action. Understanding that all language practices are positioned and interested, postmodern rhetoricians analyze and study the history of the relations between language and power. Although it is defined negatively, postmodern rhetoric nevertheless is deeply concerned with issues of justice (see Fleming; Miller and Bowden; and Jarratt, "Using Postmodern"). Classical rhetoric traditionally has had the restricted meaning of persuasive argument in civic debate. But disability activists—who actively monitor and lobby Congress and the courts (e.g., *Mouth: Voice of the Disability Nation*), reeducate the public from a disability perspective, and write and speak for change—illustrate that, from a postmodern perspective, classical and postmodern rhetorics really are not separable. From a postmodern perspective, refutation, persuasion, and action are mutually constituted out of the position and goals of the speaker/writer. Postmodern rhetoricians extend rhetorical analyses beyond an immediate text to investigate the interconnections of language and material practices. Some examples might be ethnographic studies of community literacy, studies of institutional uses of language and resulting actions, rhetorical cultural studies of media images and ads, or studies of language violence such as hate speech linked to crimes. Such studies demonstrate that understanding the materiality of discursive structures, as political philosophers Laclau and Mouffe contend, is a key step in understanding the "discursive conditions [necessary] for the emergence of a collective action" (153). Indeed, disability activists working for change have been attuned to the ways that discourse can aid collective action, for example, seizing the term *cripple* and turning it against itself into the proactive label *crip culture* (see, e.g., *Vital Signs: Crip Culture Talks Back*). Because the disabled have always been defined as deviant bodies, "corporeal feminism," which rethinks the body as a "site of the mutually constitutive interaction" between discourses and materiality (Balsamo 163), also has much to offer a disability studies analysis, as does Butler's theory of language as a social performative. Her comments on language's relation to subject/identity formation have special resonance for the disabled subject: "The terms that facilitate recognition are themselves conventional," she writes, "the effects and instruments of a social ritual that decide, often through exclusion and violence, the linguistic conditions of survivable subjects" (5). As evidence for Butler's point, consider Aristotle's command, cited above, which is at once shocking and conventional, a social ritual of exclusion and violence that the disabled are still struggling against today.

The proposition that language is constitutive of social practices becomes particularly discernible, we argue, through an analysis of disability. Nevertheless, however constitutive discourse practices are, we also recognize that language's effects are dispersed, uneven, and contradictory.[1] People wield language for many purposes, but at the same time language's effects also spill or seep out, beyond the immediate container of the situation and "intent" for which it was crafted. Language can only be partly harnessed as an instrument of agency, never wholly so, for it always carries along many other material histories and purposes and the arbitrary and differential traces of its systematic functioning. If language can be said to transform economic systems, institutions, and social practices, then its power flows diffusely in uneven currents.[2] Although the authors collected here do not all necessarily agree on what language can or cannot do or its role in the sociopolitical meaning of disability, their essays demonstrate that the work of "reassigning" meaning to disability begins with analyzing the ways the disabled have been and are inscribed in language and culture.

Disability as Exclusion

When George Bush signed the 1990 Americans with Disabilities Act, he used a metaphor engendered by the end of the cold war and the fall of the Berlin Wall to mark the occasion: "And now I sign legislation which takes a sledgehammer to another wall, one which has, for too many generations, separated Americans with disabilities from the freedom they could glimpse, but not grasp." Frankly political, cast in terms of the drama of the communist East versus the free capitalist West (not in a metaphor of the American civil rights movement, for example), Bush's rhetoric initiates a reversal in the excluded status of the disabled since Aristotle. This rhetorical move seeks to perform a coming in out of the cold, so to speak, a return from the civic, indeed literal, death of Aristotle's imperative in *The Politics,* just as the historic ADA law itself marks a start of the reversal of legal exclusion. Such beginnings are tentative, however. Linking "freedom" for the disabled with the capitalist West gestures a reversal, but it also obscures the fact that the social order of capitalism itself remains a very real structure of exclusion for those (disabled) people who cannot participate in an exchange economy by selling their labor (see Erevelles, in part one). In the present situation of worldwide capitalist culture, subjectivity and agency are generated primarily through work and consumption. Thus, economic exclusion is a very real barrier, obstructing access for the disabled not only to the means for securing their livelihood but also to the usual ways of producing subjectivity and agency.

The definition of disability as exclusion and lack of agency forms the basis of legal discourse about disability. For example, *Black's Law Dictionary,* the professional standard, defines disability as "the want of legal capability to perform an act. Term is generally used to indicate an incapacity for the full employment of ordinary legal rights; thus, persons under age, insane persons, and convicts are said to be under legal disability" (461). *Black's* extends this general definition to specific legal issues and creates a taxonomy of disability that rates degrees and kinds of exclusion: General, Specific, Personal, Absolute, Civil (or Legal), Physical, Partial, Permanent, Temporary, Total. Thus the disabled person becomes one who "lacks legal capacity to act *sui juris* or one who is physically or mentally disabled from acting in his own behalf or from pursuing occupation" (462). In its most extreme form, this denial of agency can result in what is known legally as "Civil Death."[3]

While the origins of exclusionary practices are ancient, and the forms many and sociopolitically specific, the consequences of exclusion and denial of agency, of disability as a metaphoric "Civil Death," can be seen in the material conditions of the lives of the disabled. Over two-thirds of all people with disabilities in the United States are both unemployed and living at or below the poverty line (see *Closing the Gap*). Recent statistics, including those compiled by the 1998 National Organization on Disability/Harris Survey, suggest that the percentages have actually increased since the 1990 passage of the Americans with Disabilities Act (ADA). The stated purpose of the ADA was "to provide a clear and comprehensive national mandate for the elimination of discrimination against individuals with disabilities." More than a decade later, however, most Americans with disabilities still do not enjoy full participation in school, community, and work. The walls preventing Americans with disabilities from realizing their civil rights have proved more difficult to dismantle than ones built of concrete and steel. These barriers of separation are not only physical but sociopolitical—exclusions, with a long history, codified in institutional discourses, embodied in social spaces, enacted in social practices, and deeply embedded (Bush's metaphor notwithstanding) in global capitalist economic structures. Although the ADA holds some promise of chipping away at the walls of exclusion, the extent of its power and range is still being negotiated through cases for the disabled before the Supreme Court.[4] The history of civil rights litigation for other groups suggests that the court's rulings do not always support progress toward full participation. Furthermore, as cases for the disabled are made in terms of an identity group seeking "equal" civil rights, the easier it may become for other familiar discourses embedded in our social, economic, and political culture to rebuild the walls of exclusion. For example, discourses of "cost" call forth individualistic economic and philosophic vocabularies and assumptions about pragmatism that work powerfully against inclusion (see Michalko and Titchkosky, in part three), just as discourses of "equity" are often also mobilized against the disabled. In discussing race, Carl Gutierrez-Jones notes that Americans traditionally employ "injury rhetoric" to contest equity. He notes that such rhetoric "model[s] as it does a balance of moral equivalencies, legitimat[ing] notions of harm and remedy that only make sense in reference to the norm itself—to injure may thereby be equated with displacement from the norm" (88). Concepts of universality and the norm permeate academic and work cultures. Inclusion of the disabled in higher education, as well as in the workplace, especially when it requires adapting environments, testing situations, kinds of work, and so on, is fraught with anxiety and negotiations (see Lott, in part two). Inclusion can very quickly trigger cries of reverse discrimination, exclusion, or injury from the seemingly displaced, nondisabled group that identifies itself as the norm. Concepts of universality and the norm, then, are deeply embedded in how a society defines, talks, and writes about disability per se, and these concepts also play a significant role in more general sedimented discourses and institutional practices circumscribing the place for the disabled.

Rhetoric and Disability as Embodiment

This project is founded on the belief that the field of rhetoric/composition studies can be a powerful ally of disability studies and that new perspectives and common features emerge when the two fields are brought together. One link that emerges is disability's relation to rhetoric through the mediating term of the body. In the Western humanist tradition, wherever the body is placed in a hierarchical system of value (almost always subordinated to the mind), disability is carried along but assigned to an even lower rung as "defective body."[5] Grosz reminds us that ancient Greek philosophy was founded on "a profound somatophobia" (5). She notes that Plato considered the body "a betrayal of and prison for the soul, reason, or mind" (5). Categorized within this systematic dualism and opposed to philosophy (which manifested the transcendent capabilities of mind and reason), rhetoric served the (inferior) body politic. "Aristotle describes those who require rhetoric," states Jasper Neel, as "persons 'unable to do a thing,' persons without strength or power, the disabled or incapable" (71). The concept of disability has thus been involved since classical antiquity in an enabling/disabling partnership with rhetoric, occupying the less valued side of binary oppositions necessary to defining the preferred—the "universal" (male, nondisabled) human who engages in philosophy (dialectic, not rhetoric) and who leads the incapable through the tactical application of rhetoric.

For much of the intervening two thousand years, particularly since the Enlightenment, an "embodied" position was excluded from serious consideration as "truth" or, later, as "scientific objectivity." Catherine Hobbs examines the "relationship between signification and the body" in Locke's *Essay Concerning Human Understanding* (152), reading in it a "sedimented" textuality of "normative practices producing us in various ways as bodies and as subjects" (153). In Locke, "the classical and Christian body/soul duality as well as the Cartesian split between body and mind comes to parallel the age-old conflict between rhetoric (embodied) and philosophy (intelligence/esprit)" (154) and "help[s] to construct our contemporary polarity of scientific and poetic languages" (156). This bifurcation of language is not descriptive but a question of power. To emphasize the invasive political power of scientific discourse, Grosz uses the metaphor of colonization. The body, she writes, became "colonized through the discursive practices of the natural sciences, particularly the discourses of biology and medicine" (x). Under this bifurcation, wherein scientific language renders "useful facts," art, or poetry, becomes categorized as non-useful discourse, and rhetoric becomes the subservient handmaiden in "service" to "general" discourses.[6] Thinking through the metaphor of colonization, one can see that rhetoric is both feminized and subservient, cast in the role of native servant or perhaps the colonial power's police force. Rhetoric is not the "truth," or "scientific fact," which would be rendered in utilitarian scientific discourse or aestheticized "creative art" (which makes its own separate and limited truth claims), but is conceptualized as surface embellishment, arrangement, rules, and regulations, strategically deployed, to manage and persuade the general body politic.

Since rhetoric has always been categorized as "embodied" (and thereby valued less than philosophy), it shares with disability studies and feminism a common position and interest in deconstructing this polarity and revaluing "embodied" theory and scholarship expressive of a standpoint.[7] Standpoint theory is a central tenet of feminist and most postmodern theory. As Sandra Harding explains, it acknowledges that "one must be engaged in historical struggles—not just a disembodied observer of them," and that "[t]hose historical struggles make one's argument 'embodied,' not transcendental" (*Whose Science?* 185). Harding has argued that the concept of standpoint is not about essentialism; it is not a claim that only the marginalized can produce knowledge. Rather, she argues in "Rethinking Standpoint Epistemology" that truth claims and knowledge are always related to the ways of seeing of those in power, those in the dominant position. Donna Haraway adds to this point a warning that the standpoints of the oppressed are never innocent, but they do offer critical viewpoints. Standpoint theory emphasizes self-reflexivity—the necessity of critically examining the historical assumptions and positions of power out of which knowledge is produced. Recognizing that subjects of knowledge are agents (not just objects of study), the critically self-reflexive scientist would see subjects of knowledge as a resource and have a responsibility to them for making research available for their use and critical scrutiny. Critical reflexivity asks who is speaking, to what audience, in what context, and for what purposes, uncovering the rhetorical situatedness of all knowledge making.

Rhetoric historically has been concerned with the civic tradition of political deliberation, negotiation, and debate, encompassing the study of invention, arrangement, and style of an argument for a particular audience and purpose. Although rhetoric was used for hegemonic ends for much of the preceding two thousand years, the postmodern "turn to rhetoric" (see Simons) has enlarged rhetoric's traditionally restricted terrain. Postmodern rhetoric can signify rhetoric used for refutational, contestatory, and interested political ends, as well as broader uses of the term, as the rhetoric/philosophy boundary line dissolves under postmodern deconstruction. Steven Mailloux, rereading Plato sophistically in light of deconstruction, would broaden rhetoric to include all interpretive acts, insofar as "rhetoric is based on interpretation" and "interpretation is communicated through rhetoric" (*Reception* 4). Thomas Rosteck connects rhetoric and cultural studies, arguing that a cultural rhetorical studies is more attuned to the particularities of history, especially in understanding how the "cultural practices" of discourse shape history ("Cultural" 229).[8] A postmodern understanding of rhetoric as "embodied" proceeds both from the deconstructive knowledge that figures and tropes are not mere embellishment but are a part of all argument, all discourse, as well as from historical work on rhetorical archives (see "Archivists with an Attitude"). Historical study shows that arguments emerge from particular people in specific places and are surrounded by historical and cultural contexts. "It is precisely the concept of *ethos*," write Susan C. Jarratt and Nedra Reynolds, "that theorizes the positionality inherent in rhetoric. . . . [T]his positioning is a constant awareness that one always speaks from a particular place in a social structure—an awareness common to rhetoric and to postmodern feminism" (47).

Rhetoric/composition, which has emerged as a vital discipline in the last thirty years, is concerned with literacy practices, particularly the effects of language in the production and reception of (student) texts. Composition's long history of pedagogy scholarship and its position within the academy in the nearly ubiquitous first-year literacy course set it apart from other disciplines as situated and "embodied," a field which "serves" other knowledge as the body "serves" the mind, and whose subject, student writing, is uniquely and closely aligned with its object, the student writer.[9] Composition studies is thus situated in ways that make its alignment with disability studies potentially powerful. Some scholars are already working across these two disciplinary borders,[10] but the mutual influence and dialogue between these fields can and should grow. One obstacle may be that those in disability studies know little about the history and depth of composition theory and research.

Social construction theory is one area of mutual interest. As Simi Linton states, "The need for a distinct field of disability studies is premised on the belief that disability has been socially constructed and that [such] construction serves a variety of intellectual and social ends" (151). In the last twenty years, compositionists have developed a substantial body of scholarship based on the social construction of knowledge and postmodern theories of discourse, a body of scholarship that could potentially enrich disability studies and disability pedagogy.[11] For example, critiques of the traditional humanist subject and epistemology, such as those of James Berlin, and of foundational thinking, such as those of Patricia Bizzell, have contributed to an understanding not only of how discourse constitutes and constructs subjectivity, but also how one might fashion a pedagogy that would enable students to critically analyze discursive structures and examine their particular social ends.

Compositionists have applied theory to pedagogy in ways that may be especially helpful to the teaching of disabled students. Nearly twenty years ago, Kenneth Bruffee argued that because knowledge is socially constructed teachers can create collaborative classroom activities that engage students in social interactions, which in turn will lead students to learn new discourses. Since then, collaboration and group work in composition classrooms have become widespread and the activities more complex and refined (see, e.g., Brooke, Mirtz, and Evans). Small group work and collaboration encourage student-centered instruction, orality as an alternative form of learning, and peer tutoring—all of which, Patricia A. Dunn argues, can benefit the learning disabled student. Composition theorists have also pioneered the way in new forms of assessment, such as portfolios, that potentially benefit disabled students (see, e.g., Black et al.; Yancey and Weiser).

The production of knowledge in composition studies can also be a model for disability studies. As Stephen North has written, composition is truly an interdisciplinary field comprising multiple methodological communities. Composition scholarship ranges from practical teaching lore to histories and theory making, from empirical studies and archival research to qualitative studies such as ethnographies, protocol analysis, and discourse analysis. Some of the most exciting work in composition blends a number of these approaches. New studies of literacy extend and deepen the philosophies of critical, liberatory educators such as Paulo Freire and Henry Giroux. Research on extracurricular literacy practices add to the historical archive and broaden understanding of how literacy outside the academy sustains communities.[12] Compositionists have critically analyzed the role of previously overlooked rhetorics in helping particular groups preserve their identities and give voice to their struggles (see, e.g., Hobbs; Clark and Halloran; and Peterson).

Disability studies seeks to advance the cause of the disabled and promote social change by analyzing the present social formations that contribute to maintaining the walls of exclusion. Disability studies is thus a situated discourse and expresses a particular standpoint—that of the disabled. Rhetoric/Composition's various methods of analysis, theories, and history can aid in this project; indeed, the goals of disability studies cannot be achieved without rhetoric. A studies area and an approach, disability studies is defined by Simi Linton as both "a location and a means to think critically about disability" (1). Disability studies sets aside the "natural" and medical model of disability as accidental disease, trauma, deficit, or defect, using and extending the insights of feminist, postmodern, and postcolonial theory and social and rhetorical studies of science to analyze disability as a sociopolitical construct. Considering how the disabled are—and historically have been—represented, situated, marginalized, educated, and employed, for example, yields a recognition that what it means to be disabled, indeed the very conditions of a disability, are crucially determined by the society in which one lives. Furthermore, one's location and identity within a given society in terms of race, class, and gender affect what it means to be disabled. The relationship between the categories "disabled" and disability studies is thus similar to that between "woman" and women's studies. That is, disability is not a universal category but a strategic name marking diverse differences.[13] Moreover, the term *disability* names multiple and diverse embodiments of conditions and impairments; even in cases where individuals have the "same" condition—for example, Down syndrome or spinal cord injury—the effects may be substantially different for each individual.[14]

Recognizing that disability is a strategic naming, therefore, we argue both for the broadest possible definition of disability and for the right of the disability community to debate, contest, and change their preferred definitions of disability. For how disability is defined and who does the defining have important political and social consequences to stakeholders—in receiving services, seeking protection against discrimination, or suing for compliance under ADA law, for example, and in terms of cultural and psychological constructions of disability and the creation of a disability community. Legal definitions do not end debate, but they do shape the content and scope of debate. The 1990 Americans with Disabilities Act defines disability as "a physical or mental impairment that substantially limits one or more major life activities" (ADA Document Center). The apparent broadness of this definition is being narrowed by recent court decisions.[15] And its language, "physical or mental," reinforces the separation of mind and body even as contemporary neuroscience rejects such dualistic models. The mind/body split nevertheless persists in popular thinking and has several negative effects: It reinforces the deep prejudices against disabled people with mental illness and cognitive impairments, and it pressures persons with disabilities to compartmentalize the disabled "part" of themselves as separate from some essential, nondisabled self. Most theorists of disability studies argue that disability entails the whole person, but there remains lively debate within the disability community on disability identity.

In undertaking this project, we have tried to be self-conscious about definitions of disability and explicit about our position in relation to disability, and we have asked the same of the contributors to this collection, many of whom are themselves disabled. We are parents of a disabled son whose physical and cognitive disabilities, in complex interaction, have also produced behavioral problems and mental illness. Thus our son is a prime example of the inseparability and interconnection of mind and body. Our standpoint as parents of a disabled person and our interest in language led us to this project, but long before we imagined it, our experiences had compelled us to become members of the disability community. The point we wish to make here is that a disability identity is not restricted only to persons with disabilities, just as a disability identity may not suit every person with a disability.

When our son was born twenty years ago with hydrocephalus, he was immediately inserted into a complex array of institutions and inscribed by their medical, legal, educational, and social discourses. Our subjectivity, as well as his, has been shaped by these experiences, and from this standpoint we have developed a politics of experience. We have seen the constitutive power of language shaping our son's life in countless ways. Within minutes of his birth, our son entered what Michael Berube calls the social apparatus of disability, composed of interconnecting systems and a network of institutions, each with its own well defined area of influence and each validated by a professionally codified rubric and rhetoric. Included here would be the medical, legal, social service, religious, and educational systems, all of which tend to objectify the disabled subject, though not always nor entirely. The interaction between the disabled individual and social systems is a complicated dialectic that constitutes the disabled as both subject and object.

The second point we would make here concerns the link between language and material practices. Disability provides one of the best examples of how the language of institutional discourse systems determines material practices in ways that can work to the advantage—and disadvantage—of the disabled person. For example, diagnostic labels both predict and determine outcomes by denying or providing medical treatments or educational services. Early on we encouraged, sometimes insisted, that our son speak for himself rather than being spoken for by doctors, teachers, and social workers. Rhetorical agency has helped him become his own advocate so that he might resist, with the help of others, attempts to limit his access to educational, community service, and employment opportunities. Unfortunately, attempts to limit a disabled person's rights under the ADA are not isolated instances but form part of the daily struggle of the disabled. In addition to issues of rhetorical agency and access, we have encountered other concerns: social space and literacy education, for example. If there is to be a place, a social space, for the disabled in an environment and social organization now intended only for nondisabled people, then the disabled and their advocates must develop institutional, social, and political literacy. By this we mean a politically informed awareness of the power of language to shape the social world and strategies for using language to further the inclusion and self-empowerment of the disabled.

Most encounters between the (disabled) individual and the institution tend to reinforce the unequal power relations inherent in any interaction between individual and institution. Yet it is possible for the disabled subject to use the language of the institution to secure desired services and opportunities. To do this requires knowing how to use rhetoric to shape action. In "Literacy in (Inter)Action," Ellen L. Barton demonstrated how literacy works in the clinic and hospital setting. Her research showed that medical patients who have the necessary political literacy to be effective rhetors, or who are perceived to have such, are much more likely to be treated as equals and to actively participate in decisions concerning their treatment than patients who lack rhetorical power.

Becoming a rhetor and (re)writing one's life story has the potential to counter culturally disabling narratives about disability (see Krummel, in part one). However, not all disabled people can become rhetors (see Prendergast, in part one) nor is a culture necessarily open to more than a few carefully restricted types of narrative about the disabled (see Couser, in part one). Indeed, even when narratives, such as fairy tales, actually depict the disabled positively, the familiar cultural constructions of disability may be remembered more often as negative rather than as positive (see Franks, in part three). Representations of the disabled, such as those constructed in charity campaigns, also reinforce negative and naive stereotypes, erasing the complexities of disability (see Barton, in part three). Political literacy, then, is essential in understanding how representations and narratives work to interpellate the disabled and in creating an active counter-rhetoric. A counter-rhetoric can then be shaped to resist the residual and continuing effects of common, negative cultural constructions (as in AIDS discourse) and to be more commensurate with the values and goals of the disability community (see Nye, in part three).

Aristotle's Monsters: Deviance and the Norm

Since Aristotle, the idea of the norm has legitimated exclusion of the disabled from "human" society as "abnormal" and "monstrous," even though all people who live long enough are likely at one time or another to experience disability themselves or be closely related to someone who is disabled. That is, what has been labeled "abnormal" actually occurs regularly and frequently and, yes, "normally."[16] To put it another way, the construct of an "ideal" or "universal" body is a fiction, a fantasy. As Grosz states, "Alterity is the very possibility and process of embodiment" (209).

Aristotelian and Christian intellectual traditions demonstrate the process by which a culture constructs the "norm" and, equally important, the process by which its ideology has come to inhabit and in part define (disabled) subjects. The taxonomic systems Aristotle constructs in the *Generation of Animals,* the *Nicomachean Ethics,* the *Poetics,* and the *Politics,* purport to discover the "norm " (the "average") in the discourses of biology, ethics, poetics, and politics, respectively. Rather than "finding" a norm, however, Aristotle ascribes meaning, entirely negative, to disability through classifications that create hierarchies of value through binary opposites. The typical (or normal) and the aberrant (or abnormal) are defined against one another, the typical invested with desirable characteristics and the aberrant with undesirable characteristics. Indeed, in his treatise on biology, *Generation of Animals,* Aristotle admits that difference is not "contrary to nature" in its entirety but only to nature *"in the generality of cases"* (4.4.770b).

Generation of Animals includes Aristotle's most direct comments on disability. With humans as with animals, any physical difference that "departs from type" (the able-bodied male) becomes a "monstrosity" that, by its very essence, is less than human. The "first beginning of this deviation is when a female is formed instead of a male" (4.3.767b), Aristotle claims. He goes on to say, "We should look upon the female state as being as it were a deformity" (4.6.775a). Among the most extreme cases of such "deformity" are children born with birth anomalies. "Sometimes," he states, a child "has reached such a point that in the end it no longer has the appearance of a human being at all, but that of an animal only" (4.3.769b).

Aristotle's assignment of human value based on correspondence to an imagined, privileged norm is equally explicit in *Nicomachean Ethics.* Here he defines virtue as a "mean between excess and deficiency" (2.6.5) and catalogs the three states of "moral character" to be avoided: vice, unrestraint, and bestiality. The bestial character, Aristotle writes, "is rare among human beings; it is found most frequently among barbarians, and some cases also occur as a result of disease or arrested development" (7.1.3). (Notice here that "barbarian" and the diseased/disabled are listed apart from the category of "human"). Related to the "bestial" character is the "morbid disposition," a category reserved for "those who lose their reasoning to some disease, such as epilepsy or through insanity" (7.5.6). Aristotle justifies this taxonomy of value by claiming a preexisting biological ground, or essence, and then grants "biology" a moral status: deviance from the biological norm signifies a defect in moral character.

Rosemarie Garland Thomson points out Aristotle's "conflation of disability and femaleness," but what is "more significant," she argues, "is his declaration that the source of all otherness is the concept of a norm, a 'generic type,' against which all physical variation appears as different, derivative, inferior, and insufficient" (20). The category of disabled, as it functions in the binary opposition of normal/abnormal, comprises all the excluded, different Others (including gender and racial/ethnic differences). Thus, without entering into disputes about which kind of marginalization began first (gender, race, class, or disability), one can see disability as the critical theoretical category of difference at work in these mutually constituted marginalizations. Ab/normal marks the irreducibility of otherness, the necessary gap or interval producing, for Aristotle, "humans" (free men) and deviant Others.

Aristotle endorses the desired and virtuous mean in both the *Poetics* and the *Politics*. For example, in the *Poetics* Aristotle exhibits the same intolerance for anomaly when he argues that a unified plot requires that all aberrations be excluded. In the *Politics* Aristotle establishes a biological argument for both virtue and political rights. He ranks the "composite" of citizens that together constitute the state. At the top of the political hierarchy is the male, who rules over wife and children, since "the male is by nature better fitted for command than the female. . . and the older and fully developed person than the younger and immature" (1.5.2.1259b). Below women and children are the slaves and noncitizens, who fail to possess "reason." Slavery is justified by law as well as by nature, according to Aristotle: "It is manifest therefore that there are cases of people of whom some are freemen and the others slaves by nature, and for these slavery is an institution both expedient and just" (1.2.15.1255a). Aristotle places the disabled somewhere down with slaves and noncitizens, and those born with disabilities are granted no right to material life at all. Thus the Aristotelian state is founded on the expulsion of these Others who have no political rights. Remarking that "Aristotle . . . does more harm to rhetoric than does Plato" (69), Jasper Neel concludes that "the foundation [of metaphysics] depends on slavery, racism, and sexism" (76)—and on exclusion of the disabled, we would add.

If disability is "monstrosity" in Aristotle, it is monstrosity with a purpose (namely, God's) in Christianity's rhetorical tradition. Typically, disability is presented as "affliction" in both the Old and New Testaments of the King James Bible. The *OED* defines affliction as "Cast down, depressed, oppressed in mind, body, or estate; hence, grievously troubled or distressed." The afflicted are cast down by God either as punishment for their sins or as a test to verify their faith. Thus the disabled, seen as deformed in both body and spirit, are thought to be literal manifestations of God's displeasure and/or wrath. What makes this construction so pernicious is that in it teleology becomes tautology. The disabled are disabled because they are sinful; the disabled are sinful because they are disabled! Sometimes the condemnation is total: "All the days of the afflicted are evil" (Proverbs 15:15). Sometimes affliction is cast as a test of faith, meant to purify the disabled. Job provides one obvious example of this construction, but there are many other biblical examples of disability as the "trial of affliction" (II Corinthians 8:2) or the "furnace of affliction" (Isaiah 48:10). Consider, for example, Psalms 119:71: "It is good for me that I have been afflicted; that I might learn thy statutes." The disabled, then, not only deserve but need their afflictions so that they might purify themselves.[17] In effect, the Christian rhetorical tradition demonizes the disabled.

The religious concept of affliction, casting disability as corporeal testimony of sin and punishment, was an embodied rhetoric persuading Christians of the power of God and the doctrines of the Church. As the history of disability makes clear, such constructions justify exclusionary social practices *already* in place by an implicit argument that an individual somehow has earned his or her fate of exclusion. Though it may be difficult to define oneself positively within the rhetorics of affliction, which construct the disabled as objects of pity at best, or excluded because they are deserving of punishment at worst, the disabled have had to develop strategies to contend with these constructions. In fact, the disabled have sometimes drawn upon well-known biblical narratives and a range of rhetorical strategies (especially *pathos*) for their own purposes of cultural negotiation (see Holmes, in part one).

Rhetoric, Scientific Discourse, and the Genetic Body-Text

Just as rhetoric has defined philosophy, by being paired with and subordinated to it since Aristotle, the disabled body has defined the rhetor (negatively) by its exclusion from rhetoricity. Quintilian's *Institutio Oratoria* was the most complex document about rhetoric to survive antiquity, and as such it influenced rhetorical education through the Enlightenment. In *Manly Writing: Gender, Rhetoric, and the Rise of Composition*, Miriam Brody traces the effects of Quintilian's precept (from the fourth century B.C.E.) to the eighteenth century and beyond, that good writing equates with the "good man" who is defined as a masculine body in good health (25). Brody points out the early connection in Quintilian of the most valued style with utility: "True beauty is never separate from utility" (qtd. in Brody 28). This ideology, she argues, would come to prominence in the values of scientific discourse and would "serve a developing industrial, capitalist, culture in England and in America" (4). This rhetorical tradition has influenced education in ways that have had a specific impact on the disabled. Although the disabled have, for much of history, been excluded from education, when they have been afforded opportunities for schooling, the education they were offered emphasized utility over self-expression. For example, Deaf education emphasized pragmatic communication over the development of more complex political literacy or personal growth (see Brueggemann, in part two). Educators of the deaf strove to train students to become as like the hearing population as possible (through lip-reading and speech training) on the grounds of utility (they would have to live in a "hearing" world), and many were hostile to alternative means of communication in Deaf culture like manual language (see Joyner, in part two). As Brueggemann argues ("The Coming Out of Deaf Culture"), ASL is an example of a visual, embodied rhetoric, attesting to the vibrancy of Deaf culture and enabling the agency of deaf people.

These legacies regarding disability descending from Aristotle and the Church and, later, the Enlightenment rational-empirical aesthetics of language, thought, and subjectivity sedimented into the nineteenth-century scientific discourses and practices objectifying the disabled as scientific specimens of deviancy.[18] The spectacles of medicine (such as the "hysterical" female patients Freud observed in Paris), the freak shows of the late nineteenth and early twentieth centuries (see Thomson), or the disabled patient today being visually and verbally dissected by doctors on their rounds (see Couser) all exemplify the powerful embodied rhetoric that is this legacy—the "scientific" discourses in which the deviant body is object and text.

In book 8 of the *Generation of Animals,* Aristotle had equated the "normal" with the "natural." Extending from Aristotle's "virtuous mean" through the rise of scientific discourse, this long tradition in Western intellectual history of the construction of the "normal" eventually leads to nineteenth- and twentieth-century statistical theory and the notorious bell-shaped curve, the symbol of the tyranny of the norm. Lennard Davis traces this "symbiotic relationship" ("Constructing" 14) between statistical science and eugenics. "The new ideal of ranked order is powered by the imperative of the norm," writes Davis, "and then is supplemented by the notion of progress, human perfectibility, and the elimination of deviance, to create a dominating, hegemonic vision of what the human body should be" (17). The norm becomes the ideal, which then creates the idea of the deviant, defective body that twentieth-century eugenicists tried to eliminate in the first half of the century and which twenty-first-century scientists are trying to "correct" through genome sequencing and genetic engineering. In *Exploding the Gene Myth,* Ruth Hubbard and Elijah Wald warn of the ideology that accompanies genetic testing. They cite the speech, which strikes an Aristotelian chord, made in 1971 by the retiring president of the American Association for the Advancement of Science: "The right that must become paramount is . . . the right of every child to be born with a sound physical and mental constitution, based on a sound genotype. No parents will in that future time have a right to burden society with a malformed or a mentally incompetent child" (25). That future, in which such "rights" must be negotiated, is upon us. Genetic testing, the mapping and patenting of human DNA, and its manipulation are contemporary practices demonstrating that the material body is sociopolitical. What level of genetic research and what kinds of tests and procedures will be allowed are sociopolitical, ethical, economic, and scientific questions, as are related ones, such as which genes will be allowed to remain in the human gene pool and which will not. The body has now become a genetic body-text, constituted and given significance by the discourses and technologies of encoding and decoding. The genetic body-text demonstrates that the sociopolitical meaning of disability as exclusion still persists; only now, the "wall separating Americans with disabilities from their freedom" resides inside the body, inscribed in the molecular units of matter, the chromosomes and the DNA that encode human bodies.

The project of "rewriting" disability may sound like a postmodern cliché, but scientists have already begun rewriting the genetic body-text through the manipulation of genes. If the material sociopolitics of gene "therapy" now under way is to enter public debate, the hegemony of scientific discourses will have to be challenged. This requires postmodern rhetoric, a rhetoric of political engagement, to challenge the names, the language, and the frameworks for understanding disability, to revise official histories and develop new ones. It is important to make clear that a postmodern rhetorical stance is not antiscientific, as it is often accused of being. Such accusations recirculate the traditional (de)valuation of rhetoric, which still permeates much scientific and philosophic discourse. For example, David Miller, a philosopher of science, writing in the magazine *Science* on the importance of rational skepticism to the scientific method, proclaimed, "Relativists depreciate reason, and replace it with rhetoric" (1625). In point of fact, it would be absurd for the disabled and their advocates to reject science and its related technologies, which provide many benefits to the disabled. Having been born with extreme hydrocephalus, for instance, our son depends upon science (surgical intervention, imaging technologies, drugs) for his very life.

As Elizabeth Flynn has argued, postmodernism is not the binary opposite of modernism, but a continuation of it through a criticism of its totalizing and idealizing assumptions and methods. Flynn points out that such critique, made in a context that continues to value and respect science, furthers knowledge-making. Philosopher Sandra Harding calls such critique "strong objectivity."[19]

Aristotle's concepts of norm and generic type were foundational in the positioning of traditional rhetoric as embellishment/trickery in opposition to truth or reason and in according philosophy and, later, science the status of truth. A classical rhetorical education was an education in typology; students studied models to be applied to various situations and suitable topics and kinds of arguments for all occasions. In contrast, postmodern rhetoricians argue that all knowledge-making comes from somewhere and someone in particular, from a standpoint, and thus rhetoric embodies difference. Difference, despite charges like those made by Miller is not the same as an "anything goes" relativism; rhetoric is not deracination. Every deployment of language combines the interactions of same and different. Neither wholly original nor exactly repeatable, language is a lot like the genetic body. By being the same and different at once, language produces meaning (which requires both a shared code and a particular utterance). Likewise, while each rhetorical situation is unique—language, argument, form shaped by one's particular purpose and audience—rhetors do, in part, draw on models and *topoi.*

Just as postmodern rhetoric, through the deployment of language for ethical, interested political ends, is necessary in achieving the transformative goals of disability studies, so too does disability studies contribute to an understanding of postmodern rhetoric as an embodied rhetoric of difference. Transforming disability will require transforming economic, social, ethical, and educational practices, reimagining social spaces, and rethinking ordinary habits. It will also require an understanding of embodiment as difference and the transformation of the category ab/normal and all such thinking that reads "difference" as defect and deficit and thereby lays the foundation for the many walls of exclusion. Our own experience has taught us that difference can produce delight and curiosity, as well as fear and isolation. Difference teaches us to grow, to become other than ourselves, to push beyond old identities and ways of thinking. In our lives, our son has led us along this path, as have the disability activists working for change and disability scholars engaged in creating new frameworks for reconceptualizing disability. We believe that their critiques of language and cultural practices will give rhetorical studies a deeper understanding of how difference functions.

Notes

1. "A discursive formation is not unified either in the logical coherence of its elements, or in the a priori of a transcendental subject or in a meaning-giving subject. . . . The type of coherence we attribute to a discursive formation is . . . regularity in dispersion" (Laclau and Mouffe 105).

2. The quotation marks around the word *intent* draw attention to the complex problematics of that concept. Not only are a speaker's intentions never fully knowable to self or others but language as citational practice cannot be entirely controlled by a speaker's intentions. In delineating "the limits and risks of resignification as a strategy of opposition" (38), as Butler states, "the one who speaks is not the originator of such speech, for that subject is produced in language through a prior performative exercise of speech: interpellation. Moreover, the language the subject speaks is conventional and, to that degree, citational" (39). She concludes, "Understanding performativity as a renewable action without clear origin or end suggests that speech is finally constrained neither by its specific speaker nor its originating context" (40). Language is not containable; speech or text can be subsequently cited and appropriated in unanticipated ways.

3. *Black's* defines Civil Death as "the state of a person who, though possessing natural life, has lost all civil rights and as to them is considered civilly dead."

4. In 1999 the Supreme Court heard four disability-related cases, three of which involved the definition of disability under the ADA and, specifically, whether people with "correctable" disabilities are covered by laws that bar discrimination against the disabled. In all three cases (*Murphy v. United Parcel Service,* no. 967-1992; *Sutton v. United Air Lines,* no. 97-1943; and *Albertsons v. Kirkingburg,* no. 98-591), the court ruled that people with "correctable" disabilities are not covered by disability law, a decision that Supreme Court Justice John Paul Stevens, who dissented from the majority opinion in all three rulings, called "miserly" in its interpretation of the ADA (Mauro 3A). The fourth case, *Olmstead v. L.C.,* no. 98-536, proved to be a victory for disability rights activists. The case involved two Georgia women with "mental" disabilities institutionalized in Georgia Regional Hospital in Atlanta who sued the state for failing to provide them with a less restrictive environment than a large mental hospital. The court ruled that the ADA requires states to offer alternatives to institutionalization whenever appropriate and strengthened the principle of integrating people with disabilities into the community (Mauro 3A).

5. Aristotle also categorized woman in terms of deviant body. Thus, feminist work in theorizing the body is an important tool for disability studies scholars. See, e.g., Thomson.

6. Rhetoric retains this position as servant in the college curriculum, where learning to write and speak well are seen as skills courses in service to the "real" learning of other disciplines.

7. Grosz argues that "the body functions as the repressed or disavowed condition of all knowledges" (20) and hence that rethinking embodiment

"through a range of disparate discourses" (not through the usual channels of scientific discourse) is a promising avenue for new knowledge.

8. Rhetorical studies is a lively and contested field. Some rhetoricians propose redesigning English departments around rhetorical theory, while others, both inside and outside the field, criticize postmodern rhetoric for displacing philosophy or becoming so broad as to be meaningless. See Mailloux, *Reception Histories,* ch. 8, on reconceptualizing English studies as cultural rhetorical studies; see Fleming on designing an undergraduate major in rhetorical education. For criticism of the broadening of rhetoric, see Fleming, 170; see Brantlinger for a critique of postmodern rhetoric's displacement of philosophy. For an overview of the differences in postmodern rhetorics, see Jarratt, "Using Postmodern."

9. It would be interesting to consider whether David Fleming's proposal to revive the older tradition of rhetoric as training in character and eloquence as the "course of study" for the undergraduate English major (172) would do anything to heal rhet/comp's self-division and lowly place in the college curriculum. Jasper Neel warns, "I would like to caution against the (attractive but, in my opinion, false) belief that contemporary literary theory (whether it draws its life from cultural studies, deconstruction, feminism, historicism, Marxism, or any other such matrix) offers rhetoric/composition a way to escape the role of servant" ("The Degradation" 69).

10. For example, Ellen L. Barton, "Literacy in (Inter)Action"; Brenda Brueggemann, "The Coming Out of Deaf Culture," "On Almost Passing," and *Lend Me Your Ear: Rhetorical Constructions of Deafness;* and Patricia A. Dunn, *Learning Re-Abled.*

11. See Dobrin for a brief overview of social construction and postmodern composition theory.

12. See Knoblauch and Brannon for critical literacy in the composition classroom. Some examples of extracurricular literacy studies are Brandt; Cushman; and Gere.

13. See Spivak for discussion of the category *woman* and "strategic feminism" (137–40, 162).

14. As Grosz notes, "The condition of corporeality is pure difference" (219, n. 1).

15. For a lucid discussion of definitions of disability and their consequences, see Wendell. See note 4 above for discussion of recent Supreme Court cases that narrowed the definition of disability.

16. According to the U.S. Bureau of the Census, by the mid-1990s approximately 20 percent of the U.S. population, or about 54 million people, had some level of disability, with approximately half of those disabilities classified as severe. Disability ratios rise sharply with age, with 47 percent of those from ages 65 to 79 disabled, and 72 percent of those aged 80 and older disabled ("Statistical Snapshot").

17. The self-referential notion that the disabled are sinful and thus deserving/needing their affliction leads to the more extreme position that the disabled are possessed by Satan. Margaret Winzer explains, "With the rise of Christianity came the belief in the Devil, or Satan, as the prime suspect in disabling condi-

tions" (84). One sees this in the synoptic Gospels of the New Testament, where Matthew, Mark, and Luke repeat the same curative exploits of Christ as he rids individuals of a series of disabilities including palsy, blindness, dumbness, and epilepsy. One can trace this discursive tradition, and the social practices it engenders, through the Inquisition and the persecution of the disabled as "witches." Winzer notes that Augustine "renounced any claims of disabled people for participation in the covenant of the Lord" (90); John Calvin "preached that mentally retarded persons are possessed by Satan" (94); and Martin Luther believed that "a mentally retarded child is merely a mass of flesh (*massa carnis*) with no soul" (94).

18. "The nineteenth century, particularly in France but in Europe generally," writes Henri-Jacques Stiker, "will be dominated by aid in the form of reclusion, alongside the concern for rehabilitation" (110). "[O]ne can see in these measures primarily a logic to effect social control: aid to the poor is required so that there may no longer be an excuse for begging, vagrancy, parasitism. . . . [M]edicine . . . will become the regulatory device for aberrancy" (111).

19. "Cultural agendas and assumptions are part of the background assumptions and auxiliary hypotheses that philosophers have identified. If the goal is to make available for critical scrutiny *all* the evidence marshaled for or against a scientific hypothesis, then this evidence too requires critical examination *within* scientific research processes. In other words, we can think of strong objectivity as extending the notion of scientific research to include systematic examination of such powerful background beliefs. It must do so in order to be competent at maximizing objectivity," writes Harding (*Whose Science?* 149).

Works Cited

Alcoff, Linda, and Elizabeth Potter, eds. *Feminist Epistemologies.* New York: Routledge, 1993.

Americans with Disability Act (ADA). Americans with Disability Act Document Center on-line at <http://janweb.icdi.wvu.edu/kinder/>.

"Archivists with an Attitude." Essays on the Archives of Composition Studies. *College English* 61 (1999): 574–98.

Aristotle. *Generation of Animals.* Trans. A. L. Peck. Cambridge: Harvard UP, 1979.

———. *The Nicomachean Ethics.* Trans. H. Rackham. Cambridge: Harvard UP, 1975.

———. *The Politics.* Trans. H. Rackham. Cambridge: Harvard UP, 1967.

Balsamo, Anne. *Technologies of the Gendered Body: Reading Cyborg Women.* Durham, NC: Duke UP, 1996.

Barton, Ellen L. "Literacy in (Inter)Action." *College English* 59 (1997): 408–37.

Baumlin, James S., and Tita French Baumlin, eds. *Ethos: New Essays in Rhetorical and Critical Theory.* Dallas: Southern Methodist UP, 1992.

Berlin, James. "Poststructuralism, Cultural Studies, and the Composition Classroom." *Rhetoric Review* 11 (Fall 1992): 16–33.

Berube, Michael. *Life as We Know It.* New York: Pantheon, 1996.

Bizzell, Patricia. "Foundationalism and Anti-Foundationalism in Composition Studies." PRE/TEXT 7 (Spring–Summer 1986): 37–56.

Black, Laurel, Donald A. Daiker, Jeffrey Sommers, and Gail Stygall, eds. *New Directions in Portfolio Assessment: Reflective Practice, Critical Theory, and Large-Scale Scoring.* Portsmouth, NH: Heinemann-Boynton/Cook, 1994.

Black's Law Dictionary. 6th ed. St. Paul: West, 1990.

Brandt, Deborah. "Accumulating Literacy: Writing and Learning to Write in the Twentieth Century." *College English* 57 (Oct. 1995): 649–68.

Brantlinger, Patrick. "Antitheory and Its Antitheses: Rhetoric and Ideology." Rosteck 292–312.

Brody, Miriam. *Manly Writing: Gender, Rhetoric, and the Rise of Composition.* Carbondale: Southern Illinois UP, 1993.

Brooke, Robert, Ruth Mirtz, and Rich Evans. *Small Groups in Writing Workshops.* Urbana, IL: NCTE, 1994.

Brueggemann, Brenda Jo. "The Coming Out of Deaf Culture and American Sign Language: An Exploration into Visual Rhetoric and Literacy." *Rhetoric Review* 13 (1995): 409–20.

———. *Lend Me Your Ear: Rhetorical Constructions of Deafness.* Washington: Gallaudet UP, 1999.

———. "On Almost Passing." *College English* 59 (1997): 647–60.

Bruffee, Kenneth. "Collaborative Learning and the 'Conversation of Mankind.'" *College English* 46 (Nov. 1984): 635–52.

Bush, George. Speech on Signing the ADA. *Public Papers of the Presidents of the United States: George Bush, 1990.* Book 2. Washington: Government Printing Office, 1991. 1069.

Butler, Judith. *Excitable Speech: A Politics of the Performative.* New York: Routledge, 1997.

Clark, Gregory, and S. Michael Halloran, eds. *Oratorical Culture in Nineteenth-Century America; Transformations in the Theory and Practice of Rhetoric.* Carbondale: Southern Illinois UP, 1993.

Closing the Gap: The National Organization on Disability/Harris Survey of Americans with Disabilities. Washington: National Organization on Disability, 1998.

Couser, Thomas G. *Recovering Bodies: Illness, Disability, and Life Writing.* Madison: U of Wisconsin P, 1997.

Cushman, Ellen. *The Struggle and the Tools: Oral and Literate Strategies in an Inner-City Community.* Albany: SUNY P, 1998.

Davis, Lennard J. "Constructing Normalcy: The Bell Curve, the Novel, and the Invention of the Disabled Body in the Nineteenth Century." Davis 9–28.

———, ed. *The Disability Studies Reader.* New York: Routledge, 1997.

Dobrin, Sidney I. *Constructing Knowledges: The Politics of Theory-Building and Pedagogy in Composition.* Albany, NY: SUNY P, 1997.

Dunn, Patricia A. *Learning Re-Abled: The Learning Disability Controversy and Composition Studies.* Portsmouth, NH: Boynton/Cook, 1995.

Fleming, David. "Rhetoric as a Course of Study." *College English* 61 (1998): 169–91.

Flynn, Elizabeth. "Rescuing Postmodernism." *College Composition and Communication* 48 (1997): 540–55.

Freire, Paulo. *Pedagogy of the Oppressed.* Trans. Myra Bergman Ramos. New York: Seabury, 1968.

Gere, Anne Ruggles. "Kitchen Table and Rented Rooms: The Extracurriculum of Composition." *College Composition and Communication* 45 (Feb. 1994): 75–92.

Giroux, Henry A. *Schooling and the Struggle for Public Life: Critical Pedagogy in the Modern Age.* Minneapolis: U of Minnesota P, 1988.

Grosz, Elizabeth. *Volatile Bodies: Toward a Corporeal Feminism.* Bloomington: Indiana UP, 1994.

Gutierrez-Jones, Carl. "Injury by Design." *Cultural Critique: The Future of American Studies* 40 (Fall 1998): 73–102.

Haraway, Donna. "Situated Knowledges: The Science Question in Feminism and the Privilege of Partial Perspective." *Feminist Studies* 14.3 (1988): 575–99.

Harding, Sandra. "Rethinking Standpoint Epistemology: What Is 'Strong Objectivity'?" Alcoff and Potter 49–82.

———. *Whose Science? Whose Knowledge?* Ithaca: Cornell UP, 1991.

Hobbs, Catherine. "Locke, Disembodied Ideas, and Rhetoric That Matters." Wilson and Laennec 151–62.

———, ed. *Nineteenth-Century Women Learn to Write.* Charlottesville: UP of Virginia, 1995.

Hubbard, Ruth, and Elijah Wald. *Exploding the Gene Myth.* Boston: Beacon, 1997.

Jarratt, Susan C. "Review: Using Postmodern Histories of Rhetoric." *College English* 61 (1999): 605–14.

Jarratt, Susan C., and Nedra Reynolds. "The Splitting Image: Contemporary Feminisms and the Ethics of *Ethos.*" Baumlin and Baumlin 37–63.

Knoblauch, C. H., and Lil Brannon. *Critical Teaching and the Idea of Literacy.* Portsmouth, NH: Boynton/Cook, 1993.

Laclau, Ernesto, and Chantal Mouffe. *Hegemony and Socialist Strategy: Towards a Radical Democratic Politics.* Trans. Winston Moore and Paul Cammack. New York: Verso, 1985.

Linton, Simi. *Claiming Disability: Knowledge and Identity.* New York: New York UP, 1998.

Mailloux, Steven. *Reception Histories: Rhetoric, Pragmatism, and American Cultural Politics.* Ithaca: Cornell UP, 1998.

———, ed. *Rhetoric, Sophistry, Pragmatism.* Cambridge UP, 1995.

Mauro, Tony. "Justice Calls Disability Decision 'Miserly' High Court Limits Law's Coverage." *USA Today* 23 June 1999: 3A.

Miller, David. "On Being an Absolute Skeptic." *Science* 284 (1999): 1625–26.

Miller, Thomas P., and Melody Bowden. "A Rhetorical Stance on the Archives of Civic Action" *College English* 61 (1999): 591–98.

Mouth: Voice of the Disability Nation. Vol. 10. Topeka: Free Hand P, 1999.

Neel, Jasper. "The Degradation of Rhetoric; or, Dressing like a Gentleman, Speaking like a Scholar." Mailloux 61–81.

——. *Plato, Derrida, and Writing*. Carbondale: Southern Illinois UP, 1988.

North, Stephen M. *The Making of Knowledge in Composition: Portrait of an Emerging Field*. Upper Montclair, NJ: Boynton/Cook, 1987.

Peterson, Carla. *"Doers of the Word": African-American Women Speakers and Writers in the North (1830–1880)*. New York: Oxford UP, 1995.

Quintilian. *Quintilian on the Teaching of Speaking and Writing: Translations from Books One, Two, and Ten of the Institutio Oratoria*. Ed. James J. Murphy. Carbondale: Southern Illinois UP, 1987.

Rosteck, Thomas, ed. *At the Intersection: Cultural Studies and Rhetorical Studies*. New York: Guilford P, 1999.

——. "A Cultural Tradition in Rhetorical Studies." Rosteck 226–47.

Simons, Herbert W., ed. *The Rhetorical Turn*. Chicago: U of Chicago P, 1990.

Spivak, Gayatry Chakravorty. *Outside in the Teaching Machine*. New York: Routledge, 1993.

"Statistical Snapshot." *Disability Agenda* 2.3 (Winter 1999): 2.

Stiker, Henri-Jacques. *A History of Disability*. Trans. William Sayers. Ann Arbor: U of Michigan P, 1999.

Thomson, Rosemarie Garland. *Extraordinary Bodies: Figuring Physical Disability in American Culture and Literature*. New York: Columbia UP, 1997.

Vital Signs: Crip Culture Talks Back. Dir. and Prod. David T. Mitchell and Sharon Snyder. Northern Michigan U. Videocassette. Brace Yourselves Productions, 1996.

Wendell, Susan. "Towards a Feminist Theory of Disability." Davis 260–78.

Williams, Raymond. *Marxism and Literature*. Oxford: Oxford UP, 1977.

Wilson, Deborah S., and Christine Moncera Laennec, eds. *Bodily Discursions: Genders, Representations, Technologies*. Albany: SUNY P, 1997.

Winzer, Margaret A. "Disability and Society Before the Eighteenth Century: Dread and Despair." Davis 75–109.

Yancey, Kathleen Blake, and Irwin Weiser, eds. *Situating Portfolios: Four Perspectives*. Logan: Utah State UP, 1997.

Part One

Identity and Rhetoricity: The (Dis)Abled Subject

2

Working (with) the Rhetoric of Affliction: Autobiographical Narratives of Victorians with Physical Disabilities
Martha Stoddard Holmes

The meaning of our bodies is produced in continuous, lifelong negotiations between how we see ourselves and how our culture sees us. If we have physical disabilities, we may be aware every day of our lives of these negotiations: not only with doorways or stairs but also with language, stares, assumptions, and policies. "Accommodation," that key word in the concept of legal compliance with disability rights legislation, characterizes the actions of people with disabilities as much as or more than it does the actions of people without them. This is still true in the beginning of the twenty-first century; despite the fact that disabled activists have achieved public awareness of the problems of inaccessible environments and disempowering rhetoric, daily survival for many people with disabilities requires them to work with the needs and feelings of the nondisabled.

In the nineteenth century, the challenge of living with cultural constructions of disability was incrementally more complex. If you were blind, deaf, or otherwise physically impaired in nineteenth-century England, your bodily experience was habitually described as "afflicted," "deprived," or even "defective." While disabled activism had already entered the cultural landscape (a prominent early example is the Association for Promoting the General Welfare of the Blind, formed by Elizabeth Gilbert and William Hanks Levy in 1856), most nondisabled people resisted the idea that disabled people could work, learn, or have families. Given this cultural context, how could a person with a disability build a life of economic stability, much less develop a satisfying sense of self?

If the record of such a life were examined, what could it tell us beyond confirming a history of discriminatory and stigmatizing practices?

I approach this question through Henry Mayhew's *London Labour and the London Poor,* a collection of interviews with indigent or working-class Londoners published in the *Morning Chronicle* in 1849–50 and 1851–52 and collected in a four-volume edition in 1861–62. Mayhew's interviews present a remarkable record of lives doubly slated for invisibility by poverty and physical impairment. Further, though Mayhew's questions and the narrative frames he provides have substantial control over the autobiographies, this control is never absolute. This "history of a people," despite Mayhew's interventions, does seem to issue "from the lips of the people themselves" as they speak of "their labour, their earnings, their trials, and their sufferings, in their own 'unvarnished' language" (1:xv). In the interplay between Mayhew's statements and those of his interviewees, we can see both the rhetoric of affliction and the ways in which people with impairments worked within its constraints.

As in our time, the people Mayhew interviews are diverse both in their bodily configurations and in their life circumstances. They have several things in common, however, including an experience of cultural and economic discrimination and the proven ability to accommodate the disabling effects of their culture. Above all, these autobiographical narratives remind us that physical impairment has always occasioned exceptional capabilities. In all centuries, people with disabilities have developed particular skills for negotiating buildings, attitudes, and social systems, as well as particular intelligence about human interdependence and collaborative strength.

> Few there are, if any, who have entered the walls of this Institution without emotion, at the sight of so many of their fellow-creatures deprived of that blessing, without which, *every other* appears empty and insignificant; and although the gloom of their once lonely and dependent condition is happily cheered . . . still present to the mind is the lamentable conviction of their dark and benighted state, for which no relief can be found on this side of the grave. . . . Your compassionate assistance is now implored.—Extend a helping Hand to raise their drooping Hearts,—to cheer their gloomy paths. (School for the Indigent Blind, Liverpool [n.p.])

Nineteenth-century writing about physical disabilities often tells us more about feelings than it does about bodies. In Charles Dickens's *Cricket on the Hearth,* for example, we know nothing of the cause of the "Blind Girl" Bertha Plummer's visual impairment or how (given that she does all the housework) her father manages to convince her that their hovel is a cozy cottage. For paragraphs on end, however, her character is developed through public unburdenings of joy and (mostly) misery. In George Meredith's *Diana of the Crossways,* similarly, Emma Dunstane's emotional strength in the face of invalidism and her husband's philandering is one of the flagships of the novel, but we never have a clear idea of how she is impaired or where on her body the surgeons cut in a crisis midway through the book.

Not only fiction writers but also educators, social reformers, journalists, and even physicians habitually characterized people with disabilities in terms of their melancholy, spiritual, or suspicious tendencies, in some cases with scant attention to the causes, sites, and practical effects of their bodily impairments. A focus on feeling and the use of affect-laden language characterizes the settlement work of individuals like "Sister Grace" Kimmins, whose turn-of-the-century "Guild of the Brave Poor Things" had as its motto "Happy in My Lot" (Vicinus 235). Contemporary medical constructions of disability are similarly melodramatic: From a twentieth-century perspective, they are as literary as they are clinical. Physician William Lawrence, for example, introduces a series of lectures on "the nature and treatment of diseases of the eye" with the statement that "blindness is one of the greatest calamities that can befall human nature short of death; and many think that the termination of existence would be preferable to its continuance in the solitary, dependent, and imperfect state to which human life is reduced by the privation of this precious sense . . . their existence reduced to a dreary blank—dark, solitary and cheerless—burthensome to themselves and to those around them" (145).

Before he reaches his ultimate focus on eye inflammations, Lawrence quotes from *Paradise Lost* and (erroneously) cites Milton as "always" writing of his blindness "in a tone of anguish and despondency characteristic of recent misfortune" (145).

A letter to the editor of a prominent social reform periodical, the *Charity Organisation Reporter,* similarly supports a training institution for "crippled persons" in terms of its emotional benefits rather than its material effects, only alluding to the material world in an awkward postscript: "The undeserved misery which such persons suffer, not merely from actual want, but from enforced idleness, with its concomitant evils, would melt the hearts of the hardest; its relief . . . would command the sympathy of everyone capable of feeling for another's distress, and would involve . . . the violation of no economic principle" ("The Crippled" 55).

While most medical writers eventually return to clinical discourse, writing about disabilities in other disciplines frequently submerges bodily, economic, and other material details in discussions of the emotions that physical impairment is supposed to produce. In the process, people with disabilities are often made to exist more in various emotional states than in the infirm body that is the putative cause of such "affliction."

The emotional lives of the whole diverse population of people with disabilities, moreover, were collapsed into a limited set of affective states: Either they were innocent sufferers—afflicted children grateful for charitable assistance—or they were embittered, suspicious, and emotionally and morally degraded, begging impostors willing to counterfeit suffering in excess of reality in order to gather alms. Imagining people with disabilities as emotionally limited made it easier for nondisabled people to react in similarly limited, uncomplicated ways: They could feel pity, or they could feel outrage.

Characterizing the impaired body as an emotional entity can minimize the importance of material and social circumstances and maximize personal responsibility for rehabilitation (and by extension, for the impairment itself). The physician John Fosbroke's assertion that "the chief impediment which stands so much in the way of the deaf, in the most favourable cases for treatment, [is] . . . the vice of despondency," demonstrates how the emotional rhetoric of affliction could position people with impairments as exemplars of the failure to perform the "self-help" of a positive outlook (70–71).

Despite their emphasis on personal emotion and volition rather than on disabling social conditions, however, there is a decidedly interpersonal element to nineteenth-century constructions of impairment. As both the opening quote from the Liverpool School for the Indigent Blind and the *Charity Organisation Reporter* excerpt demonstrate, many texts posit an emotional exchange system in which currents of feeling, stimulated by the presence of a corporeally "different" body, connect people who are not disabled and people who are. The texts construct emotional identities for both kinds of people and model the feeling relationships that should exist between people on the basis of their bodies.

The dynamics of this economy are anything but stable. The feelings generated by disability circulate from person to person with no clear logic, and the identity of the "feeling person" is anything but consistent. Overpowering suspicion, for example, is said to characterize blind men's feelings toward their sighted wives, the mutual feelings of the blind and sighted, and deaf people's feelings toward the world at large. Suspicion is also glaringly evident in social reformers' treatment of the disabled poor—as they ferret out "that scandal of the blind, the blind beggar and his debauched dependents" ("Co-operation Among Societies for the Benefit of the Blind" 123).

Similarly, emotional "affliction" circulates from person to person with the same disturbing randomness that characterized conflicting nineteenth-century theories about the genesis of physical impairment. In the decades before the rise of bacteriology in the late 1800s, debates raged between contagionist and anticontagionist views of the transmission of illness; theories of hereditary transmission of traits were also very different from those accepted today. Within this theoretical context, physical impairment might result from an infant's contact with "morbid secretions" in the birth canal or from a pregnant woman seeing a person with a disability; it could be the product of a weak constitution's meeting with a miasmic environment, or simply arise from within a "scrofulous" or otherwise unsound constitution inherited from a parent (see Hamlin, Lomax).

Scientific uncertainty about physical "affliction" has its parallel in the verbal shiftiness of descriptions of affliction as an emotional condition. For example, while deaf children are habitually described as "stricken" beings, they are also accorded substantial power to harm others; one educational institution asserts that "the uninstructed Deaf and Dumb must be causes of unceasing sorrow to their afflicted parents and friends, and in most cases useless and burdensome, often dangerous and injurious, members of Society" (*Historical Sketch* iv). Another school report assures gentlefolk that they "need not be apprehensive of seeing anything which can hurt their feelings" when they visit (*Account* 8). The family afflicted by a disabled child, the charitable donor who sees an impaired person on the street or in a school, or even the reader of an emotionally moving representation of physical disability is in many texts invested with as much or more narrative energy as people with disabilities themselves. In fact, like so many twentieth-century narratives of disability, the stories of feeling written on the bodies of nineteenth-century people with impairments seem written to express and manage the feelings of the nonimpaired. More than anything, they address the issue of how to feel about physical disabilities and people who have them, a problem that people today find so disturbing that they tend to avoid it until their own inevitable disablement makes that avoidance impossible.

In the nineteenth century, as in our own, the issue that produced the greatest volume of written discourse was how to feel about people who were not only physically impaired but also economically needy. Nineteenth-century writing often articulates the need to find out how people with disabilities feel not only in order to find out how to feel about disability but also in order to decide, in a century of frequent, often severe unemployment, which individuals with disabilities deserve public or private help.

This project is central to *London Labour and the London Poor*'s interviews with the "afflicted" classes. Because Mayhew's overall objective is not simply to catalog the varieties of work that poor Londoners do but also to distinguish the "energetic" from the "anergetic" segments of society, his questions always prod interviewees to comment on the significant question of how much emotional misery they are in. Like Oliver Sacks, he inquires into the experience of disability from a stance of eager interest and gears his questions to the interests of nondisabled readers. The interviews are atypically particular about the bodies of physically disabled people; *London Labour* sometimes renders them from three perspectives: seen and described by Mayhew; seen and described by the interviewees themselves; and shown in daguerreotypes. There is a clear purpose underlying Mayhew's "scientific" explorations, however; his questions and his narrative frames inscribe both the rhetoric of affliction as an emotional state and its particular function for middle-class nondisabled people concerned with the "afflicted and neglected" as social problems, as "the minor streams which ultimately swell the great torrent of pauperism" (*Report* xii). With each interview, Mayhew supplies an implied or direct evaluation of the authenticity of emotional suffering in the subject and, by extension, a judgment on whether this person is deserving or undeserving of financial help, an afflicted child or a begging impostor.

Despite Mayhew's ostensible control over the purpose and meaning of the narratives, what emerges from the interviews is as informative about the position of people with impairments as it is about the stance of nondisabled culture toward them. These coached narratives may not accurately reflect the subjectivity of Victorian people with disabilities. They do provide ample evidence of the difficulty of authenticating one-self within the rhetoric of affliction, as well as the range of strategies "afflicted" people used to negotiate the social judgments that hinged on emotional constructions of disability.

In their material facts, the lives of many of Mayhew's interviewees are unremittingly difficult. At the same time, however, these people's accounts of their lives are often surprising for their *lack* of sentiment. This becomes especially noticeable when Mayhew establishes the narrative as a melodramatic story of affliction, and then the subject of the story counters with a story that is grounded in material facts rather than feelings, or a story that mingles unhappiness with joy and accomplishment. A fascinating interplay ensues between Mayhew's diagnosis of a person's degree of suffering, the interviewee's own treatment of the facts of his/her life, and the reader's response.

While pain is not necessarily a component of physical disability, Elaine Scarry's comments on pain are pertinent to the continual project of assessing suffering that *London Labour* enacts in its pages and encourages in its readers (the same project that is a significant component of social agencies' "diagnosis" and classification of applicants for aid). Scarry writes, "When one hears about another person's physical pain, the events happening within the interior of that person's body may seem to have the remote character of some deep subterranean fact, belonging to an invisible geography that, however portentous, has no reality because it has not yet manifested itself on the visible surface of the earth. . . . [T]he pains occurring in other people's bodies flicker before the mind, then disappear" (3–4). Bodily pain has the ironic status of being both undeniable and unconfirmable, depending on one's perspective; "to have pain is to have *certainty*; to hear about pain is to have *doubt*" (13).

Because the emotional suffering attributed to people with disabilities is as unconfirmable as bodily pain, Mayhew's stance is subject to shifts from pity to suspicion, based on the fluctuations in the performance of affliction he observes and Mayhew's sense of its authenticity or falsehood.

The crippled street-seller of nutmeg-graters is an example of an emotional expression of disability that passes muster through its understatement of sorrow (fig. 2.1). This man, who has multiple congenital limb impairments and must navigate the streets on his knees, seems absolutely to merit Mayhew's assessment as the ultimate in suffering, given the accumulated abuse to body and spirit he has experienced. The man's rendition of these events, however, seems anti-emotional at times. His mother, a woman of "weak intellects," bore him out of wedlock, paid a fellow-servant to take care of him after her marriage, and saw him only once a year until her death. The street-seller's explanation of what could certainly be called abandonment, however, is nonjudgmental and appreciative: "No mother couldn't love a child more than mine did, but her feelings was such that she couldn't bear to see me." He emphasizes only her generosity to him, and at one point says (as if in response to a probing, incredulous Mayhew), "Oh, yes; I used to like to see her very much" (1:331). It is the reader (and presumably Mayhew) who supplies the heart-wrenching frame for this story, not the interviewee.

At other times, the man seems on the verge of characterizing himself as a helpless, afflicted child, as in this passage: "I feel miserable enough when I see the rain come down of a week day, I can tell you. Ah, it *is* very miserable indeed lying in bed all day, and in a lonely room, without perhaps a person to come near one—helpless as I am—and hear the rain beat against the windows, and all that without nothing to put in your lips." This melancholy, lyrical construction of disability, however, is essentially thrown away by the matter-of-fact assertion that follows it: "I've done *that* over and over again where I lived before; but where I am now I'm more comfortable like" (1:330). The image of misery is ephemeral, not something the man expands to define his entire life. Similarly, although he says he was suicidal when his mother and guardian died, because "I was all alone then, and what could I do—cripple as I was," the question immediately becomes rhetorical, as he details the many things that he *can* do: read and write, build and renovate furni-

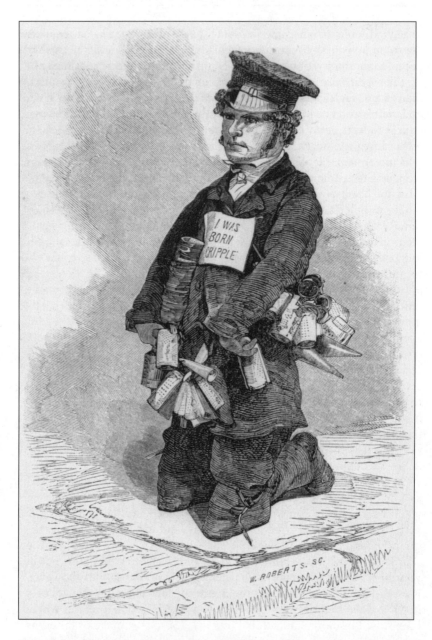

Fig. 2.1. "The Crippled Street-Seller of Nutmeg-Graters." From Henry Mayhew, *London Labour and the London Poor* (1861–62), 1:168.

ture, and trade in household items (1:331). At one point he had his own shop; after his inability to collect debts caused him to lose it, he hawked kitchen goods. It was illness, not his limb impairments, that sent him to the workhouse, and he left it with five shillings (hard-won from the Poor-Law Guardians) to buy stock and try to make his own living. While this venture was not entirely successful, the street-seller believes that "[w]ith a couple of pounds I could . . . manage to shift very well for myself. I'd get a stock, and go into the country with a barrow, and buy old metal, and exchange tin ware for old clothes, and, with that, I'm almost sure I could get a decent living. I'm accounted a very good dealer" (1:332). The last thing the man says of himself emphasizes his business ability, not his incapacity. It is worth noting, however, that the final image Mayhew gives us—via an interview with one of his friends—is of an "utterly helpless" creature, hurled into the streets by his arms and legs and left shivering against a lamp-post for not paying his rent (1:333).

Other interviewees collaborate with Mayhew's tendency to characterize the disabled as helpless, suffering children. The blind needle-seller, despite fifteen years of increasing visual impairment, seems not to have adapted at all to his blindness:

I go along the streets in great fear. If a baby have hold of me, I am firm, but by myself, I reel about like a drunken man. I feel very timid unless I have hold of something—not to support me, but to assure me I shall not fall. . . . [I]f I missed [the bannister], I'm sure I should grow so giddy and nervous I should fall from the top to the bottom. (1:344)

He further emphasizes his physical and emotional delicacy by describing wonderful, colorful dreams that "so excite me that I am ill all the next day" (1:343). Unlike the nutmeg-grater seller, he describes his emotional affliction as encompassing his whole existence: "Oh, ours is a miserable life, sir!—worn out—blind with over work, and scarcely a hole to put one's head in, or a bit to put in one's mouth. God Almighty knows that's the bare truth, sir" (1:341).

The needle-seller's lyric lament is at times disrupted by Mayhew's eager questions about blindness, producing statements like this one:

Oh, yes; if I had all the riches in the world I'd give them every one to get my sight back, for it's the greatest pressure to me to be in the darkness. God help me! I know I am a sinner, and believe I'm so afflicted on account of my sins. No, sir, it's nothing like when you shut your eyes. . . . I see a dark mass before me, and never any change-everlasting darkness, and no chance of a light or shade in this world. But I feel consoled somehow, now it is settled; although it's a very poor comfort after all. (1:343–44)

In this last passage, we can almost hear Mayhew interrupting the flows of lamentation in order to pose more questions about what blindness feels like. In contrast to his verbal prods to the nutmeg-grater seller to bemoan his existence, Mayhew seems here to want to rein in what he considers an excessive display of emotion.

This characterizes his interview with the crippled street-seller of birds as well. This man looks and feels healthy, is never in pain, and sleeps well. He has a regular place to lodge, with his married sister, and has mostly avoided the workhouse. He maintains himself through a business he enjoys. He discusses, at length, the characteristics and diets of the various birds he sells, accounts himself "a very good judge of birds" and a knowledgeable manager of them, and is confident that "[i]f I had a pound to lay out in a few nice cages and good birds, I think I could do middling" (2:69).

In regard to his disabilities (as well as having no ankle, he has impaired speech), the bird-seller says, "I am quite reconciled to my lameness, quite; and have been for years. O, no, I never fret about that now." At the same time, he repeatedly gives his life a melodramatic frame, in the form of an overriding narrative of affliction that cancels out all conflicting information (2:68). He collapses his beginning and end into the fact of his disability, making himself into a disabled "type": "I was born a cripple, sir," he said, "and I shall die one." While he says that he likes reading, he has no interest in the newspaper because "there'll be no change for me in this world" (2:67). Both he and his birds are "prisoners." His narrative, like the needle-seller's, culminates in woe:

> I think of the next world sometimes, and feel quite sure, quite, that I shan't be a cripple there. Yes, that's a comfort, for this world will never be any good to me. I feel that I shall be a poor starving cripple, till I end, perhaps in the workhouse. Other men can get married, but not such as me. . . . I never was in love in my life, never.

Mayhew, who has termed the man "poor fellow" and "poor cripple," and authorized his misery in various ways, seems to run out of patience at this. He comments, "Among the vagrants and beggars, I may observe, there are men more terribly deformed than the bird-seller, who are married, or living in concubinage" (2:68).

Mayhew's response to what he seems to consider excessive emotional displays recalls Evangelical minister Thomas Chalmers's cautionary words to charitable donors: "Many applications will end in your refusal of them in the first instance; because *till they have had experience of your vigilance, the most undeserving are likely to obtrude themselves*" (qtd. in Young and Ashton 72; emphasis added).

If the undeserving are the most stimulating spectacles, then the truly deserving never present themselves to the eye at all, or at least do not "obtrude" themselves. This model for distinguishing the deserving from the undeserving is a particularly effective way to reduce charitable giving. If being seen and/or heard is usually a prerequisite of being helped, Chalmers's theory allowed donors to entertain the fantasy that there were no deserving poor in the vicinity, only visible, audible impostors, and thus that no help was required. Within this model of the charitable relationship, it becomes nearly impossible for the needy person to hit the right level of emotional distress in his or her tale of suffering; too little emotion seems safe, but may run the risk of being ignored; even a hair too much (as gauged by the listener) tends to classify the pain as too extreme to be real and the complainer as a potential malingerer.

Every one of Mayhew's interviewees has experienced physical and emotional misery. At the same time, narratives like those of the crippled bird-seller and the blind needle-seller make clear that what is at stake for a person telling his or her story is not only to tell the truth but also to tell it plausibly enough to generate support from the nondisabled. The needle-seller's lament ends with a mention of Day's Charity, a clear indication that he sees Mayhew's interview as his best chance to publicize and authenticate his need and thus find assistance outside of the workhouse.[1] For a poor person with a disability, nondisabled beliefs about "affliction" could not be resisted or avoided without serious financial consequences.

Mayhew generally manages to remain the proprietor of the master narrative of emotion and disability in most of these autobiographical narratives, guiding, controlling, and correcting. One of his most extended interviews, however, with a blind boot-lace seller (fig. 2.2), elicits a narrative with such complicated relationships to disability and affect that it utterly confounds Mayhew's control. The interviews with the boot-lace seller produce Mayhew's most elaborate discourse on disability, revealing not only his complicated attitudes toward blind people, begging, and work, but also his utter fascination with blindness. This lively, loquacious informant gives Mayhew several pages of material regarding the life and character of the blind in general and the London street blind in particular. He confirms some stereotypes (spirituality and love of music) and counters others (blind men's asexuality; blind women's inability to keep house). He describes the street folk who are blind as a warm and hospitable community, and suggests what we might now call blind culture. Perhaps most provocatively, his comments about the blind beggar—one of the most emotionally invested stereotypes of blindness— exceed Mayhew's capacity to supply a unitary narrative framework.

The blind boot-lace seller offers the strongest testimony of the communities that are built among disabled people on the streets of London. His account of street life is a combination of harsh environmental condi-

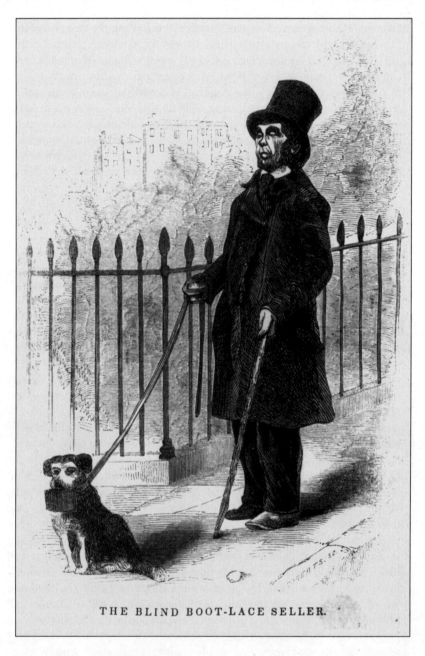

THE BLIND BOOT-LACE SELLER.

Fig. 2.2. "The Blind Boot-Lace Seller." From Henry Mayhew, *London Labour and the London Poor* (1861–62), 1:176.

tions (including treatment by the nondisabled middle classes) and warm relationships among people on the street who are visually impaired:

> The blind people in the streets mostly know one another; they say they have all a feeling of brotherly love for one another, owing to their being similarly afflicted. If I was going along the street, and had a guide with me that could see, they would say, "Here's a blind man or blind woman coming"; I would say, "Put me up to them so as I'll speak to them"; then I should say, as I laid my hand upon them, "Holloa, who's this?" they'd say, "I'm blind." I should answer, "So am I." "What's your name?" would be the next question. "Oh, I have heard tell of you," most like, I should say. . . . [T]hen we say, "Do you belong to any of the Institutions?" that's the most particular question of all; and if he's not a traveller, and we never heard tell of one another, the first thing we should ask would be, "How did you lose your sight?" (1:398)

This sense of community, it is important to note, is far less evident in the life writings of wealthier Victorians with physical impairments.[2]

Most disabled interviewees define themselves against the beggar (of necessity, as this is the identity most likely to be clapped on them). The bird-seller would rather be twice as lame than beg; the nutmeg-grater seller would rather starve. The boot-lace seller, in contrast, details his "fall" into mendicancy with what I can only call delight. After fifteen years successfully gathering and selling coal, he decided to "shake a loose leg" because of a conflict with his father. Contacts at the low lodging-houses persuaded him to use his blindness to make a living; over time he became, as Mayhew puts it, "heart and soul, an ingrained beggar" (1:407). Now he perambulates the streets of London, "selling" boot-laces as a cover story for begging. It is a life he calls "dreadful slavery," but one which makes him "a comfortable living—always a little bit in debt" (1:399).

The boot-lace seller's acumen as a professional object of charity in many ways confirms him as exactly the kind of person the Charity Organisation Society blind registers were designed to thwart. He demonstrates a prodigious memory for the names, addresses, and pensioning habits of upper-class Londoners, unfurling a charter that would have been invaluable to other blind people in search of aid. He himself receives several small pensions despite his begging (in theory, a disqualification). His skill at tapping the flows of systematic and casual charity establishes him as much too capable to be an "acceptable" beggar.

In terms of his relationship to sentiment, however, the boot-lace seller confounds the stereotype of a beggar/impostor. In the first place, the really scandalous beggar would seem by definition a creature devoid of feelings. He cheats the feelings and alms from others, and eventually hardens their hearts through his abuse of the sacred and emotional charitable compact, but he feels neither affliction nor gratitude, only greed and malicious amusement.

The blind boot-lace seller, however, seems to confirm his own description of the blind as "persons of great feeling" (1:401). His accounts of his first travels as a beggar are fervently emotional (albeit toward an unorthodox object). The narrative is suffused with a sense of naïve enthusiasm, attractive enough to make it an advertisement for begging:

> You see I'd never had no pleasure, and it seemed to me like a new world—to be able to get victuals without doing anything—instead of slaving as I'd been with a couple of carts and horses at the coal-pits all the time. I didn't think the country was half so big, and you couldn't credit the pleasure I felt in going about it. . . . [At one lodging-house] I found upwards of sixty or seventy, all tramps, and living in different ways, pattering, and thieving, and singing, and all sorts; and that night I got to think it was the finest scene I had ever known. I grew pleaseder, and pleaseder, with the life, and wondered how any one could follow any other. There was no drunkenness, but it was so new and strange, and I'd never known nothing of life before, that I was bewildered, like, with over-joy at it.

In terms of more "appropriate" responses, the man weeps while recounting the death of his dog and is "affected, even to speechlessness, at the remembrance of his family troubles." He is similarly moved by Mayhew's stories of other disabled street-sellers (1:406).

Even more provocatively, the boot-lace seller's feelings extend beyond what we might call his "personal" life (he is intriguing in part because he does not separate his personal feelings and his professional ones). His appreciation of the emotional capital of blindness is not only business-like and distanced but *also* sentimental and engaged. His attitude toward his pattering lament (one of the tools in the trade of a professional "afflicted child") exemplifies this doubleness. The lament itself, as the man delivers it to Mayhew, is a combination of avowed feeling and professional notes:

> You feeling Christians look with pity,
> Unto my grief relate—
> Pity my misfortune,
> For my sufferings are great.
> I'm bound in dismal darkness—
> A prisoner I am led;
> Poor and blind, just in my prime,
> Brought to beg my bread.
> When in my pleasant youthful days
> In learning I took delight,
> (and when I was in the country I used to say)

And by the small-pox
I lost my precious sight.
(some says by an inflammation)
I've lost all earthly comforts,
But since it is God's will,
The more I cannot see the day,
He'll be my comfort still.
In vain I have sought doctors,
Their learned skill did try,
But they could not relieve me,
Nor spare one single eye.
So now in dismal darkness
For ever more must be,
To spend my days in silent tears
Till death doth set me free.
But had I all the treasures
That decks an Indian shore,
Was all in my possession,
I'd part with that wealthy store,
If I once more could gain my sight,
And when could gladly view
That glorious light to get my bread,
And work once more like you.
Return you, tender Christians dear,
And pity my distress;
Relieve a helpless prisoner,
That's blind and comfortless.
I hope that Christ, our great Redeemer,
Your kindness will repay,
And reward you with a blessing
On the judgment day.

(1:399)

This is a performance of affliction, presented in the exact terms that will elicit sympathy without suspicion. As in the document produced by the School for the Indigent Blind, blindness is constructed as a "dark and benighted state, for which no relief can be found on this side of the grave." The *disinterest* in money that seems, ironically, so central to the charitable exchange is displayed as well; the beggar would give untold riches only to see *and work*. At the same time, he has something substantial to transfer to the benevolent donor: his own intimacy with God.

Much of this, of course, contradicts what we have heard of the man's real feelings. He is anything but dismal, devoid of earthly comforts, or desirous of traditional work. His comment that the lamentation is "a very feeling thing," however, is impossible to view with irony alone when it seems so heartfelt.

> Many people stands still and hears it right through, and gives a halfpenny. I'd give one myself any day to hear it well said. I'm sure the first time I heard it the very flesh crept on my bones. (1:399)

Further, as Mayhew's remarks confirm, the boot-lace seller's awareness that he is manipulating public emotions for gain has not hardened him to the pleas—or manipulations—of others:

> [T]here was, amid the degradation that necessarily comes of habitual mendicancy, a fine expression of sympathy, that the better class of poor always exhibit toward the poor; nor could I help wondering when I heard *him*—the professed mendicant—tell me how he had been moved to tears by the recital of the sufferings of another mendicant—sufferings that might have been as profitable a stock in trade to the one as his blindness was to the other; though it is by no means unusual for objects of charity to have *their* objects of charity, and to be imposed upon by fictitious or exaggerated tales of distress, almost as often as they impose upon others by the very same means. (1:407–8)

Finally unable to categorize the boot-lace seller as either an innocent afflicted child or (despite his practices) a reviled begging impostor, Mayhew presents the man as a sort of demonic child, "a strange compound of cunning and good feeling; at one moment . . . weeping over the afflictions of others . . . the next minute . . . grinning behind his hand, so that his laughter might be concealed from me, in a manner that appeared almost fiendish" (1:407).

The boot-lace seller is among the very cheeriest of Mayhew's disabled interviewees. Of all of them, he seems the only one whose relationship with popular stereotypes of blindness has an expansive, not constrictive, effect on his sense of self. His business is to embody both the beggar and the child, and yet he is neither of these figures; he occupies multiple positions within the emotional economy of disability, weeping freely and making others weep, receiving alms and passing them on. Rather than resisting the emotional stereotypes of his time, he puts them to work.

One of the dangers in uncovering the cultural history of discrimination against people with physical impairments is that the story we piece together is a narrative of villains and victims that effectively re-enshrines disabled people as incapable of speaking or acting for themselves. While it is crucial to make it clear just how that discrimination took place and how thorough it was, it is equally crucial to recover the subjectivity, voice, and agency of people with disabilities who survived discrimination.

These Victorian narratives have a lot to tell us about the motivation to see physical impairments in emotional (and largely negative) terms. They let us measure how the enculturation of physical disability has changed since the nineteenth century and how much it still needs to change. While words like *affliction* have gone into semiretirement, the end of the feelings behind these terms is much less certain. We may laugh at nineteenth-century theories of heredity and disease, but still act as though physical and emotional "affliction" were catching.

The most important message of narratives like those in *London Labour,* however, may be to remind us that the main site of change since the nineteenth century has been in the behaviors of nondisabled people rather than in the capabilities of people with disabilities. One of the key gaps in cultural concepts of disability is the failure to recognize the practical strengths it occasions in people. Living at odds with your culture because its physical and social environments are designed with other bodies in mind almost always catalyzes the development of mental, emotional, physical, and social capabilities, including exceptional problem-solving skills. These strategic abilities are not solely features of Supercrip or "overcoming disability" narratives, but strengths that persist in anyone who has learned to get to work in a wheelchair, raise a child while chronically ill, or accommodate the feelings of nondisabled culture. These Victorian stories tell us that even when people with disabilities had limited power to determine the policies or language that shaped their lives, they still created their experience beyond the limits of "affliction."

Notes

1. In the 1830s, Charles Day, of the city firm Day and Martin, left to blind charity a legacy of £100,000, which Chancery elected to deploy in small pensions (Owen 173).

2. For Elizabeth Gilbert, as for many sighted middle-class women, social activism was a route to greater autonomy, mobility, and life satisfaction within Victorian beliefs about proper behavior for gentlewomen; see Vicinus 22–23. Gilbert's daily involvement with the blind workers whose cause she championed, however, was even more significant, because it allowed her to join the community of other blind people, an opportunity few middle-class blind women would have enjoyed. MP Henry Fawcett's story provides a striking contrast; while he spoke (with difficulty) on behalf of the blind, he did not himself identify as blind, pointedly spoke as if he could still see, and advised others to "do what you can to act as though you were not blind" (Stephen 68). As much as this strategy of "passing" was promoted and necessitated by his culture, following it left him with no way to experience the particular social ties and collaborative strength that other blind and visually impaired people enjoyed in his time and enjoy in our own.

Works Cited

An Account of the School for the Indigent Blind, in St. George's Fields, Surrey. London: Philanthropic Society, 1830.

"Co-operation Among Societies for the Benefit of the Blind." *Charity Organisation Reporter* 3 July 1872: 123.

"The Crippled." *Charity Organisation Reporter* 14 Mar. 1878: 55.

Dickens, Charles. *The Cricket on the Hearth.* 1845. Christmas Books. 1852. Oxford: Oxford UP, 1954.

Fosbroke, John. "Practical Observations on the Pathology and Treatment of Deafness: No. VIII." *Lancet* 16 Apr. 1831: 69–72.

Great Britain. Royal Commission on the Blind, the Deaf and Dumb, &c., of the United Kingdom. *Report.* London: HMSO, 1889.

Hamlin, Christopher. "Predisposing Causes and Public Health in Early-Nineteenth-Century Medical Thought." *Social History of Medicine* 5 (Apr. 1992): 43–70.

An Historical Sketch of the Asylum for Indigent Deaf and Dumb Children, Surrey. London: Edward Brewster, 1841.

Lawrence, William. "Lectures on the Anatomy, Physiology, and Diseases of the Eye: Lecture I." *Lancet* 22 Oct. 1825: 145–51.

Lomax, Elizabeth. "Infantile Syphilis as an Example of Nineteenth-Century Belief in the Inheritance of Acquired Characteristics." *Journal of the History of Medicine* 34 (1979): 23–39.

Martin, Frances. *Elizabeth Gilbert and Her Work for the Blind.* London: Macmillan, 1884.

Mayhew, Henry. *London Labour and the London Poor.* 4 vols. 1861–62. New York: Dover, 1968.

Meredith, George. *Diana of the Crossways.* 1885. New York: Modern Library, 1971.

Owen, David. *English Philanthropy, 1660–1960.* Cambridge: Belknap-Harvard UP, 1964.

Scarry, Elaine. *The Body in Pain: The Making and Unmaking of the World.* New York: Oxford UP, 1985.

School for the Indigent Blind, Liverpool. *School for the Blind.* 1818.

Stephen, Leslie. *Life of Henry Fawcett.* London: Smith, Elder, 1886.

Vicinus, Martha. *Independent Women: Work and Community for Single Women, 1850–1920.* Chicago: U of Chicago P, 1985.

Young, A. F., and E. T. Ashton. *British Social Work in the Nineteenth Century.* London: Routledge and Kegan Paul, 1956, 1967.

3

On the Rhetorics of Mental Disability

Catherine Prendergast

Schizophrenia never had an easy access code.
—Avital Ronell, *The Telephone Book*

When Barbara[1] said that she was aware of her mind as having been reconstructed by the discipline of psychiatry, I started listening. Barbara at this point had not been on the inside of a lockdown ward for five years, hadn't been living in a halfway house for over four years, and was working, though not steadily. She was talking to me from her own (albeit heavily subsidized) apartment. At the time of our conversation, I was completing a dissertation in the field of composition and rhetoric. My specialization often involves tracking the effects of social formations—disciplines, institutions, texts—on the creation and management of knowledge. Her comment reminded me of Lucille McCarthy and Joan Gerring's analysis of the revision of the American Psychiatric Association's [APA] *Diagnostic and Statistical Manual of Mental Disorders* [DSM] into a fourth edition and their conclusion, which I have much admired, that the resulting document is largely an artifact of the professionalization of psychiatry. To have Barbara, an "insider" to the psychiatric system, validate the impact of disciplinary formations on the construction of her thoughts was perhaps part of the reason I perked up at her statement. In all honesty, however, I really started listening because, to me, her statement made sense, and I above all wanted Barbara to make sense.

Barbara and I have been close friends all my life. I would like to be able to say that mental illness has done nothing to shatter that closeness, but it has, perhaps in greatest part because of our inability to broker a shared understanding of it. Her comment offered me schizophrenia in a way I could understand it. In short, it was to *my* mind an index of sanity, and I had developed an ear for indexing where Barbara was concerned. I reasoned her condition had been steadily improving over the course of the seven years since her original diagnosis; she had passed into progressively less restrictive settings to receive care. But in the year after that phone call Barbara was admitted to her county's psychiatric hospital four times in the course of six months, and I have been forced to reconsider the value of one of our few shared insights—its utility if not its validity. As I reflect on the trajectory of her life since her diagnosis, it seems to me that both our lives and our relationship have been shaped by multiple ideological currents (not simply disciplinary ones) and by biological forces, the nature of which seems to surpass anyone's understanding.

Just to be clear, at this point I believe, along with the National Alliance for the Mentally Ill [NAMI], that schizophrenia is no less a brain disorder than Alzheimer's disease or multiple sclerosis. This is apparently a belief that puts me on a collision course with many of my colleagues in rhetoric, English literature, and cultural studies, colleagues with whom I generally share—along with office space, Xerox machines, and hours of conversation—a number of basic epistemological assumptions. I've noticed that if I mention mental illness in the company of many of these colleagues, I become suddenly culturally unintelligible. As Carol Neely, literary scholar of madness, observes, in the present theoretical climate "contradictions within the subject are inscribed by institutions, social formations, representations, and discursive practices" (786); she suggests that this theoretical orientation has the effect of rendering insanity at once "ubiquitous and irrelevant" (786). For an academic like myself with generally poststructuralist leanings, to think of schizophrenia as a "disease" makes me sound at best conservative and at worst theoretically unsound. I am therefore left wandering far from my usual terrain to find language with which I can address the dilemmas and gaps in understanding that mental illness presents. The growing literature on disability would seem a natural place to turn to find such language, yet it seems that disability studies, with its emphasis on the body and not the mind, creates fissures through which attention to the mentally disabled easily falls. One might ask if there are any discourses in which people with severe mental illness might comfortably reside. I proceed with that question in the hope of identifying the rhetorical slippages that left many of the mentally ill of the 1990s in as poor straits as those of the nineteenth century, despite the advent of antipsychotic medicines and the institution of formal rights; specifically, I am hoping to discover how it happened that in the 1990s to be mentally ill was practically a crime.

A Short Disclaimer

This account will resemble a pastiche more than a teleological argument. This is not to enact stylistically my conception of schizophrenic thought patterns. Such mimicry is problematic because schizophrenics are, by virtue of having been diagnosed schizophrenic (or "SZ"), in a distinct and complex relationship to "audience" that I am not in, by virtue of not having that diagnosis. This, then, is my own account, my own trek through case studies, textbooks, theoretical essays, films, manuals, and memoirs—texts that treat the same subject from radically divergent perspectives and with widely variant rhetorical sensibilities. In the absence of an all-encompassing grand narrative, I trace recurrent tropes and ironies that slide between the public discourse on insanity, the scholarly discourse, and my own personal experience in the hopes that charting this movement will bring about a kind of coherence. I have as a result many more questions than answers. Barbara, by the way, is quite capable of telling her own story. However, as I observe in the following pages, since the diagnosis of schizophrenia necessarily supplants one's position as rhetor, Barbara may tell her story, but no one can hear it.

Paperwork: Part One

A poststructuralist perspective suggests that insanity is a discursive construct, expressed, reinforced, and sometimes subverted by public discourse, the discourse of experts, and by institutional structures which themselves can be viewed as discursive constructs.

Barbara has been perpetually in the midst of paperwork, hanging on by the thread of unfilled-out forms in her refusal to be declared officially "disabled," a designation she doesn't particularly enjoy but one that she is entitled to according to the provisions set forth in the Americans with Disabilities Act. Among other things, the designation of disability is facilitated by a diagnosis in line with the DSM IV. Like most of the mentally ill, Barbara's diagnosis has migrated among the categories of severe mental disorders outlined by the DSM IV, and her numerous medications have changed with each diagnosis.

I asked her recently, between her third and fourth trip to the hospital this year, what the "diagnosis du jour" was:

"They have me down as bipolar with psychotic features."

"What happened to the diagnosis of schizophrenia?"

"That was a leftover from that doctor years ago who decided I had sufficient thought disruptions to be diagnosed schizophrenic. I have no use for her, so I can't remember her name."

"Oh. So it's bipolar with psychotic—with psychotic what?"

"Features."

I got stuck on that word *features* because images of cartoon characters with their tongues hanging out in zigzags or their eyes turned into gyroscopes started flying through my mind. I wondered silently just what "feature" of Barbara is psychotic, and perhaps she wondered that, too, because we both laughed. Nonetheless, that I can so easily reconfigure Barbara as a cartoon character, two-dimensional and fragmented, is symptomatic of a certain perceptual problem that has evolved on my part either as a result of dealing with symptoms of the disease (e.g., "flattened affect," "pressured speech") or with the "side effects" of the drugs used to suppress symptoms of the disease which have disturbing symptoms of their own, or perhaps as a consequence of the oft-noted depersonalizing effects of the psychiatric system. Under the weight of all these effects and affects I search for ways in which I can think of Barbara without first recategorizing her in my mind as a mass of misfiring molecules.

The categories of disorders presented by the DSM IV have been indicted by rhetoricians on the grounds that they contribute to such perceptual distortion. The APA's urtext has been viewed by many as an illness-constructing document of incredible rhetorical power. Carol Berkenkotter and Doris Ravotas suggest, for example, that as a result of the discursive tools of categorization provided by the DSM IV nosology, "In effect, the client becomes the sum of his or her symptoms" (271). Another rhetoric-oriented denouncer of the DSM, Theodore Sarbin, charges that "schizophrenia, originally a metaphor created to help communicate about crazy behavior, is now regarded as a disease entity by most medical practitioners," completing what he calls the "metaphor-to-myth transformation" (313). McCarthy and Gerring point to the proliferation of disorders in the DSM IV and suggest, "The DSM classification system adopts the biomedical assumption that there are clear boundaries between diseases and between the sick and the healthy" (183). For McCarthy and Gerring, the DSM IV is the psychiatric profession's main vehicle for maintaining dominance over other mental health disciplines, firmly entrenching the biomedical model of mental disorder.

Coming from a perspective of wholehearted endorsement of the biomedical model and the very assumption of a clear boundary between sick and healthy in particular, NAMI's favored spokesperson/professional, E. Fuller Torrey, is no less critical of the DSM IV and no less willing to grant the document rhetorical force as an constructor of illness. Torrey, however, concludes the reverse of McCarthy and Gerring: that the proliferation of disorders that characterizes the present incarnation of the DSM is problematic because it dissolves the boundaries between the sick and the healthy. Torrey argues that the document enacts an expansion of the definition of mental illness to include everyone. He suggests that the present proliferation of disorders ("the Woody Allen Syndrome," he calls it) allows psychiatrists to devote their attentions to "the wealthy and worried well"—those Torrey believes are in a different category of need altogether from the severely mentally ill. If everyone is sick, Torrey complains, no one is, and funds originally ear-marked for the most needy are spread thin to accommodate everyone (*Shadows* 182). Torrey nevertheless does not assign the APA complete blame for what he sees as misdirected attention and funding. He sug-gests the Woody Allen Syndrome is connected to wider social and po-litical trends, not simply to the actions of a particular discipline or or-ganization. It would seem that for Torrey, as for Neely, mental illness is—discursively speaking—at once everywhere and nowhere.

Progress

One might argue that this is a good way to remove the burden of stigma from the mentally ill, to contextualize them within the vast spectrum of mental health and hygiene, to make them "not other." Ironically, other attempts to improve the lot of those with severe mental illness have re-lied on viewing the mentally ill as a distinct group. The concern for rights of the mentally ill in this century came not a moment too soon after dec-ades of appalling treatment. Enforced lobotomies and sterilizations, the use of aversive conditioning and uncontrolled medical experimentation, and the scandalous conditions in asylums led many to demand reform. And wide-reaching reform has been a fairly recent phenomenon. In *Is There No Place on Earth for Me?* Susan Sheehan documents that "Creed-moor" State Hospital's 1952 annual report referred to lobotomy as "fur-ther evidence of the desire here to keep up with the modern trend in the care of patients" (10). Every day I am grateful—especially when Barbara is in the hospital—that psychosurgery is now discredited and illegal.

According to Sheehan, sociologists' accounts of the horrible and overcrowded conditions in asylums were routinely attacked by New York State's Department of Mental Hygiene until the advent of anti-psychotics made the possibility of relieving some of the overcrowding a reality. Then, she suggests, "the department's every pronouncement agreed with its critics: State hospitals were hazardous to the health of men-tal patients" (12). In the wake of mass deinstitutionalization, the Dor-othy Dix–style reform of asylum conditions gave way to a more inte-grationist approach in which the emphasis was placed on defending the rights of inpatients and, increasingly, outpatients. By the late seventies, "litigation to correct inhumane institutional conditions had turned to advocacy for the development of community-based services as a means to advance social justice for people with mental disabilities" (Levy and Rubenstein 3). The rise of identity politics helped make possible the application of the rhetoric of rights to situations facing the mentally ill. The irony of this development is that while the presence of a diagnosis would be the very thing that would "identify" the mentally ill, the thrust of identity politics—to end discrimination—effectively recasts the mentally ill not as "ill," not as being in need of treatment, but as being in need of social empowerment and liberation, much like other historically excluded groups (e.g., Native Americans, African Americans).

"Liberation" in terms of the discourse surrounding mental illness, though, necessarily involves addressing the practice of involuntary commitment, a practice which allows for the holding of people against their will under special legal circumstances. The legal standard for involuntary commitment is that a person be deemed "likely to cause serious injury to himself or others" (Levy and Rubenstein 353). This phrase, and the word *likely* in particular, is vague enough that to make that call is to create and re-create dramas of diagnosis and doubt. Almost always, it seems, the practice of involuntary commitment invokes scripts of oppression. Many of the mass-market images of involuntary commitment center around malevolent family members or government agents trying to control free-thinkers or get a grip on someone's assets (e.g., *Terminator 2* and *The Madness of King George*). Barbara has at times compared the managed care organization that handles her outpatient treatment to the Gestapo, forcing her into "voluntary" commitment. As she puts it, the managed care representatives ask if you want to go to the hospital when they really mean, "You're going to the hospital." Sociologist Erving Goffman's critique of mental asylums, published in the early sixties, employs the Gestapo analogy as well; he compares (with a weak qualifier regarding intentions) the "betrayal funnel" relatives help construct to facilitate "the prepatient's progress from home to hospital" to the coaxing of concentration camp victims toward the gas chambers (137).[2]

It is quite possible that Goffman's study was one of those reports Sheehan refers to that were routinely ignored until antipsychotic medicines began to be seen as the biochemical equivalent of physical restraints. Indeed, Foucault's *Madness and Civilization,* another blast at institutionalization, became popular around the same time. More to the point, however, is that neither Goffman's ethnomethodological account of the dynamics of commitment in the 1950s, nor Sheehan's journalistic account of her subject's experiences with institutionalization in the late 1970s, nor, for that matter, Foucault's meditation on confinement throughout the ages is well poised to represent the current conditions under which the mentally ill are held involuntarily. Now, in the 1990s, it is more and more the case that the mentally ill will progress from street to jail, or from homeless shelter to hospital as Barbara initially did. For most, however, there aren't that many hospitals left to progress to as mental institutions have become a thing of the past. In 1955, the year Goffman conducted his study, there were 559,000 patients in state mental institutions (an all-time high). As of 1995, there were 69,000 (Butterfield). Where are the rest?

Too Vast

> This book does not discuss rights in the criminal process. Although these rights are important, the subject is simply too vast to be included in this small volume. (Levy and Rubenstein 13)

> The [Los Angeles County] jail, by default, is the nation's largest mental institution. On an average day, it holds 1,500 to 1,700 inmates who are severely mentally ill, most of them detained on minor charges, essentially for being public nuisances. . . . On any day, almost 200,000 people behind bars—more than 1 in 10 of the total—are known to suffer from schizophrenia, manic depression or major depression, the three most severe mental illnesses. (Fox Butterfield, *New York Times,* 5 March 1998)

A 1998 investigation by the Federal Justice Department of the Los Angeles County jail revealed that a significant proportion of prisoners are severely mentally ill. According to the investigation, the mentally ill upon admission were "issued yellow jumpsuits, which made them easy targets for guards or other inmates. They might be locked 23 hours a day in dirty isolation cells. And any medication they had would be confiscated until a jail psychiatrist saw them—which could take weeks" (Butterfield). Recordkeeping was so inconsistent that many of the inmates either were misdiagnosed or were given the wrong medication. Understandably, many others who had been admitted before were loathe to "identify" themselves as mentally ill, knowing what treatment they would receive, and so they received no medication at all. The federal investigation led to improved conditions in the Los Angeles jail, mostly brought about by moving the mentally ill to another facility; in effect, a mental hospital was created *within* the prison system, but one where inmates seldom stay long enough to receive adequate care or to plan for follow-up care after their release. After years of working toward integration into the wider community, it seems that the mentally ill are being segregated again, even within the already institutionalized community of the prison system.

Los Angeles may be the worst case scenario of a nationwide problem. Following a period of deinstitutionalization in which states slashed their budgets by closing mental hospitals but started shelling out for prisons, jails have become one of the only "asylums" open to the mentally ill around the clock. Managed care policies and the legal gymnastics that must be undertaken to prove that someone is "likely" to injure him or herself make hospital admissions difficult. It is much easier to arrest someone, particularly if that barrier of injury is crossed, which

Torrey and others have argued convincingly is that much more "likely" to happen the longer someone remains untreated. The deinstitutionalization of the mentally ill has therefore resulted in transinstitutionalization. Through legal and economic policy, mental illness has become increasingly criminalized, and the mentally ill increasingly are housed, if housed at all, in jails instead of the dwindling state hospitals. In Los Angeles, a startling 70 percent of the severely mentally ill have been arrested at some point (Butterfield).

In a sense this transinstitutionalization should have been predictable. The penitentiary is quickly becoming the repository for other historically excluded identity groups whose rights have been formally recognized (e.g., Native American, African American). As for Barbara, she has not—to my knowledge—spent a night in jail but has always been referred to the hospital. This I attribute at least in part to her being white, young, pretty, and not particularly aggressive. Even at her worst she looks "likely" to have insurance. These attributes have not saved her, however, from spending quite a few nights on the street or in homeless shelters, the other fast-growing repository for the mentally ill.

There are such things as "mercy busts," arrests officers make to subvert the bureaucratic machinery and shelter people like Barbara from the perils of homelessness. The usual perils the homeless face are in fact multiplied for the mentally ill, who are at greater risk of injury and death and, particularly in the case of women, rape. One survey of 529 homeless people revealed that the prehospitalized participants were three times more likely to eat out of garbage cans and much more likely to use garbage cans as a primary food source (Torrey, *Shadows* 19). I actually haven't asked Barbara if she ate out of garbage cans during the six months she was homeless in New York City; the details she has revealed to me about that period are sketchy on actual events, or perhaps what I would call events. She has recalled voices guiding her this way and that, into certain peril or into protected spaces. She has recalled her first thought in the morning often was to wonder whether she had been raped. I asked her once what she was doing during all that time, and she explained that she was making connections; she would find things, like a bullet hole in a pane of glass and then ride the subways around until she found another bullet hole in a pane of glass.

For Barbara, this constituted her work. Although she was aware she was in danger, she does not to this day think of her time on the streets with as much regret as she thinks of her time in the hospital. Right now she is writing a spy thriller, based on her experiences on the streets, in which a government investigator asks a mental patient with mystical insight to help solve a case.

Insight

> It sounds nice. . . . Who could be against insight? Who could be against motherhood? But clinically, it has zero effectiveness. (Mark Vonnegut, author of *The Eden Express,* a biographical account of his descent into psychosis [quoted in Wyden 84])

> She's a fine mind, but no insight. (One of Barbara's doctors)

Historically, the severely mentally ill have been granted either no insight or insight of an enhanced and often creative or spiritual nature. Having "no insight," in clinical terms, means that a patient does not recognize that he or she has a disease. Schizophrenics, generally having religious inclinations of some kind, have a very different definition of insight. To many schizophrenics, impaired insight is what you get from taking antipsychotics.

In the genre of creative nonfiction written by relatives of schizophrenics, there seems to be an awareness that any impaired insight the mentally ill might have is at least matched by our own incomplete understanding of mental illness or the experience of madness. The title of Robin Hemley's memoir of his schizophrenic sister, *Nola: A Memoir of Faith, Art, and Madness,* seems to place all forms of insight on the same level. "She was a good person. She was a holy person. She was deluded. She was pompous, self-important. . . . I am reminded that whatever I say condemns her, romanticizes her, lies about her, idolizes her, but never, never recreates her in all her complexity," he writes, his portrait of his sister retaining the complexity that the word *and* in his title suggests (121). Author Susan Neville observes of her mother's speech, "When there are recognizable words but no one else can make sense of them, they call it 'word salad.' No one ever thinks to call it music" (214). I include this last statement because I'm not sure that I agree with it. It seems to me that after "word salad," "music" is the next inevitable descriptor. Thinking of popular movie portrayals of the mentally ill, I notice that there isn't a whole lot of gray area there between *Psycho* and *Shine.*[3] I sense from reading Foucault that the position of mad poet is to be regarded as preferable to the position of mental patient. I would argue, however, that these polarized positions effectively place the mentally ill and schizophrenics in particular in a rhetorical black hole. Whether it is music or word salad, one never has to think about "it" at all.

Paperwork: Part Two

> Patients' own writings were included in the record only at the discretion of clinicians. This was done in order to exemplify psychopathology. Sometimes poetry was included as evidence of patients' creativity but writing

which merely displayed rational thinking or logical planning was not actively sought by clinicians to be included. (Barrett 267)

Barrett's observation suggests that clinicians use something like the word salad/music filter to sort patients' writings and that the psychiatric gaze functions as a kind of "terministic screen" (Burke 1035); it is blind to any kind of writing that might be evidence of complexity, of sanity intermingled with insanity. Berkenkotter and Ravotas, too, note in their study that case records as a genre tend to screen out complexity. They compare client accounts of states of being with therapists' written translations of the initial accounts to demonstrate how emic (deeply contextual) descriptions are translated into DSM-speak, largely for purposes of establishing credibility and billability. "The resulting written account supports a billable diagnosis thereby fulfilling its institutional purpose. It fails, however, to serve another important purpose to many therapists, which is helping the therapist to guide the therapy process by providing a record of the client's perspective of his or her lifeworld" (256). They repeatedly note the loss of "richness" in the translation of "the client's rich lifeworld account" (269), "the client's richly descriptive narrative" (271). In doing so they echo Barrett's earlier lament over the loss of "nuance" in clinicians' writing: "They attempted to record what they saw as the essential meaning of the conversation but in doing so, much of the radiant meaning, ambiguity, and nuance was eliminated" (Barrett 272).

I can see how these rhetorical analyses are attempting to demonstrate the dehumanizing effect of the DSM IV and the biomedical model, as well as the bureaucratization of therapy. What seems missing in these rhetorical analyses is some sense of the significance of the loss of the descriptive account, besides the loss of descriptiveness in and of itself. Without such analysis it seems that the real failing of the biomedical model is that it turns clinicians into unimaginative literary critics, translating poetry into psychopathology. Except to note that there is loss in translation, the rhetorical analyses cited above don't engage with "it," the sense of what the patient is saying or writing, any more than the clinical analysis does. The lack of analysis of "it," that which is lost, and what "it" might possibly mean only reassigns the mentally ill to the rhetorical black hole and furthermore avoids engaging in what to me is the most complex rhetorical quandary of all: How or maybe when does one honor schizophrenics as rhetorically enabled subjects?

This is not an easy question. Barbara's "rich lifeworld" accounts have over the course of time I've known her involved CIA drug-testing at parties she's been to, visions of Jimi Hendrix visiting ward B3, and detailed descriptions of thoughts that have been projected into her head by outsiders. They consist of a number of things I don't believe in, though more significantly her doctors don't believe in them. Initially, talking to her about these subjects, I felt the privilege of suspending my disbelief long enough to consider that, well, she might be right. She might be a canary in the mines, more sensitive to the vagaries and possibilities of the technological, political, and spiritual present than I am. At the very least she has an experience of certainty I can't even approach.[4] The writing teacher in me would be drawn to this wealth of unusual, raw description, although I would think of her input as underdeveloped ideas and rough "first drafts" and I would await the kind of clarification that never arrived. Then I read in manuals like *Surviving Schizophrenia, Conquering Schizophrenia,* and the disarmingly entitled *Understanding Schizophrenia* that one of the most characteristic marks of SZs is that they claim that thoughts are being projected into their heads. Schizophrenics by the score testify to being followed by the CIA. Noting the similarity between Barbara's accounts and the accounts of others, I found myself feeling a little schnuckered, as if I'd been taken in by a plagiarist. Lately I've come to think of that initial pedantic reaction as wishful thinking on my part. It's hard to think of anyone you know as a textbook case, especially when the revelation comes so literally.

All this has led me to wonder about the therapeutic value of rich, descriptive, and ambiguous narratives; too often their value is assumed. I think it is worth noting, however, that the assumption that rich, descriptive, nuanced, and ambiguous narratives have therapeutic value harkens back to Freud, who had no patience with the severely mentally ill and no interest in treating them. He crafted a distinction between neurotics and psychotics and devoted his attention to the former, barely even thinking of the latter as human. Furthermore, when American Freudians who didn't acknowledge Freud's self-imposed limitations still dominated the psychiatric profession, recordkeeping and diagnostic features took on a more narrative and nuanced, but nonetheless dehumanizing and invasive character, as Goffman observed: "Current psychiatric doctrine defines mental disorder as something that can have its roots in the patient's earliest years, show its signs throughout the course of his life, and invade almost every sector of his current activity" (155). Thus, Goffman notes, clinicians are justified in invading every sector of the patient's past. Nothing is without relevance. From Goffman's reported data we find this record of a patient which is quite rich and descriptive, though obviously not representative of the patient's perspective:

> Armed with a rather neat appearance and natty little Hitlerian mustache this 45 year old man who has spent the last five or more years of his life in the hospital is making a very successful hospital adjustment living within the role of a rather gay liver and jim-dandy type of fellow who is not only quite superior to his fellow patients in intellectual respects but

who is also quite a man with women. His speech is sprayed with many multi-syllabled words which he generally uses in good context, but if he talks long enough on any subject it soon becomes apparent that he is so completely lost in this verbal diarrhea as to make what he says almost completely worthless. (Qtd. in Goffman 157–58)[5]

This passage is a stark contrast to the post-rise-of-APA case records Barrett and Berkenkotter and Ravotas studied. It is short on nominalization and devoid of jargon. Nevertheless, in its reluctance to report the "sense" of what this man was saying, it stubbornly refuses to let him into the world of rhetoric, and through extension implies that he shouldn't be allowed into the world at all. This patient may have had a narrative of his own, but neither Goffman nor the clinician could render it.

A Multiple Choice Test

Barbara once thought it would be interesting to write down every instance in literature where a narrator invoked the phrase "I heard a voice inside" and then present this list to her psychiatric evaluators.

If I transcribed a passage from Deleuze and Guattari's *A Thousand Plateaus* here and a passage from Avital Ronell's *The Telephone Book*—both of which were written to enact rhetorically the experience of schizophrenic thought—and a passage from a letter Barbara wrote to me from the hospital, you might be hard-pressed to distinguish them, one from the other. If you saw the first two in their published form and Barbara's letter as it reached me, on a rectangle of unlined paper, written in green pencil cramped scribbles that looked as if she had written it in a moving vehicle, your task would be a lot easier. Of course, what stops me from actually conducting this test is that I have noticed that anything a person with a severe mental disorder on their record writes is that much more liable to be appropriated in any number of medical and legal contexts. I would love to cite here the many passages from Barbara's writing: the logical ones, the incoherent ones, the poetic ones. Unfortunately, given this possibility of selective appropriation, she and I both thought it best that I did not.

Suffice it to say that there is a moment at which something or someone is granted what I'll call "rhetoricability"—a moment that has little to do with syntax, grammar, or vocabulary. Nowhere has this moment been more clearly dramatized than in Ted Kacyzinski's pretrial hearings in which teams of psychiatrists examined Kacyzinski in order that it might be determined whether he was to be considered a rhetorically enabled subject capable of defending himself—a status for which he was willing to risk the death penalty. Were his words to be presented in defense of his actions or as evidence that his condition rendered any defense of his actions irrelevant? The latter was eventually decided to stave off a trial that almost certainly would have ended badly for him (Finnegan 61). And so he was put in a bizarre situation—your rhetoric or your life—whereby his own journal was offered paradoxically as evidence that his testimony should be inadmissible.

To be disabled mentally is to be disabled rhetorically, a truth Barbara knows as well as any. Her definition of disability she has phrased at times as "a life denied significance." In the field of rhetoric her statement might be translated into "a life denied signification." Given the present configuration of discourses on mental illness, the writing of schizophrenics can only be seen as arhetorical, the test, the record of symptoms, Exhibit A. At best it is seen as music, as poetry, as some personal expression that has no bearing outside of itself, no transactional worth. It shares much in this respect with the writing of first-year composition students (cf. Miller). That the mentally ill are treated as devoid of rhetoric would seem to me to be an obvious point: If people think you're crazy, they don't listen to you. But I wonder about the implications of that phenomenon as I confront them frequently, as friend, as researcher, as scholar of rhetoric. Specifically, if, as anthropologist Renato Rosaldo offers, we have much to learn from the way the oppressed analyze their own condition, the question of how one listens to the mentally ill in an age in which they have been oppressed by the effective criminalization of their condition becomes vital. Does some kind of al/chemical transformation need to occur before the mentally ill can be heard? And in whom does it need to take place?

Illogical Fear

As a public relations dilemma, schizophrenia was ever a disaster. "Illogical fear," as Senator Domenici had put it, was only one of the barriers giving the illness a reputation as dreaded as leprosy. Other obstacles were resignation that engendered hopelessness; and a near-total ignorance—a NAMI poll found that fifty-five percent of the American public denied that mental illness existed. Denial was rooted in intense repugnance. (Peter Wyden, Conquering Schizophrenia 200)

As Wyden points out, the mentally ill are the most reviled of the disabled: Schizophrenia has no poster child. There is no Special Olympics for institutionalized patients. Nobody runs telethons to raise money for "the cure." Despite all the lip service paid to integrating the severely mentally ill into society (of which I think the newest label "consumer" is the most revealing of greater cultural values), the repugnance Wyden speaks of is palpable and the analogy to leprosy is apt. Tellingly, when Goffman described the five categories of total institutions, he divided the physically disabled, those he classified as incapable of caring for themselves and harmless, from the mentally ill, those he classified as incapable of taking care of themselves and a threat to the community. The other groups Goffman included under this heading were TB patients and lepers. Schizophrenia, it seems, is contagious.

Barbara senses this. She has said that she feels like a red light goes off every time her brain gets too close to someone else's brain. Back when she lived in a halfway house, the very small child next door came up to her and said, "I hate you," a clear translation of "My mommy told me not to talk to you." Founding and maintaining the kind of community enterprises like halfway houses that are so essential to the treatment plans of many outpatients is difficult in the face of frequent hostility from the community.

Of course, this kind of repugnance is meted out to the physically disabled as well. The late anthropologist Robert Murphy, who suffered from ever-deepening quadriplegia, noted that the physically disabled are reviled by the able-bodied because the able-bodied feel themselves at threat: "The disabled serve as constant, visible reminders to the able-bodied that the society they live in is shot through with inequity and suffering, that they live in a counterfeit paradise, that they too are vulnerable. We represent a fearsome possibility" (117). But while it is the visible aspect of the physically disabled that poses a threat, for the mentally disabled the threat is in speech. As historian of perceptions of schizophrenia S. P. Fullinwider has observed, "Certain sorts of people—those the profession learned to call schizophrenics—place an almost unbearable perceptual strain on the psychiatrist. As the doctor confronts the patient he feels his world break apart. He begins to lose perceptual control over his environment" (4).

Perhaps this illogical fear is what accounts for the present banishing of the severely mentally ill to steam grates, dumpsters, jail cells, and isolation tanks. Perhaps in our most closeted imaginations we fear schizophrenics as the most able rhetors of them all. Sadly, though cultural constructions of mental disability have varied widely in the last two hundred years, gone through several crises of categorization and rigorous rhetorical shifts, this banishing, this inability to treat sufferers with humanity or often to treat them at all has remained a cultural constant. The criminalization of the mentally ill has at this point effectively negated many of the gains made over the past fifty years toward more humane treatment. Whether viewed theoretically as acts of faith, art, or madness, the present reality is that the acts of many of the mentally ill are viewed as criminal and the actors are treated accordingly. I wonder about the utility of a rhetoric of rights without a corresponding rhetoric of public responsibility. I wonder how a rhetoric that renders mental illness irrelevant can contribute to healing. I wonder if there will

ever be a rhetoric of mental disability that the mentally disabled themselves will have the greatest part in crafting.

Postscript

As of the spring of 2000, as this article goes to press, Barbara is in
the process of getting a master's degree in recombinant DNA technology at a prominent research university. Maintaining a 3.9 average, she
is planning to pursue a doctorate in biomedical research. She credits her
recent successes to three things: a stable support network of friends,
the therapeutic effects of returning to school, and two new drugs,
Olanzapine and Venlafaxine, which make it possible for her to study.

Notes

I would like to acknowledge the invaluable comments of Cynthia Lewiecki-
Wilson and James Wilson, who patiently read and thoughtfully responded to
several previous versions of this essay. I also thank Gale Walden and David Eng
for their thoughtful comments. Most especially I would like to thank Barbara
for her continuous engagement and support.

1. All efforts have been made to conceal Barbara's identity, including the use
of a pseudonym.

2. Ironically enough, given the Gestapo analogy, the hospital Goffman studied was, at the time he was studying it, shielding from trial one of this country's
most renowned anti-Semites, Ezra Pound, by exaggerating his condition (Torrey,
Roots).

3. The award-winning documentary *Jupiter's Wife* presents a more realistic
portrayal of mental illness in which the narrator's desire to either believe or
discount everything his schizophrenic subject says is itself foregrounded and
examined. The film was not a popular success, however.

4. I am indebted to my colleague Lori Newcomb for the phrase "experience
of certainty," which she used to describe Joan of Arc's zealousness.

5. In the library book from which I took this excerpt, a previous reader had
written next to the last line, "Sounds like a professor."

Works Cited

American Psychiatric Association. *Diagnostic and Statistical Manual of Mental Disorders*. 4th ed. Washington: American Psychiatric Association, 1994.

Barrett, Robert J. "Clinical Writing and the Documentary Construction of
Schizophrenia." *Culture, Medicine, and Psychiatry* 12.3 (1988): 265–99.

Berkenkotter, Carol, and Doris Ravotas. "Genre as Tool in the Transmission
of Practice over Time and Across Professional Boundaries." *Mind, Culture,
and Activity* 4.4 (1997): 256–74.

Bizzell, Patricia, and Bruce Herzberg, eds. *The Rhetorical Tradition: Readings
from Classical Times to the Present*. Boston: St. Martin's, 1990.

Burke, Kenneth. "Language and Symbolic Action." Bizzell and Herzberg 1034–41.

Butterfield, Fox. "Prisons Replace Hospitals for the Nation's Mentally Ill." *New York Times* 5 Mar. 1998: A1+.

Deleuze, Gilles, and Felix Guattari. *A Thousand Plateaus: Capitalism and Schizophrenia*. Trans. Brian Massumi. Minneapolis: U of Minnesota P, 1987.

Finnegan, William. "Defending the Unabomber." *New Yorker* 16 Mar. 1998: 52–63.

Foucault, Michel. *Madness and Civilization: A History of Insanity in the Age of Reason*. Trans. R. Howard. New York: Vintage Books, 1965.

Fullinwider, S. P. *Technicians of the Finite: The Rise and Decline of the Schizophrenic in American Thought, 1840–1960*. Westport, CT: Greenwood Press, 1982.

Goffman, Erving. *Asylums: Essays on the Social Situation of Mental Patients and Other Inmates*. Chicago: Aldine, 1961.

Hemley, Robin. *Nola: A Memoir of Faith, Art, and Madness*. Saint Paul: Graywolf, 1998.

Keefe, Richard S. E., and Philip D. Harvey. *Understanding Schizophrenia: A Guide to the New Research on Causes and Treatment*. New York: Free Press, 1994.

Leary, David, ed. *Metaphors in the History of Psychology*. New York: Cambridge UP, 1990.

Levy, Robert M., and Leonard S. Rubenstein. *The Rights of People with Mental Disabilities*. Carbondale: Southern Illinois UP, 1996.

McCarthy, Lucille Parkinson, and Joan Page Gerring. "Revising Psychiatry's Charter Document DSM-IV." *Written Communication* 11.2 (1994): 147–92.

Miller, Susan. *Textual Carnivals: The Politics of Composition*. Carbondale: Southern Illinois UP, 1991.

Murphy, Robert. *The Body Silent*. New York: Holt, 1987.

Neely, Carol T. "Did Madness Have a Renaissance?" *Renaissance Quarterly* 44 (1991): 776–91.

Neville, Susan. *Indiana Winter*. Bloomington: Indiana UP, 1994.

Ronell, Avital. *The Telephone Book: Technology, Schizophrenia, Electric Speech*. Lincoln: U of Nebraska P, 1989.

Rosaldo, Renato. *Culture and Truth: The Remaking of Social Analysis*. Boston: Beacon Press, 1989.

Sarbin, Theodore R. "Metaphors of Unwanted Conduct." Leary 300–330.

Sheehan, Susan. *Is There No Place on Earth for Me?* New York: Vintage, 1983.

Torrey, E. Fuller. *Out of the Shadows: Confronting America's Mental Illness Crises*. New York: Wiley, 1997.

———. *The Roots of Treason: Ezra Pound and the Secret of St. Elizabeths*. New York: McGraw-Hill, 1984.

———. *Surviving Schizophrenia: A Family Manual*. New York: Harper and Row, 1988.

Vonnegut, Mark. *The Eden Express*. New York: Praeger, 1975.

Wyden, Peter. *Conquering Schizophrenia: A Father, His Son, and a Medical Breakthrough*. New York: Knopf, 1998.

4

Am I MS?

Miriamne Ara Krummel

*To Yetta Papish Pomeranz and Jeremy Richard, whose
courage I recall when I search for my own*

The four seasons of the year resemble our lives. . . . Our bodies always
transform: we are not now what we have been nor what we will be
tomorrow."

—Ovid's *Metamorphoses* (translation mine)

April 1995. A Wednesday evening. My companion is driving me to
my office. It is a harrowing time for both of us because we are trying to move our studies to another university. Having been admitted to
seven doctoral programs, I try to discuss my choices with him. We are
busy and find little time to relax. We stop talking, opting instead for
silence as a form of relief from the effort to communicate. Halfway
between our home and my office, my companion makes a complete stop
at an intersection so that a number of students can cross. When he applies the brakes, my head bends forward slightly; as my chin approaches
my chest, I experience this weird pulling up/electrical sensation inside
of my body.

I am writing seminar papers for two courses. I am particularly involved in my analysis of Thomas Hoccleve's *Stabat Mater Dolorosa,*
which I have been drafting on my office computer. The mother board
on my six-month-old PC no longer works, so I find myself spending a
considerable amount of time writing in my cold office and drinking even
colder coffee. Dealing with the idiosyncrasies of technology has become
necessary and almost natural to me, but I am unprepared for the unnatural and unnecessary—weird—feeling that continues to present itself. I blame my office computer and the chair I use, thinking that the
strange, inner electrical sensation is work related. My mother thinks I
am pregnant. Being in my twenties and immortal, I neither change my

sleeping habits nor alter my diet in any way. I continue to sleep five or so hours a night and to be lax about remembering to eat breakfast or even lunch. But, as always, I try not to interrupt my exercise regimen, which includes step aerobics, the stair master, and brisk walking.

In one week, my legs are numb and tingling. Having Raynaud's phenomena (a circulatory disease that affects my ability to stay warm but in the winter affects the circulation in my fingers and toes), I attribute the numbness to some malfunction related to Raynaud's. I continue thinking about my work (as opposed to my health) and writing about Thomas Hoccleve. But the numbness spreads, up and up, taking over my legs and traveling into my hips. I know something is wrong when my arms also register the tingling sensation. I admit (some) defeat and visit the health center.

There I describe my symptoms. When questioned about having other illnesses, I mention the Raynaud's. Then I am dismissed. The health center person remains in the room while I gather my things.

As I finish buttoning my overcoat, I add, "I must be experiencing a new form of Raynaud's."

"Why do you think that?" she asks.

"Well, my legs are numb and a little stiff," I respond, also wondering why I need to repeat myself because I had mentioned this numbness earlier.

"Oh, really? Numb, you say? Let's take a more involved look. Why don't you undress. Put on this gown, and when I return, we'll run further tests."

Thinking—even at this point—that not very much could be wrong with me, I become overwhelmed by this person's response after she runs the tests (pricking my legs and toes with a broken tongue depressor). She does not hide her worried look from me and immediately schedules an emergency visit to a local neurologist.

Together, my companion and I journey to a new part of town. By now, the numb limbs are becoming weak. Both walking and writing have slowed a bit. We don't know very much about neurology, and the other patients who approach the building in wheelchairs and hold canes in the waiting room heighten our anxieties about the unknown.

The neurologist himself is neither calm nor disturbed. He is in this special mode that I will later characterize as "the good doc," wry and willing to wait, not pushy, not demanding, not an alarmist. He subjects me to more tests, again the broken tongue depressor. But I am also asked to walk a straight line, stand erect with both feet together, and touch my index and second fingers to my nose (first the right hand and then the left). Like an intoxicated person pulled over for driving under the influence, I fail. I become a wobbling, swaying mass of molecules that cannot locate its nose with its digits. The neurologist continues with the next battery of tests, checking my sensory responses to external stimuli—the visual response to light and the aural response to sound, as well as my legs' responses to a tuning fork. At this moment—when prompted with a question—I realize that I have lost my sense of taste.

I am asked to dress and then meet the neurologist in his office, where he discusses with me and my companion his desire to perform more tests at the hospital.

"Are further tests necessary?" I ask, both worn out and troubled by the sequence of events.

"Yes," he answers kindly. "We need to rule out a brain tumor. Only an MRI exam can help us rule out many possibilities and help us locate what is causing the numbness."

He pauses. Silence. "Are you claustrophobic?" he then asks. "If you are, I can prescribe a drug that will help you deal with the confines of the MRI machine."

I do not know whether I am claustrophobic, so emergency magnetic resonance imaging (MRI) exams are planned, as well as a battery of blood tests, without any prescribed drugs. I have no idea what an MRI is, and the neurologist's questioning me about whether I have claustrophobia alarms me. As it turns out, instead of suffering from claustrophobia in the machine, I wrestle with insomnia at home.

I spend the following two mornings (7–10 A.M.) confined to the MRI machine while my companion paces the halls outside. Having been told to bring a tape of my own choice of music, I make the mistake of choosing a Beethoven symphony. Both the banging and screaming of the cement coffin—otherwise known as an MRI machine—prevent me from hearing most of my Beethoven tape. (Some MRI machines have a sound system, I later learn, but my first experience of imaging occurs in a machine without a sound system, so I only have earphones that never—not by any stretch of the imagination—could compete with the noise of the machine.) Since I believe I can defeat this noise, I bring a tape of The Who along with me to the second day of testing. Even so, being confined to the small cylindrical container, I am still only able to hear a small portion of *Quadrophenia*. On this second morning, I am injected with gadolinium, "a chemical compound that can be administered to a person during magnetic resonance imaging to help distinguish between new lesions and old lesions" ("Glossary of Terms" 9).

Two days pass, and I return to the hospital for more tests, accompanied by my companion and my parents. This time the tests (known as visual evoked potentials, brain stem auditory evoked potentials, and sensory evoked potentials) involve electrodes and monitors. It's Friday, so I will have to spend the weekend wondering what the tests will tell me . . . us. On Monday, my companion and I return to the neurologist's office. There he shows us the X ray–like sheets of my thoracic spine and cervical cord. He points to one spot in particular.

"This is what concerns me," he remarks, pointing to a white spot in an otherwise gray area. He, more aware of the future than I am, has read the "impression" from the physician's report sent to him from the local hospital's diagnostic imaging department:

> Isolated focus of increased signal in the posterior cervical cord at C5 that enhances following Gadolinium injection. This is a nonspecific finding. Additional criteria for diagnosis of MS would require imaging of the head, CSF, and clinical evaluation. (Persic, 27 April 1995)

The neurologist—by far the best part of the entire experience—shares with me what he knows, what he has learned, what he has read. Still pointing to the white spot, he expounds upon the results of the MRI. We have ruled out a tumor.

"The demyelinated areas suggest to me the possibility that you may have multiple sclerosis. Only time will tell. Should you have more symptoms at a later date, we will need to reconsider the diagnosis and take MRIs of your brain. Until then, I would like to stay away from taking more MRIs and administering steroids. For now, this experience can be considered a onetime event, so I will diagnose you as having transverse myelitis."

"Super," I think. "What the hell's transverse myelitis?" I am reassured that transverse myelitis can be a passing illness but that a repeat of the illness or something related to it can signify multiple sclerosis (MS). I will need to wait.

And so in a matter of weeks, I walk away from that neurologist, that office, and that university—after having had the most bizarre experience in my twenty-eight years of life—with no answer. All the excitement and all the tests end very unclimactically: I do not know what is wrong with my body. And I wait.

My family and I choose (not) to deal with the diagnosis in a variety of ways. I think about my body and the numbness often. My father encourages me to play more tennis with him, supposing—I think—that exercise will sweat out the infection. My mother concludes that I am experiencing something as ordinary as the common cold. One of my brothers only discusses with our father the possibility that I may have a disease, and the other brother chooses our mother's route—namely, completely denying the neurologist's ability to diagnose what has happened to my system. My companion remains the same—somewhat demanding, somewhat exasperated, somewhat attentive. Each in our own way, we ignore the diagnosis.

June, July, August 1995. Throughout the summer, I continue to feel spots of numbness upon exertion (when I am walking quickly or running briefly). I am studying French at Yale in an intensive course, and I devote a great deal of time to my studies. I love sitting in the Quad surrounded by the old architecture, French books, and new peers. I talk about my "whatever-it-is" with my summer Francophiles.

It was easy to talk about transverse myelitis. But it is not easy to talk about multiple sclerosis. And now it is so much more important to me to believe that people trust the information I give them; it is so important to me that people understand me and what I fight daily. Nonetheless, what happened to me at the health center will later become an all-too-familiar (and by now despised) experience. People look at me (a physically fit person) and immediately assess me as "fine."

When I was able-bodied, I could never have imagined how meaningful a long-term disability would, could, and has become to my construction of my own identity. I feel that I—in some uncharacterizable way—belong to an undifferentiated group of people whom I do not know and whom I have never met. Louis J. Rosner and Shelley Ross's *Multiple Sclerosis* tells me, "No one knows what actually causes MS, but we do know that it is an acquired disease—you are not born with it. Multiple sclerosis is also an exogenous disease, meaning that it is contracted from the outside. And fortunately, it is not contagious" (5). Only 1 percent of husbands and wives share the disease, Rosner and Ross are careful to point out (5). I imagine that this statistic about spousal sharing is probably a result of having experienced similar environmental or genetic circumstances as children. We know so little.

Multiple sclerosis is mysterious. As a medievalist, I often consider how much more we know today about the Black Plague than those who actually suffered from the disease. We know, for instance, that the Black Plague was caused by bites from fleas disposed to dwell on rats. I imagine that at some point in the future, we will all look like fools for not having gathered more information about or made some critical link among the data collected in the studies of MS.

So what causes MS? According to Rosner and Ross, "Most evidence suggests that exposure to MS occurs before age eighteen, followed by a latency period (before symptoms appear) of twenty-one years" (9). Since my first bout befell me when I was twenty-eight, something might have happened to me when I was seven and living on Long Island. Already my self-discovery begins: I feel I can trust Rosner and Ross's statistics because they cite a study that explores a population and a culture from which I am drawn:

> In Israel, scientists recorded every single case of MS—and the age of onset, where each patient came from, at what age he or she immigrated, and

the latency period. They found that MS was unknown among native-born Sabras and immigrants from North Africa and Yemen but high among immigrants from western, northern, and eastern Europe. In fact, the MS frequency among immigrants matched the incidence rates in their native countries. (Rosner and Ross 9)

Where do I place myself in regard to this study? How do I categorize my (MS) identity? I begin searching for a mirror that will speak to me about who I am. At the same time, I am afraid that people will guess from my looks, gestures, and walking patterns that I am afflicted with MS.

"Are there any other incidents of transverse myelitis, demyelinating disease, or multiple sclerosis in your family history—something that afflicted your grandmothers?" each of the four neurologists has asked.

How would I know?

What I know is that my native country is the United States: I am a second-generation American because both of my parents were born in New York City. But I have always felt tied to a legacy that my grandmothers left me. When I think of my heritage, I hear klezmer music and the stories of the Schtetl—the pogrom (the Jewish ghetto) in Poland and in Russia—where my Bubby (grandmother) Yetta Pomeranz, neé Yentl Papish, grew into her teenage years. I have the strength and severity of my Lithuanian grandmother, Grandma Teresa, neé Tesse Jaffe. I carry a German or maybe Danish last name. People see the Tartar eyes and Finnish cheekbones. Suddenly, my identity and my self-definition become the driving influence in my life. Am I a Jewish-American woman, I wonder? A Russian-Polish-Lithuanian-Finnish-Danish-American woman (with some Tartar) who has MS? A woman with MS whose Jewish roots link her to eastern and northern Europe? I begin to feel that I am a person, genderless and without culture, who has MS.

Still the disease is so much bigger than my needs—sometimes a foe, sometimes a secret-sharer, sometimes my portable home. It's all mine. I know no one else who has MS. I know only myself.

I reread the letter that first linked me (in print) with multiple sclerosis:

> This is a brief letter on Miriamne Krummel, a patient that I have known since April of 1995, when she presented with numbness from the waist down. An MRI revealed a demyelination plaque at C5. . . . I elected not to treat her at that point. . . . Since that initial visit, she has [had] some spells of diplopia and scattered numbness in other body areas. My feeling is that Miriamne probably has multiple sclerosis and I have been frank with her about this. She is geographically removed from me now and I understand she is seeking some neurologic care in your area. If I can be of any assistance, please contact me. (Parry, 15 Oct. 1996)

This letter, sent both to me at my home address and to (another) disbelieving health center doctor at school, was the culmination of my first real battle with a new health center in my attempt to hook up with a new neurologist. Met with disbelief about my symptoms at the local health center, I had to produce a letter from the neurologist who had diagnosed me as having demyelinating disease. By the time the health center doctor received (and ratified) this letter, I found myself in the advanced stages of my third episode.

I consider this letter my first notification of MS because the correspondence marks the beginning of my new and very different life. I am now receiving (or acquiring, as the case may be) letters that introduce the MS language to me: demyelination, "a loss of myelin [a substance that forms a sheath around the nerves of the central nervous system] in the white matter of the central nervous system (brain, spinal cord)" and diplopia, "double vision, or the simultaneous awareness of two images of the same object that results from a failure of the two eyes to work in a coordinated fashion" ("Glossary of Terms" 6). Doctors write to each other about me and use the words "multiple sclerosis." I am not particularly disturbed by being referred to in the third person; I realize that I have internalized Miriamne Ara Krummel as "patient."

My first neurologist was hoping that my multiple sclerosis would be "benign"—"mild or completely remitting attacks with long symptom-free periods" (Holland)—and that a long time would pass before I might experience a second attack. His wishes are now outmoded, for "benign," as an operative mode of MS, is no longer considered efficacious ("New Names" 1). Today, one attack of MS constitutes something more complicated than the diagnosis of "benign."

I liked this first neurologist, and I enjoy remembering my associations with him, recalling his manner. Nevertheless, later letters demand that I envisage another neurologist—the doctor who scheduled an MRI of my brain—as the neurologist who made the official diagnosis: "This letter is to let you know that Miriamne Krummel is a patient under my care with a diagnosis of multiple sclerosis of relapsing type. This diagnosis was made earlier in 1997" (Rae-Grant, 14 Nov. 1997). According to this letter (a verification of my multiple sclerosis diagnosis for the disabilities specialist at the university), the medical field directs itself toward a neurologist who subjected me to more MRIs, who elected to treat me (read: to push drugs, expensive drugs that cost over $1,000 a month, composed of chemicals which may—or may not—be what my body lacks). "I recommend strongly that you start thinking about beginning one of the available drug therapies, one of the intramuscular interferon injections. My nurse will provide you with the appropriate literature.

It is important to remember that the drugs will extend the number of ambulatory years that you have ahead of you."

The one office visit that I attend alone meets with these words. The neurologist who expresses these thoughts is considered the one who first identified my MS (because he conducts the MRI exams of my brain and discovers demyelination there), although another neurologist (whose diagnosis is based upon MRIs of my thoracic spine and cervical cord and what I physically present) is the one who first introduced *me* to the reality of my having multiple sclerosis.

When I suffer from fatigue and walk slowly, the discouraging news reverberates in my mind, and I am overcome by lack of hope, which is even more devastating than the disease itself. "A patient's expectation of improvement is also crucial. Researchers know that across a wide range of illnesses, patients who think they will feel better are more likely to do so" (Brown 93). I remember starting up my car after leaving the office of the neurologist who officially diagnosed my MS and contemplating whether I should buckle up my seat belt. Why use a seat belt? After all, it's only a matter of time before my legs will be useless.

The inevitable distrust of my body has made my mind become more and more important to me. On the other hand, my search for the activities and depictions of Jews in the Middle Ages and in the sixteenth century has ironically motivated me to take better care of my physical self. I now eat a diet low in fat and sugar (as suggested); I militate against products that include unnatural preservatives (after a meeting with a homeopath). The time allotted to food shopping increases by half an hour. I walk religiously for an hour five days a week, even when I am fatigued. The walks reinvigorate my fatigued body. At times, I cannot distinguish between whether my personal care is a sort of defiance against the diagnosis or an attempt to deny it, but I love walking and thinking now more than I did when I was still immortal.

September 1995. My neck gets stiff. I feel as if I cannot turn my head properly, smoothly, gracefully, without pain. We students in the "Introduction to Teaching Freshman Composition" seminar are visited by a stress specialist. I share my thoughts that stress makes my neck stiff (because my neck has been stiff of late, and I elect to consider the stiffness as stress rather than related to MS). The stress specialist looks concerned. I wonder.

In a week or so, my vision becomes watery. In the course of the next few weeks, the wateriness turns into blurred vision that becomes double vision that transforms into an intense double vision that—at its peak—seems to produce a third image. "Since that initial visit, she has [had] some spells of diplopia and scattered numbness in other body areas. My feeling is that Miriamne probably has multiple sclerosis and I have been frank with her about this" (Parry).

I am now a composite of diplopia and "other body areas." I am a fragment of parts. *Cogito, ergo sum.* I am numb and see things funky; therefore, I am MS. And neurologists can be "frank" with me. I belong to a new club. On my vita, I will place "Frank With Me" next to other memberships in, for instance, the Modern Language Association, National Council of Teachers of English, and the New Chaucer Society.

I am new to this doctoral program, so I keep my double vision a secret. I don't trust anyone, and I don't know what will happen if I speak out. So I keep quiet. I sit in seminars, isolated and silent, so that no one will notice my diplopia, my disability. And yet I feel very noticeable and a little larger than the other students, although I am 5'2". I teach my composition class—the best class that I have had in my eight years of teaching writing. (I cry when that class ends.) I continue to lead the class even though I have double vision for two weeks. I wonder whether the students notice that anything is amiss.

November 1996. I wake up Thanksgiving morning with numbness that is a little different, a little more severe than usual. And with each morning until the middle of December, the numbness increases. This episode marks a change in the way my body unleashes the MS exacerbation, for now my episodes climb step by step to a peak and then retrace the steps back downward toward normalcy. After a few days of a numbness that spreads up my limbs, I then notice the appearance of L' Hermitte's sign, "an abnormal sensation of electricity or 'pins and needles' going down the spine into the arms and legs that occurs when the neck is bent forward so that the chin touches the chest" ("Glossary of Terms" 11)—the electrical sensation that I had experienced during my first episode in April 1995. Next, there is a tight band around my chest, which causes me to fear that my breathing will shut down. (But a neurologist explains—on the telephone during an emergency call—that the experience is sensory and not motor, and he offers intravenous steroids, which I refuse.) As the episode peaks, I can hardly use my hands. I begin to walk so, so slowly. I feel disabled. For the first time, I feel diseased.

More MRIs, this time of the brain. I write the seminar papers that are due (I have been studying *Beowulf* and Marie de France), and I teach my composition class. I start using martial metaphors to describe myself. I soldier on. I ask for no incompletes. I ask for no special favors.

And no one offers any. The professors do not know what is happening to me. What seems so screamingly obvious to me is invisible to others. Or at least others choose not to notice how slowly I walk up the flight of stairs to my office or how crookedly I walk in an otherwise direct path from one place to another. My invisibility during a serious episode, I learn, is even stranger and more discomfiting than the waiting in between episodes. I am plagued by invisible "signal abnormalities," "lesions," and "mild disk bulging." Only an MRI *machine* can really see *me*. I have become a disability that is an unknown quantity. I have an enemy inside of me who hungers after my myelin, "a soft, white coating of nerve fibers in the central nervous system, composed of lipids (fats) and protein. Myelin serves as insulation and as an aid to efficient nerve fiber conduction" ("Glossary of Terms" 13).

Suddenly, the summers on the Cape with my uncle, Bernie Siegel, seem like kismet. I recall how he used to encourage his daughter Carolyn and me to kick all of the bad things out of our bodies while we listened to his charming and relaxing voice with our eyes closed. He would hypnotize his daughter and me in order to instruct us on how to dispel the harmful contaminants from our systems. While Carolyn and I sat on her bed in a wood home on the Cape, Bernie would ask us to close our eyes and imagine a beautiful and safe place. As he counted slowly and spoke softly, I used to imagine—superimposed upon the appropriate happy site with babbling brooks and green conifers—my Bubby's apartment on Manhattan's Amsterdam Avenue. My Bubby alive and running around, as she always did, and my Uncle Kal alive and young and preposterously obsessed with mathematics as he almost always was, talking to Bernie Siegel, and my Zeydeh, my grandfather (just a cut out from a picture because I never knew him as a living man). There was also a young, cautious, thin, small, pale girl playing the piano, wanting praise while the whole household yelled. They yelled because they loved her music, but she did not know. She thought they could not hear her, and she also thought that even if—by some miracle—they could hear her music, their loud voices were purposely drowning out what she played. This girl is my mother.

"Now, open your eyes," I hear Bernie remark gently as I leave this secret happy place.

> Miriamne returned for reevaluation of multiple sclerosis. The diagnosis seems to be fairly confirmed with the findings on the MRI scan showing periventricular white matter changes. This in association with previously described spinal cord white matter changes and her clinical history of at least three episodes of neurologic events including the more recent one of gait difficulties, L' Hermitte's sign and a sensory band-like sensation in the abdomen. (Redenbaugh, 20 Jan. 1997)

I neither understand nor recognize myself in this description of me. I feel alienated and concerned. The neurologist, I sense, does not see me as a human being; he sees me as a disease. Our conversation is dull, and his questions imply that he doesn't believe my descriptions of my symptoms. My father joins me for my first visit. My father is becoming involved in his own way, immersing himself in the mystery of MS. I have become my father's retirement project. My reading of this doctor (and my father's sense as well) is that he doubts my emotional stability and believes in the possibility that I am a little "on edge." I sense some level of distrust.

I attempt to obtain a second opinion:

> She is a very pleasant, articulate woman in no acute distress. She is understandably anxious. She did not appear depressed. Discs were flat without pallor. There is a mild APD OD but her Ishihara plates are 14/14 OU. Extraocular movements are full without nystagmus. Face is symmetric. Facial sensation intact. There is a 1+ jaw jerk. She still has prominent L' Hermitte's phenomenon. There is no drift or altered tone, power or dexterity. She was able to do Romberg and tandem Romberg and I would judge gait as normal at present. There was full strength in all muscle groups tested. She has intact vibration and light touch sensation. Coordination of finger-to-nose and heel-shin-knee rapid toe tap was excellent. Deep tendon reflexes were 2+ in the arms, 3+ in the legs, but not pathologic. The left toe was down-going. The right may have been up to Bing, but this was equivocal. . . . I would prefer to have her on preventative medication. She is still not convinced about this. I gave her the Avonex videotape to look at and told her to consider the situation and to fit it in as conveniently as possible in the exam schedule. . . . I shall be happy to follow her however she wishes. (Pruitt, 28 Feb. 1997)

The most clinical of the neurologists I have seen. Her comments read like warning signs of what is to come. Her intelligence and personality—so much fun in an office visit—make for a good read in that she writes "but this was equivocal" as if the entire experience and diagnosis are not equivocal. So, so unreal to me. But to her, there are answers and there are solutions. She can quantify the test results in numbers—2+ and 3+. She can judge the movement of my body according to standards of measurement invented by other doctors—Bing and Romberg. She evaluates physical movement as if my limbs and body are foreign objects. She is very intelligent and observes disease.

I am beginning to understand MS through all of my neurologists' letters. I am beginning to realize that my visits are my own way of researching my disability. My visits are the way in which I unpack what multiple sclerosis means to me.

My visits are also a way to connect with this unknown quantity. I want answers rather than intramuscular interferon injections.

"How can they suggest such serious drugs when they know so little about multiple sclerosis?" I ask myself over and over again, lost in an iteration of disability and diagnosis.

As the neurologist observes my movements, she speaks to me of her interest in Rashi, her love of her cat, and the music she creates with her cello. There are two sides to these neurologists—a hidden complexity not unlike the disease they chart in their fellow humans. For a few minutes—as we discuss our cats, our musical instruments, and medievalia—this neurologist becomes a friend who understands the chaos that has taken over my life, and I seek ways to prolong my visit with her. But the inevitable discussion about the drugs leaves in its wake a doom that is irrecoverable. So I leave. At lunch, my mother and I sob while my father sits still, controlled, contained, with eyes that speak of desperation.

November 1997. Still have not gone on the drugs. I just don't trust them—that is, the drugs. I am also in search of a neurologist who will refrain from badgering me about injection. I am in search of my first love, my first neurologist, who was humorous and sad and apologetic. I have an appointment.

When I arrive in his office, I am presenting vertigo problems. My balance is a little unsteady. In a few days, my vision changes: things begin to shake and appear on a slant. The stages of death and dying according to Elisabeth Kübler-Ross start all over again: Denial and Isolation > Anger > Bargaining > Depression > Acceptance. For three weeks, the episode progresses until I peak, spending an evening without a compass in my cerebellum, uncontrollably vomiting whenever I slightly move my head. I sit up all night in a chair with my head stationary and elevated. Days later—when I can again lie in bed—I sleep with four big pillows as bolsters for my disabled cerebellum. One morning I sleep late, and my cat, Teaser Girlie, kisses me on the lips, hoping I will wake up. I do.

The composition class I am leading, like the composition class of the fall of 1995, has created a democratic community of writers, and I continue to meet with them despite my vision disability. But I cancel one meeting with my composition class this time. Only one class.

On Thanksgiving, my brothers and one of their friends drive three hours to my place with food prepared. My parents are in Portugal on a planned vacation. They had called me from JFK the evening that I had peaked; I made them promise me they would go and not cancel.

> Miriamne Krummel is a patient under my care with relapsing multiple sclerosis. She has had a recent exacerbation in the brain stem, with severe vertigo, and continues to have significant weakness. She has problems processing due to the interference with the scanning of her vision. . . I would suggest that she be given 3 hours for her examinations. I think this is medically appropriate for her definitely significant multiple sclerosis. (Rae-Grant, 28 Nov. 1997)

I like my new neurologist. I have fallen in love again. He is concerned and sees me as a human body. I am a "brain stem"—a "body part"—

rather than an "extra ocular movement." I begin to realize that I prefer the former over the latter. And I can now identify my MS as relapsing-remitting.

In the past there has been a distinction between the two forms of relapsing MS: relapsing-remitting, one form, involves "periodic acute onset of symptoms followed by partial or complete recovery, with plateaus of stable impairment" (Holland) whereas relapsing-progressive, another form, is a bit more serious, presenting "exacerbations with modest recovery and significant residual impairment. There is a slow 'step-wise' deterioration of function" (Holland). But researchers are trying "to develop standard definitions and terminology for MS types," so both forms of relapsing have now been fused as relapsing-remitting (RR), meaning "clearly defined disease relapses (flare-ups) with full recovery or with sequelae (resulting conditions) and residual deficit upon recovery; periods between disease relapses characterized by a lack of disease progression (gradual worsening)" ("New Names" 1). The categorical difference makes choosing patients for drug-involved trial runs more efficacious, I now know, although there is some satisfaction for the MS person as well who knows what label to adopt to describe her/himself, I believe.

I also discover that most healthy people find it difficult to understand their neighbors with MS because of a probable stigma attached to people with disabilities and diseases. I am convinced of this. Having MS is something that no one outside of the family or my close companion will consider real. I absolutely hate the phrase, which I have heard twice this fall of 1997, "Oh, you look so well." (Read: "Where are the crutches? You are fine!") The implication, to me, is that were I to don a prop, such as an eye patch or a cane, I would be taken more seriously. At the same time, I also understand that most people have a need to say something encouraging which—once spoken—can be received wrongly. The years of vigorous exercise, which I have continued albeit with much less vigor, have left me with a strong muscular system. My tripping while I walk might be another MS person's falling, for instance.

MS is a confusing disease that requires attention from others; casual relationships become more frustrating than they are worth. Now all of my relationships are intense, personal, and honest. Acquaintances have become tiresome and upsetting. Imagine, can there be anything worse than someone's forgetting that you almost lost complete use of your hands?

Rosner and Ross insist that MS "is best kept a private matter, not a public tragedy. The fewer people you tell, the easier it will be to diminish the importance of MS in your life" (148). I disagree. One of the most serious problems associated with being diagnosed is that one has to decide how to explain that only 15 percent of the people with MS are "chronic-progressive," meaning "continuous functional deterioration over months or years with risk for life-threatening complications" (Holland). I believe that it is neither emotionally nor psychologically nor even socially healthy to ferret away a disease and disability to protect oneself from possible discrimination. We all must fight the horrors of racism, sexism, and ageism. Fear of the disabled must also be fought.

I begin to realize that I have lived too many years haunted by—and scarred by—the racial assaults of my childhood and adolescence (when my security blanket went up in flames because of an arsonist's attempt to burn down the synagogue to which my nursery school was adjoined or when the boy who sat behind me on the school bus would hold his silver crucifix in front of my eyes in an attempt to exorcize me or later when I would be called "Jewish pinko" by an unknown voice in the street).

For half of my life, I chose to pass. But as I begin to speak about my MS and to explain to others what having MS entails, I recognize a look that I thought I had forgotten: disgust tempered by a wide-eyed expression of gentle innocence. My recognition of that look sends a shimmer down my spine as I realize how thin the lines are between racial and disability Otherness. I vow that I will no longer pass. I will try to accept—and maybe even like—myself. Suddenly I am liberated from the suffocating weight of years of personal neglect, psychological indifference, and cultural embarrassment. Teaching my students about respecting themselves and Others becomes more real as our classroom transforms into a discovery zone of sorts.

Recently, I told my father that I have come out of the closet. And I have. I am willing to explain what MS is to someone who does not understand and wants to know. And just as a peer might tell me she was vomiting all weekend or that she has a fever because of the flu, I will share what I am experiencing because of my MS. People feel very free to discuss ailments associated with the everyday illness. I have discovered that people with MS should not conceal their episodes because others will imagine very strange things. And fear, I find, is caused by the unknown whereas knowledge breeds familiarity and acceptance (to some extent). People must learn to understand Otherness whether it be related to race or disability.

> There is no personality profile of a person who will cope best with MS. For many, adversity—such as an MS diagnosis and subsequent battles with the disease—helps promote personal growth. . . . MS is a kick in the gut that will no doubt change your life. You may feel a loss of innocence, a lot less carefree, but there's a positive side to the drama too. MS forces you to look at what your true goals are. . . . You've learned that nothing should wait until tomorrow. Crazy things will make you happy. . . . The only loss to prove a real tragedy would be the loss of your sense

of humor. It has been said that in MS, your sense of humor may not be the first to go, but it's the toughest to live without. (Rosner and Ross 147)

My companion clips an article from the *Connecticut Post* entitled "Fighting MS." Through this article I meet Judy Rahmani, whose collection of more than forty canes includes one with a *Magen David,* the star on David's shield that now occupies a central position on the Israeli flag. The *Magen David* is just visible in the photo. I covet this picture as another kernel that has helped me to find myself. Rahmani's eccentricity, her 40-plus cane collection, speaks to me as a living example of what Rosner and Ross call "crazy things" that make us "happy," maintaining a "sense of humor" despite and to spite the horror of MS.

In two years I too have metamorphosed the scary into the ironic through my own developing eccentricity. I am beginning to understand the medical rhetoric about the patient; I can read the differences in their words. My family and my companion worry too much at times, but their worrying—oddly enough—makes me less frightened about my future. MS is all about waiting gracefully, and I think each of us has confronted the horror of waiting without something to do and without someone to do that something with.

Today a professor on my dissertation committee and I discuss fairness and justice. He often refers to how unfair it is that I have MS, and I appreciate his honesty and questions. He and I enjoy using the martial metaphors. One of my brothers who will receive a Ph.D. in biology calls me up to tell me the most recent thoughts about what might cause MS (still no real sense of what it is that makes my T-cells hunger after my myelin). My father volunteers in an MS research lab. My companion warns me, while driving, that he will need to take a sharp turn.

I have learned a great deal about disability and my disabled students. My initial reaction to time-and-a-half with breaks for the doctoral exam was that I would have more than enough time to compose the necessary essays, but during the written exam, I soon learn that I now work a bit slower and need ten-minute breaks to prevent the throbbing headaches and fatigue from presenting themselves. Alert to the unsteadiness of my balance system, I work hard to avoid moving my head during the orals.

I have changed physically and emotionally, and sometimes I do not recognize the woman named Miriamne Ara Krummel. But I am relapsing; therefore, I am. Acceptance.

Yesterday, I felt an overwhelming wave of happiness when a peer told me that she was pregnant. I thought, "Life is growing in my friend!"

"Excellent," I remarked joyously and carefully hugged her as if I were the expectant father. She had waited to tell me because in the past I had disparaged children. Now as I write, there are plants surrounding me, sharing the sun's rays with me in this window-filled apartment. I can hear Teaser Girlie snoring in her favorite chair (which I do not need today). I can recall the sounds of my students laughing at my jokes. And next semester (having passed the doctoral exams), I will begin work on my dissertation proposal about the Jews in the Middle Ages (and academically march toward candidacy). In an oddly poignant way, my life before MS was not as meaningful as my life after has been. What I am and what I have become—a soldier who is proud of her heritage and who wants her students to love learning—is (on most days) worth the trip.

I have taken the occasion to study myself to clarify what cannot be completely clarified. I have attempted this process for all of us with MS who often find themselves at a loss for the words to explain what we undergo. I have used the rhetorical and theoretical skills honed by graduate school and a lifetime of studying texts to attempt to understand what has happened to me both psychologically and physically, although the placebo effect leads me to believe that the physical and the mental cannot be separated through some outmoded dualism of mind and body. While I have no intention of implying that either having MS or being temporarily able to overcome a disability has been an event that has positively changed my life or converted me in some special way, I do find that I have tapped (and in some ways discovered) a personal reserve of a courageous fighting spirit that had lain dormant between my teenage years and 1995. I do not regret the rediscovery of this spirit, for I have been able to meet myself and to recognize my courage. Years ago I would have despaired much more easily after having met some of the barriers I have faced and overcome.

There are many days now when I recall a childhood book, *The Little Engine That Could*. I suppose the sense that "we shall overcome" is hope, yet I remain uncertain about what hope is. While I have internalized the social-epistemic that hope is a strong force in survival, my inability to define hope forces me to see hope as enigmatic. We will not all pull through the terror caused by a fluctuating disability on hope alone, even though some of us will. As Kübler-Ross points out, "Children in Barracks L 318 and L 417 in the concentration camp of Terezin maintained their hope years ago, although out of a total of about 15,000 children under fifteen years of age only around 100 came out of it alive" (122). What compelled those 100 children to survive? Writes Kübler-Ross, "It is the hope that occasionally sneaks in, that all this is just like a nightmare and not true" (123). Hope demands a supportive community of family, friends, and doctors: "It might be helpful if more people would talk about death and dying as an intrinsic part of life. . . . I am convinced that we do more harm by avoiding the issue than by using time and timing to sit, listen, and share" (125).

Even someone like me, who prefers not to be drug-bound, has hope. Scarily, what Kübler-Ross refers to as "hope" sounds like a strategic denial, but there is no mistaking an acceptance of a disability that includes the hope that maybe this year I won't have an episode that will take four months of living well away from me. Hope and the placebo effect are uncanny events in the life of the disabled and not to be discounted. The drug trials are filled with people who improve even though they are being administered a placebo rather than the drug therapy (Brown 90). And while I would never imply that disabilities can be overcome with hope alone, I can say (after what I have lived through) that with a little help, understanding, and acceptance, any of us (not only the disabled) would perform much better if encouraged to share the strength that helps us march onwards.

Works Cited

Brown, Walter A. "The Placebo Effect." *Scientific American* Jan. 1998: 90–95.
"Glossary of Terms for MS." 11 Dec. 1996. 1–22. National Multiple Sclerosis Society. 5 Dec. 1997. <http://www.nmss.org/msinfo/glossary.html>.
Holland, Nancy J. "Basic Facts." *Clinical Bulletin*. National Multiple Sclerosis Society, New York. Jan. 1995: EG 101.
Kübler-Ross, Elisabeth. *On Death and Dying*. New York: Macmillan, 1969.
"New Names for Types of MS." *Current Research Highlights*. 1996. 1–2. National Multiple Sclerosis Society. 5 Dec. 1997. <http://www.nmss.org/msinfo/current_research/highlights/newnames.html>.
Ovid. *Metamorphoses*. Ed. William S. Anderson. Leipzig: B. G. Teubner, 1977.
Parry, J. Kevin, M.D. Letter, "To Whom It May Concern." 15 Oct. 1996.
Persic, Louis A., interpreting physician. "MRI Scanning: Final Report for J. Kevin Parry." 27 Apr. 1995.
Piper, Watty. *The Little Engine That Could*. Uhrichsville, OH: Barbour, 1997.
Pruitt, Amy, M.D. Clinical evaluation note. 28 Feb. 1997.
Rae-Grant, Alexander D., M.D. Letter to Cheryl A. Ashcroft. 14 Nov. 1997.
———. Letter, "To Whom It May Concern." 28 Nov. 1997.
Redenbaugh, James E., M.D. Office note. 20 Jan. 1997.
Rosner, Louis J., M.D., and Shelley Ross. *Multiple Sclerosis: New Hope and Practical Advice for People with MS and Their Families*. New York: Simon and Schuster, 1992.
Talan, Jamie. "Fighting MS." *Connecticut Post* 1 Jan. 1998: B3.

5

Conflicting Paradigms: The Rhetorics of Disability Memoir

G. Thomas Couser

To marginalized people, autobiography may be the most accessible of literary genres. It requires less in the way of literary expertise and experience than other, more exalted genres. It seems to require only that one have a life—or at least one considered worth narrating—and sufficient narrative skill to tell one's own story. Most literary scholars would agree that autobiography has served historically as a sort of threshold genre for other marginalized groups. Within the American literary tradition, witness the importance of autobiography to African Americans, Native Americans, and women, for example. Presumably, it might serve disabled people this way as well. It is not just the apparent accessibility of autobiography—a kind of negative qualification—that recommends it but also something more positive: the notion that autobiography by definition involves self-representation. If marginalization is in part a function of discourse that excludes and/or objectifies, autobiography has considerable potential to counter stigmatizing or patronizing portrayals of disability because it is a medium in which disabled people may have a high degree of control over their own images.

Yet there are serious obstacles in the way of realizing the counter-hegemonic potential of the disability memoir. Obstacles can be found at three distinct junctures: having a life, writing a life, and publishing a life. Like minority racial or ethnic status, disability may disqualify people from living the sorts of lives that have traditionally been considered worthy of autobiography. Insofar as people with disabilities have been excluded from educational institutions and thus from economic opportunity, they will be less likely to produce the success story, perhaps the favorite American autobiographical subgenre from Benjamin Franklin on. That their disqualification lies not in individual incapacity but in social and cultural barriers does not change the fact that people with disabilities are less likely to live the sorts of lives considered narratable and less likely to be encouraged to display themselves in autobiography. One aspect of this discrimination, shared with other minorities, is the internalization of prejudices. Those who accept society's devaluation of them are less likely to consider their lives worthy of autobiography. Stigma serves to silence the stigmatized.

Writing a life is an aspect of accessibility that may seem secondary, but it is pertinent here because it is peculiar to disability. Despite important recent developments in assistive technology (such as voice-recognition software), the process of composition itself may be complicated by disability. People who are blind, deaf, paralyzed, or cognitively impaired are disadvantaged with regard to the conventional technologies of writing, which take for granted visual acuity, literacy in English, manual dexterity, and unimpaired memory. For people with many disabilities, the process of drafting and revising a long narrative may be too arduous. At this juncture, people with disabilities may be disadvantaged in ways that do not apply to racial and ethnic minorities and in ways that may not be immediately apparent to those who are not disabled. If a disability is such that it requires collaboration in the production of an autobiography, questions arise as to the agency, authority, voice, and authenticity of the self-representation.

Furthermore, it is not enough to produce a manuscript. Publishing—as distinct from printing—a life involves negotiating access to the marketplace through intermediaries who may have their own agendas. A third problem, then, may be located in the genre as defined by the literary marketplace, which may impose hegemonic scripts on a disempowered group. It is here that "rhetoric" and "disability" crucially intersect. In effect, people with disabilities may be granted access to the literary marketplace on the condition that their stories conform to preferred plots and rhetorical schemes. What characterizes these preferred rhetorics is that they rarely challenge stigma and marginalization directly or effectively. Indeed, their appeal to the reading public may vary inversely with the degree to which they threaten the status quo. This essay will distinguish a few of the most common rhetorical patterns of autobiographical disability narrative with reference to some recent examples, moving from rhetorics that reinforce conventional attitudes—the rhetorics of triumph, horror, spiritual compensation, and nostalgia—to a rhetoric that contests received attitudes about disability—the rhetoric of emancipation.[1]

The first of the common rhetorics is so obvious as to require little comment. Because disability is typically considered inherently "depressing," it is most acceptable as a subject of autobiography if the narrative takes the form of a story of triumph over adversity. In this formula, a successful individual takes pride in, and invites the reader's admiration for, a recounting of his or her overcoming of the obstacles posed by disability. Needless to say, the lives that fit this paradigm misrepresent the experience of most people with disabilities. This paradigm nominates as the representative disabled person the Supercrip, who is by definition atypical. These may be "true stories," but they are not truly representative lives. This rhetoric tends to remove the stigma of disability from the author, leaving it in place for other individuals with the condition in question. In any case, this scenario, like the other preferred scenarios, is entirely congruous with the medical paradigm, which locates disability entirely within a "defective" or "abnormal" body. Disability is presented primarily as a "problem" that individuals must overcome; overcoming it is a matter of individual will and determination rather than of social and cultural accommodation.

Another rhetoric frequently employed in the representation of disability is Gothic rhetoric, or the rhetoric of horror. Here, disability is characterized as a dreadful condition, to be shunned or avoided. At worst, Gothic rhetoric encourages revulsion from disability; at best, pity for the "afflicted." Such rhetoric might seem unlikely to be used in first-person discourse, such as disability memoir, because it would reflect negatively on the author-narrator. But this deterrent vanishes when impairment is corrected or "transcended." From the standpoint of those who are cured or rehabilitated—or who otherwise destigmatize themselves—it is common to look back upon a period of disability as a Gothic horror. In this rhetoric, narrators represent their former condition as grotesque. Readers are invited to share narrators' relief at escaping marginalization.

An example of this scenario is *A Leg to Stand On*, in which Oliver Sacks recounts his experience of temporarily losing the use of one leg after a climbing accident. The following passage may serve as a synecdoche of the book-length narrative:

> I had imagined my injury (a severe but uncomplicated wound to the muscles and nerves of one leg) to be straightforward and routine, and I was astonished at the profundity of the effects it had: a sort of paralysis and alienation of the leg, reducing it to an "object" which seemed unrelated to me; an abyss of bizarre, and even terrifying, effects. I had no idea what to make of these effects and entertained fears that I might never recover. I found the abyss a horror, and recovery a wonder; and I have since had a deeper sense of the horror and wonder which lurk behind life and which are concealed, as it were, behind the usual surface of health. (13–14)

Written from the perspective of complete recovery—which he narrates as a mysterious conversion experience—his account reinscribes, rather than erases, the line between disability and nondisability.[2]

Used this way, Gothic rhetoric tends, of course, to confirm the worst stereotypes about disability, to reinforce stigmatization. But such rhetoric is sometimes also used in accounts that do not culminate in the removal of the narrator from the condition in question. When the source of horror is not the condition itself but the treatment of the condition, Gothic rhetoric has some counterhegemonic potential. Julia Tavalaro's account of the six-year period following her two strokes, during which she was assumed by hospital staff to be completely unaware of her surroundings, is a good example of the latter form of Gothic rhetoric— a medical horror story of inattention, indifference, and abuse. In *Look Up for "Yes,"* then, Gothic rhetoric serves to indict the medical care of the severely disabled, those who are presumed to be unconscious or beyond rehabilitation.

When Tavalaro is discovered, by a speech therapist, to be cognizant, her treatment improves radically, and what ensues is a narrative of rehabilitation. But even when, as here, Gothic rhetoric is used to generate outrage at ill-treatment, rather than revulsion at a disfiguring or disabling condition, it is entirely consonant with the medical or individual model of disability and leaves conventional attitudes in place. It does not challenge the idea that disability resides in the individual body; at most, it calls for more attentive treatment of such individuals.

The rhetoric of spiritual compensation has also frequently been used to narrate experiences of disability.[3] Ruth Cameron Webb's *Journey into Personhood*, a recent memoir by a woman with cerebral palsy, is a particularly interesting example of this, in part because the rhetoric of conversion was not the only, or even the most obvious, rhetoric available to her. Given the outlines of Webb's life, one might expect her narrative to employ the rhetoric of triumph. For despite delays in her education, Webb got a Ph.D. in clinical psychology and had a successful career counseling people with disabilities. Indeed, because the major obstacle to her eventual success was not her cerebral palsy but blatant discrimination—she was repeatedly expelled from schools and colleges because her disabilities were considered unmanageable—and because she was professionally involved with disabled people, the circumstances of her life might have impelled her toward a more aggressive political rhetoric.

Webb does not, however, narrate a secular success story—much less question the medical paradigm—because of a deeply ingrained sense of inferiority associated with her disability. In therapy she traces these feelings to being examined, naked, by physicians at her first boarding school. Her sense of invalidity is so great that it challenges her religious faith: "Often I wonder why God allowed me to be injured at birth. Have I done anything to deserve cerebral palsy? Why can't I walk and talk like everybody else?" (70) Here we see a biblical view of disability, that it is a mark of sin or God's displeasure with an individual. Her double bind is that though her faith contributes to her sense of inferiority, it also condemns her anger, which she finds hard to quell nevertheless. Her religion does hold out some promise of relief, but she has an ambivalent response to faith healing. On the one hand, at a Christian summer retreat, she feels humiliated and angry when enthusiastic evangelicals form a circle around her and pray for her healing without asking her permission or cooperation. On the other, after volunteering to be healed by Oral Roberts, she sinks into depression when her condition does not improve. (The most that faith healing seems to be able to accomplish for her is to suppress her recurrent suicidal impulses.)

There are tantalizing moments when she moves toward a more social and political paradigm of disability. For example, becoming friends with a biracial couple, she recognizes their kindred marginalization—"Then I'm not the only side show, I think" (79)—and learns to ignore stares. Later on, through an experience with an African American colleague, she has another glimmer of minority consciousness: "As a member of a social minority group, she has been discriminated against and excluded. I understand her anger because, after all, I, too, belong to a minority" (140). Through experiences like these, Webb approaches the brink of consciousness of disability as a socially constructed condition, but she always stops short.

Only late in life does she resolve these issues, through a transfiguring visitation in which a voice tells her to give up her anger and accept God's love:

> Then, suddenly, these words come into my mind. "Ruth, you have a special mission from the Lord, the Great Spirit. Your mission is similar to that of the man born blind about whom John, the gospel writer, wrote. You, too, are asked to reflect God's glory in your disabled body. Without knowing your assignment, you have faithfully pursued this mission by helping everyone you met on your journey. The time has now come for you to pursue this mission actively. To do this, you need to review the battles you have won. Remember, with each victory, you have taken another step on our journey into personhood."
>
> During the next several months, I often awake around four o'clock in the morning and watch as a panorama of triumphal scenes passes rapidly through my mind. (180)

Webb can regard her life as a success only with the help of faith. Indeed, she can only be certain of her personhood—which for her is somehow compromised by her disability—when it has been conferred and confirmed by divine authority.

Only through spiritual compensation can she find a comic plot in her life. Part of the implicit "purpose" of her disability, then, is to make her a better Christian. She finds solace finally in her sense of value to God, who has assigned her a special mission on earth. Indeed, the book might as well have been called "Journey into Sainthood" (in the Protestant meaning of the sainthood of all believers) in that the resolution of her lifelong feeling of inferiority comes from a sense that she has success-fully borne her personal cross. Such rhetoric invites readers to assent to the conditions of Webb's validation as a person. In her view, disability is her problem—a challenge given her by God for his own inscrutable reasons—not a social or political issue. But skeptical readers will see her religious schema as part of the problem, rather than as an ultimate or generalizable solution. The effect of her mystical validation is not to remove stigma from disability as a condition but from her as an indi-vidual. Her resorting to God for validation precludes any attempts to find remedy in worldly efforts toward reform, short-circuiting any movement toward the competing political paradigm of disability.

A third rhetorical schema, the rhetoric of nostalgia, is illustrated in pure form by a recent memoir that was greeted by extensive press cov-erage and positive reviews: Jean-Dominique Bauby's *The Diving Bell and the Butterfly*. Written by the editor-in-chief of *Elle* magazine after a massive stroke to the brain stem left him almost completely paralyzed, this memoir was translated and published in the United States in 1997. Bauby's paralysis was so extensive that it left him deaf in one ear and mute, able to move only his left eye. Nevertheless, he managed to com-pose a memoir by blinking to select letters, one by one, as an attentive collaborator, Claude Mendibil, recited the alphabet for him.

Partly as a result of this extremely labor-intensive method of com-position, the book is very short; it consists of a series of brief vignettes. The chapters range over a number of topics, but typically recount iso-lated memories of his life before the stroke. This is a memoir in a par-ticularly literal sense. It is far from a full-life narrative. Bauby makes no attempt to recount his life as a chronological narrative of becoming. The severity of his disability seems to have played a role here. By the time he undertook his narrative, he was past the initial phase of denial, dur-ing which he continued to believe he might soon return to work. Aware that he would never recover, though he might improve in certain lim-ited respects, Bauby ceased to orient himself toward the future.[4] Partly, then, because his condition did not allow for his reintegration into the world of the nondisabled, he minimizes the narrative of rehabilitation. If the book hints at any narrative progression, it is one of recession: "I am fading away. Slowly but surely. Like the sailor who watches the home shore gradually disappear, I watch my past recede. My old life still burns within me, but more and more of it is reduced to the ashes of memory" (77).[5] As a result, there is no consideration of issues of accessibility.

Other biographical circumstances reinforce the rhetoric of nostalgia. Bauby died of a heart attack only two days after the French publication of his book. Thus, by the time the book was available in translation to the American public, readers knew—from the book jacket—that its author was dead. This knowledge confirms Bauby's characterization of himself as already a dead man. There is a strong undercurrent of morbidity in the book, an implicit equation of severe disability with death. This undercurrent is part of a Gothic or grotesque subtext that surfaces— sometimes in the form of black humor—when Bauby looks at himself through others' eyes. Thus, when he sees his image—the face of a "man who seemed to have emerged from a vat of formaldehyde"—reflected in a stained-glass representation of the patroness of the hospital, he experiences a frisson and then a moment of euphoria: "Not only was I exiled, paralyzed, mute, half deaf, deprived of all pleasures, and reduced to the existence of a jellyfish, but I was also horrible to behold. There comes a time when the heaping up of calamities brings on uncontrollable nervous laughter—when, after a final blow from fate, we decide to treat it all as a joke" (25).[6] An interesting variant of the Gothic occurs in a dream in which Bauby visits a wax museum where his orderlies and nurses are on display. Here the tables are turned: It is the staff who are immobilized, exposed, and objectified. A passage like this exemplifies the Gothic's potential for political critique, but Bauby draws back, concluding ambivalently, "I realized that I was fond of all these torturers of mine" (111).

Bauby's account of an earlier touristic visit to Lourdes makes clear that his present disablement realizes a deep fear of becoming an invalid. Having become one of "them," however, he does not reevaluate, but rather acquiesces in, the stigmatization of disability. Instead of questioning it, he deflects his attention away from his present condition to his "normal" life, which now seems all the more precious and poignant. Thus, although Bauby writes from a position of nearly total paralysis, disability provides not the subject of his narrative but only its motivation.

For this reason, one could argue that his book is not truly a disability memoir. In some significant respect it is not one, but it demands discussion here because of the way its rare compositional circumstances (its being "eye-typed" and its having been written in a short interval between traumatic injury and death) trigger a response characteristic of much disability memoir. In one blurb, for example, Sherwin B. Nuland, author of *How We Die*, exclaims, "To read this most extraordinary of narratives is to discover the luminosity within a courageous man's mind. His incomparable final gift to us is a heartbreaking and yet glorious testament to the wrenching beauty of the human spirit." Cynthia Ozick's endorsement is even more enthusiastic: "Jean-Dominique Bauby's extraordinary narrative testifies to the infinitude of the human imagination, to the resilient will that drives boundless courage. The heroic composition of *The Diving Bell and the Butterfly* renders it the most remarkable memoir of our time—perhaps of any time." Such extravagant responses are encouraged by the purely nostalgic and virtually postmortem perspective of the narration. Since the author did not live long with disability, there is no question of his using his position as a prominent editor to offer personal testimony on behalf of others with disabilities. Rather, he earns praise in part for having undertaken, in forbidding circumstances, to create a book and for having written a book that is not "depressing" but "uplifting" because, rather than raising disturbing questions about the status of people with disabilities, it offers poignant accounts of pleasures and pastimes no longer available to him.

The diving bell is Bauby's image for his confinement in a kind of hermetic zone removed from the world of "ability." The butterfly is an image of the compensatory liberation of his mind so that it may float freely over his past, as his eye surveys the souvenirs and snapshots surrounding him in his room (3). The emphasis throughout is much more on the freedom of the butterfly than on the confinement of the diving bell.[7] Indeed, one might say that, despite its occasional Gothic passages, the text tends to idealize Bauby's condition as one freeing him from mundane constraints to reminisce, fantasize, and "travel" (103): "There is so much to do. You can wander off in space or in time. . . . You can visit the woman you love, . . . realize your childhood dreams and adult ambitions" (5). In effect, then, Bauby treats his disability not as an experience of the body but as an experience of being "out of the body." Indeed, the memoir has aspects of the near-death narrative insofar as his life passes slowly before his eyes during his months of post-trauma hospitalization. Knowledge of his ensuing death frees readers from the impulse to pity him, allowing them to enjoy the fantasy of being able to range back over one's life in memory, without having to contemplate the present or the future. The effect is not to challenge or erase but to mark a distinction between past and present, function and dysfunction, ability and disability, living and remembering. Although there is little that physicians can do for him other than to stabilize his condition and minimize his discomfort, his narrative in no way challenges the medical paradigm. Compared with the rhetoric of horror, the rhetoric of nostalgia seems benign, and yet it too tends to marginalize disability insofar as it is rooted in an equation between severe disability and the end of life.

In contrast to the preceding memoirs and their rhetorics, my final example realizes some of the counterhegemonic potential of disability narrative. *I Raise My Eyes to Say Yes,* by Ruth Sienkiewicz-Mercer and

Steven B. Kaplan, is the story of a woman with cerebral palsy so severe that she has never been able to walk, feed herself, speak, or write. After spending some time as a child in rehabilitative facilities, she was sent to a state hospital in Belchertown, Massachusetts, because her father changed jobs and his new insurance did not cover private hospitals. Upon entering this new facility at the age of twelve, Sienkiewicz-Mercer was misdiagnosed as mentally retarded, and she was then "warehoused" with people who were either cognitively impaired or mentally ill.[8] Eventually, her abilities were recognized and gradually recultivated. In her midtwenties she was able to move out of the hospital into an apartment and to marry a fellow former patient—both beneficiaries of the new approach to disability that favored deinstitutionalization.

In her new environment, she was presumed to be a body without (much of) a mind. Though toilet-trained early on, she was diapered, dressed in a hospital johnny—all for the convenience of the staff—and supervised, rather than educated or rehabilitated. It was thus not her own severe impairments but the disabilities of her physicians that threatened to limit her development.[9] What saved Sienkiewicz-Mercer from languishing in the institution was her ability, using very limited means, to connect with those around her. Virtually the only moving parts of her body under her control were her eyes and her vocal cords. By making eye contact with other inmates and staff members, she was able to establish vital connections with them; by gesturing with her eyes, and coordinating nonverbal vocalizations with those gestures, she was able to communicate ideas and emotions about life around her in a kind of private language to receptive others. The most receptive were the captive audience of other similarly misdiagnosed patients. It was only through eye contact and private language that she and a few peers could establish that there was intelligent—and intelligible— life within them. In this initial bonding with other inmates we can see the beginnings of political consciousness shared with others in the same predicament, an element that distinguishes her account from those of Bauby and Webb.

The role of her "gaze" in self-construction, then, is crucial. Whereas the disciplinary medical gaze had sized her up (or rather, down) as mentally deficient, through her own inquisitive and aggressive gaze she managed to challenge or defy her misdiagnosis—and, not incidentally, to have a social life. Once her consciousness and intelligence were recognized, she was able to expand on and refine this method of communication, but she could never abandon it. In order for her to communicate with the staff and move herself beyond the limits assigned to her, she needed to make them respond to her gaze as well.

The writing of her text is only a more deliberate and extensive application of this means of self-creation. The medium of autobiography is an elaboration of the process of self-possession and self-assertion through manipulation of her gaze. Collaborative self-inscription is the means for releasing herself from the institution. Personal narrative is thus crucial to her physical and psychological emancipation. Rather than accepting her dependency as disvaluing, she exploits interdependency as a means of self-assertion. While not achieving independence (or subscribing to the ideology of personal autonomy), Sienkiewicz-Mercer moves herself through reciprocity to a position of greater power and mobility. (The reciprocity of her self-construction is attested to by the way in which her narrative vividly individualizes others also consigned to near-oblivion in the hospital.)

Although, like most personal narratives of illness and/or disability, the narrative has an undeniably comic plot, it is not a story of overcoming disability—at least not in the usual sense. It is not what Arthur Frank calls a "narrative of restitution"—a narrative of complete healing in which a physician would play a transformative role (77). Nor is it primarily a narrative of rehabilitation. Although she does learn to use various assistive technologies to communicate, Sienkiewicz-Mercer never manages to walk or talk, nor does she achieve autonomy. Her rhetoric is thus not that of triumph. Rather, she manages, with a great deal of help, to work around her impairment. The comic resolution is not a function of removing or correcting her impairment but of getting the world to accommodate her irreparable impairments, of removing the physical, social, and cultural obstacles to her integration into "mainstream society." In that sense, her narrative demonstrates what we might call the rhetoric of emancipation.

Indeed, *I Raise My Eyes to Say Yes* has interesting affinities with slave narrative. The narrative is reminiscent of a slave narrative both in the sense that, on the level of plot, it traces a movement from virtual imprisonment to relative freedom, and in the sense that her emancipation is a function of a broader movement to deinstitutionalize disabled people. Like many, if not all, slave narratives, it defies the ascription of mental deficiency to the body of the Other and exposes the confinement of those bodies as a contingent social phenomenon rather than a "natural" one. It has particular affinities, then, with those slave narratives elicited by sympathetic abolitionists, for Sienkiewicz-Mercer's account is in effect promoted and sponsored by individuals seeking to liberate people with disabilities and even to abolish their "institutionalization." In this case, however, neither the disabled subject nor the nondisabled collaborator has made the narrative especially polemical—except, perhaps, in the afterword, where Sienkiewicz-Mercer is quoted as giving a speech that calls for the abolition of institutions like the one in which she was confined.

One of the striking things about *I Raise My Eyes to Say Yes* is that it represents, by implication, many lives that generally go unrepresented, uninscribed because of disability.[10] In that sense, it suggests not the limitations of people with disabilities but those of autobiography as an accessible medium of self-representation. That is, it suggests that autobiography as traditionally conceived, with its inherent valorization of individualism and autonomy, presents its own barriers to people with disabilities. The book communicates both the limitations of language and the liberation of access to it. Some of the best parts of the book suggest that subjectivity is not entirely a linguistic construct; at least, it offers a glimpse of life being lived and communicated in gestures, looks, and sounds—beyond or without the resources of what we usually recognize as language or autobiography.

To associate this disability memoir with slave narrative alone, however, would be perhaps to limit its resonance. It might also be considered a form of autoethnography, as Mary Louise Pratt defines the term: "instances in which colonized subjects undertake to represent themselves in ways that *engage with* the colonizer's own terms. If the ethnographic texts are a means by which Europeans represent to themselves their (usually subjugated) others, autoethnographic texts are those the others construct in response to or in dialogue with those metropolitan representations" (7). This narrative does display a kind of postcolonial impulse—the impulse to define oneself in resistance to the dehumanizing categories of the medical and health-service institutions (see Frank 7–11). It's autoethnography, too, in that it is a first-person account of what Erving Goffman calls the "underlife of a public institution," the inmates' view of the asylum—the gossip, the games, the inside dope. Both as individual and institutional history, it supplements, challenges, and indicts official discourse, which assumes that standardized testing can adequately indicate the inner life of the subject in question.

To characterize it as standing in for other unwritten, perhaps unwriteable, accounts is to suggest its affinity with a more current first-person genre: testimonio. In an incisive discussion of testimonio, John Beverley has distinguished it from autobiography as follows: "*Testimonio* represents an affirmation of the individual subject, even of individual growth and transformation, but in connection with a group or class situation marked by marginalization, oppression, and struggle. If it loses this connection, it ceases to be *testimonio* and becomes autobiography, that is, an account of, and also a means of access to, middle- or upperclass status, a sort of documentary *bildungsroman*" (103). In this text we have a disability memoir that moves toward, though it may not fully occupy, the position with regard to the disability rights movement that testimonio occupies with regard to the movement for the rights of indigenous peoples. *I Raise My Eyes to Say Yes* is testimonio to the (considerable) extent to which its narrator speaks not as a unique individual but for a class of marginalized individuals, in ways already suggested. My term "rhetoric of emancipation" should perhaps be qualified here, then, insofar as it overstates the position from which Sienkiewicz-Mercer composes her memoir.[11] To be sure, she is liberated from the confining state hospital, but she narrates her account from within the context of an ongoing personal and collective struggle for recognition of the value and rights of people with disabilities. While the political critique within the text is muted, her story decisively represents disability not as a flaw in her body but as the prejudicial construct of a normative culture. It thus suggests the way in which personal narrative of disability may articulate and advocate the political paradigm of disability and thus align itself with testimonio as deployed in other modern liberation movements.

One of the arguments made against *narrating* disability would seem to apply to all forms of narrative, including autobiography: "[B]y narrativizing an impairment, one tends to . . . link it to the bourgeois sensibility of individualism and the drama of an individual story" (Davis 4). Given the examples I have cited here, there is no question of exempting first-person discourse from this critique. Indeed, most of my examples suggest that the conventional rhetorics for representing disability in autobiography do tend to individualize the condition and, worse, to reinforce its stigma. Thus, although autobiography may offer a degree of access that other literary genres do not, and although it may offer a degree of control over representation that other media may not, various cultural constraints limit the counterhegemonic potential of disability memoir. Culture filters and manipulates even seemingly "self-generated" texts in various ways, protecting its interest in marginalizing and ignoring disabled lives.

At the same time, there are signs of promise in some recent texts—narratives from hidden corners, some of which may actually connect with each other in ways that challenge and undermine the limited medical paradigm of disability. Such narratives not only attest to but advance the work of the disability rights movement. In their consciousness of their own condition as culturally constructed and as shared by others, their authors may move beyond the familiar formulas of disability memoir and point the way to broader critiques of the construction of disability in America today.

Notes

1. These different rhetorics are often combined within single memoirs, but in most cases one pattern dominates. My examples are chosen to exemplify particular rhetorical appeals.

2. For a more sustained discussion of this book, see my *Recovering Bodies*, 186–89.

3. See *Recovering Bodies*, 192–98, for a discussion of the use of paradigms of spiritual autobiography in disability narratives by Reynolds Price and John Callahan.

4. It also lacks any confessional dimension. Bauby may have been deterred from a more confessional mode because his stroke occurred at a time of great instability in his life; he had just moved out of the house he shared with his wife and two children. Writing memoirs, rather than a more self-exploratory autobiography, he worked around rather than through this life crisis.

5. At the same time, his writing of letters to friends and of the book—his letter to the world—is an act of resistance against this seemingly inevitable recession. As his letter to friends seeks to counter the rumor that he is a "vegetable," his book seeks to establish that there is yet intelligent life within his immobilized and silenced body.

6. For a similar moment in Tavalaro, see 150–53; on one of their rare visits, her daughter and her mother "make her over." Even though Tavalaro acquiesces to their desire to beautify her, she finds the resulting image as alien as her previous appearance. Indeed, she describes herself in the third person: "Even all gussied up, I didn't know the person in the mirror. If I had known her, I'd have felt sorry for her. She was skin and bones, a few teeth, some sagging flesh, and fake color. Her hands were like a baby's, always held in a fist. Her head lolled from side to side, and the wig looked awful. I had no idea how much I'd aged in six years. Instead of Judy's mother, I could have been her grandmother" (153).

7. The organization of the book around these two opposing images suggests that it, too, participates in the rhetoric of spiritual compensation, even though it is utterly devoid of explicitly religious language.

8. Given her treatment, or mistreatment—her leg was once broken by a careless and clumsy aide and not immediately attended to—Sienkiewicz's story, like Tavalaro's, has Gothic potential, but the Gothic remains a minor element in her account, as in Bauby's.

9. Reading Sienkiewicz-Mercer's and Tavalaro's accounts against Bauby's exposes the role of social class in the ascription of disability. For Bauby, though he never leaves the institution, the hospital is not a site of oppression in the way that it is for her. This is in part because of his socioeconomic status, with all the clout and connections it entails. For him, the major problem is his locked-in condition; for Sienkiewicz-Mercer and Tavalaro, it is the institution's (mis)treatment of their condition, which they have no powerful advocates to question.

10. Of course, new technologies may quite literally write new lives, but in Sienkiewicz-Mercer's case, high-tech methods did not ultimately prove superior to the low-tech word boards.

11. Although I do not have the space to explore it fully here, I cannot entirely omit a discussion of the mediation of the collaborative narratives under discussion. For the collaboration of a disabled subject with a nondisabled agent to produce an "autobiographical" text raises the same political and ethical questions that pertain to testimonio. In any collaborative account, the "rhetoric" in question may not be entirely attributable to the subject; indeed, it is generally the case that the "writers" of collaborative accounts will be more conversant with conventional narrative rhetorics. This is, after all, one reason that they are used.

In the case of Bauby, who was highly educated and sophisticated about print media, it is probably safe to assume that his collaborator functioned mostly as a scribe—active in prompting him with recited letters, but probably largely passive in the composition of the memoir. With Tavalaro and Sienkiewicz-Mercer, who were far less highly educated, their collaborators probably played much more active roles in the solicitation and composition of the memoirs. In both cases, the narratives contain texts attributable solely to the women themselves; in both instances, the disparity between the style of those texts and that of the collaborative text suggests that the voice of the memoir is not really that of its subject and putative narrator—regardless of the *accuracy* of the accounts, which both women were apparently able to ensure.

Works Cited

Bauby, Jean-Dominique. *The Diving Bell and the Butterfly*. Trans. Jeremy Leggatt. New York: Knopf, 1997.

Beverley, John. "The Margin at the Center: On *Testimonio* (Testimonial Narrative)." Smith and Watson 91–114.

Couser, G. Thomas. *Recovering Bodies: Illness, Disability, and Life Writing*. Madison: U of Wisconsin P, 1997.

Davis, Lennard J. *Enforcing Normalcy: Disability, Deafness, and the Body*. London: Verso, 1995.

Frank, Arthur W. *The Wounded Storyteller: Body, Illness, and Ethics*. Chicago: U of Chicago P, 1995.

Goffman, Erving. *Asylums: Essays on the Social Situation of Mental Patients and Other Inmates*. Chicago: Aldine, 1961.

Pratt, Mary Louise. *Imperial Eyes: Travel Writing and Transculturation*. London: Routledge, 1992.

Sacks, Oliver. *A Leg to Stand On*. New York: Summit Books, 1984.

Sienkiewicz-Mercer, Ruth, and Steven B. Kaplan. *I Raise My Eyes to Say Yes*. Boston: Houghton Mifflin, 1989.

Smith, Sidonie, and Julia Watson, eds. *De/Colonizing the Subject: The Politics of Gender in Women's Autobiography*. Minneapolis: U of Minnesota P, 1992.

Tavalaro, Julia, and Richard Tayson. *Look Up for "Yes."* New York: Kodansha, 1997.

Webb, Ruth Cameron. *A Journey into Personhood*. Foreword by Albert E. Stone. Iowa City: Iowa UP, 1994.

6

In Search of the Disabled Subject
Nirmala Erevelles

> To speak within these classical contexts of *bodies that matter* is not an
> idle pun, for to be material means to materialize, where the principle of
> that materialization is precisely what "matters" about that body, its
> very intelligibility. In this sense, to know the significance of something is
> to know how and why it matters, where "to matter" means at once "to
> materialize" and "to mean."
> —Judith Butler, *Bodies That Matter*

Any attempt to reconceptualize a critical social theory of disability
necessitates an engagement with poststructuralist readings of the
material body, given its recent predominance in theorizing oppositional
subjectivities. Critical of the Cartesian dualisms of mind/body that have
characterized theories of the subject in western philosophical thought,
poststructuralists have argued that "bodies cannot be adequately understood as ahistorical, pre-cultural, or natural objects in any simple way"
(Grosz x). They have therefore theorized the body as the local site where
the micro politics of power are disrupted so as "to release [it] into a
future of multiple significations, to emancipate it from the [normative]
ontologies to which it has been restricted, and to give it play as a site
where unanticipated meanings might come to bear" (Butler, "Contingent Foundations" 50). Such reconceptualizations of the body have
opened up transgressive possibilities for posthuman bodies to establish
themselves—where posthumanity "marks a solidarity between disenchanted liberal subjects and those who are already disenchanted, those
that seek to betray identities that legitimize and delegitimize them at too
high a cost" (Halberstam and Livingston 9).

In many ways, the transgressive possibilities of posthuman bodies
would initially appear to be most useful in the retheorization of the disabled subject. After all, as Susan Wendell has described, disabled subjects are assumed to inhabit bodies that are feared, ignored, despised,

and/or rejected in society and its culture (85). Thus, in a context where disabled people are constructed as de-authorized subjects, it would appear that the rhetorical interventions of poststructuralism would suggest the ironic and blasphemous (re)writing of the disabled body in order to (re)invent alternative emancipatory subjectivities.

While I acknowledge the contributions of poststructuralist feminist theory to disability studies, I argue in this essay that these rhetorical interventions will need to extend their analyses to include a historical materialist analysis of disability. I view this extension as essential especially at this historical moment because of the real material effects that the expansion of transnational capitalism (globalization) has had on the disabled subject—effects that I argue cannot be easily brushed aside by transgressive discursive interventions. In saying this, I am referring to the social and economic transformations that globalization has generated—the shifting of production processes to offshore locations in search of cheaper wage labor, accompanied by rising unemployment and sizable cuts in public spending. These transformations have had adverse effects on the lives of disabled people, not only in the United States but also globally.[1] In fact, the 1995 World Summit on Social Development held in Copenhagen reported that disabled people now constitute one of the world's largest minority groups facing poverty and unemployment as well as social and cultural isolation ("Copenhagen Declaration on Social Development" 15-h).

At the same time, I would like to add that the adverse effects of the current global economic crisis have affected not only disabled people but other marginal groups marked by race, class, gender, and sexuality. However, while these other marginal groups have attempted to support coalitions of resistance against oppressive structures,[2] they have often experienced a paralysis when faced with the overwhelming physiology that disability represents and embodies. Moreover, their attempts to include disabled people, citing their common experiences of marginality, are merely discursive gestures reminiscent of the add-and-stir policy that used to haunt race, gender, and queer studies.[3] Alternatively, I argue here that it has become necessary to move beyond this obvious commonality and treat disability as a critical theoretical category—one that can also account for the challenges posed by the other constructs of difference. Therefore, in this essay I ask the question: In what ways can we, from the vantage point of disability, rewrite the terrain occupied by race, class, gender, and queer theory within the context of transnational capitalism?

In a context of economic crisis and conservative social policy, theories that locate emancipation solely in the transformation of meaning systems ignore the reality that disabled people's lives are also bounded by oppressive social and economic conditions that are much more difficult to transcend. I propose, therefore, a theoretical shift from the "metaphoric" to the "material," by turning to a materialist reading of the disabled body that will render visible the historical, political, economic, and social interests that have supported debilitating constructions of disability in the current context of transnational capitalism. I will argue here that it is essential to (re)theorize the disabled subject in such a way that it would enable us to explain where disabled people are located within the prevailing social relations of production, why it is that this location has produced conceptualizations of disability that are exclusionary and exploitative, and how such a location benefits capitalism in particular ways. By doing so, I hope to demonstrate that it is only through such an analysis (why disability?) that we can seek to transform the material structures that have rendered it imperative to constitute "disabled" bodies as bodies that do not matter.

Reading the Postmodern Body: Disability as Discourse

Almost all subjects of difference who have posited an oppositional politics against normative traditions have begun these struggles from within the liberal humanist tradition. Humanist discourses have their historical roots in the Enlightenment, where the God-given, socially fixed, free subject of the feudal order was transformed by the secular capitalist state to become the free, rational, self-determining subject of modern political, legal, social, and aesthetic discourses. It is through the recognition of this essential humanity that the individual has been guaranteed the universal rights of freedom, equality, fraternity—ideals that emerged from the historical context of the French and American Revolutions.[4]

Notwithstanding the claim to the universality of these human rights, large sections of the population that included women and children, gays and lesbians, the poor, non-Europeans, and disabled individuals have historically been denied such guarantees, based on the presumed deviations from the prescribed norm as embodied by the bourgeois, heterosexual, able-bodied, European male. Both First and Second Wave Feminism as well as the Civil Rights Movement were among the first social movements to take issue with Enlightenment discourses that explained the social, economic, and political subjugation of marginal populations by judging their bodies through their "natural inequality" (Grosz 14). Disabled people and their advocates, also anxious to debunk the absolute nature of disability as rooted in biology, have argued that the deviance ascribed to their physiological differences are in fact social constructions of reality.[5] They have, therefore, sought to establish their humanness in the social sphere by claiming the space, the voice, and the power to write themselves into the social world, and they have deployed various rhetorical strategies to displace normative constructions of truth, power, knowledge, history, self, and language in an attempt to reconstruct emancipatory subjectivities.[6]

At first glance, it would therefore appear that disability theorists would have much to gain from poststructuralist attempts to deconstruct normative notions of humanness and offer alternative constructions of normality. Yet, even though poststructuralists have celebrated the transgressive and deviant body, they have seldom bothered to articulate a theory of disability. In fact, rather than face "the nightmare of the [disabled] body—one that is deformed, maimed, mutilated, broken, diseased," poststructuralist theorists have focused on "the fluids of sexuality, the gloss of lubrication, the glossary of the body as text, the heteroglossia of intertext, the glossolalia of the schizophrenic . . . [b]ut almost never the body of the differently abled" (Davis 5). Even poststructuralist feminists who have been most sensitive to the nuances of difference as inscribed on the gendered body have refrained from theorizing disability in relation to gender. Instead, though feminist anthologies have integrated most constructions of difference with gender analyses, they have "relegated disabled women to a realm beneath their intellectual and political ken" (Fine and Asch 4). Yet, despite these marked absences in feminist theory, I am suggesting here that possibilities exist for alliances between both feminist theory and disability studies when examined in critical relationship to each other. Therefore, in this section, I take up the arguments of Judith Butler and Donna Haraway, in order to critically explore the possibility of theorizing the disabled subject through poststructuralist feminist theory.

Poststructuralist feminists have struggled to represent the "peculiar temporality" of the category "woman" (Riley 6) so as to account for the multiple ways in which social difference has marked the female body. Following in this tradition, Butler in *Gender Trouble* has sought to subvert the humanist logic that bodies possess essential and coherent identities by exposing the signs through which culture polices sexuality and marks its normative limits. By drawing on Foucault's study of the hermaphrodite Herculine Barbin, Butler argues that through the coping strategy of parodic performance (which both contests and replicates privilege and both confuses and redistributes the coherent elements of categories of identity), subjects of difference demonstrate that identity is no more than an effect variably produced in response to the exigency of the moment. In this way, Butler describes how gendered categories (we can replace gender by disability here) are themselves neither stable nor transcendental but are in fact always constructed and reconstructed through historically specific discursive practices.

However, in her second book, *Bodies That Matter*, Butler explains that in exploring the possibilities of "parodic performance," she has not intended to reinvoke humanism's free and autonomous subject. In other words, she claims that she does not presume as a viable theoretical option "a willful and instrumental subject" (x) who decides on its gender but who fails to realize that its existence is already decided by gender. On the other hand, she argues that the ideological social constructions of our reality serve as "constitutive constraints" such that material bodies are compelled to negotiate with "not only the domain of intelligible bodies [bodies that matter], but produce as well a domain of unthinkable, abject, unlivable bodies [those that do not matter in the same way]" (xi). Butler is quick to point out that the latter domain does not constitute the distinctive binary "other" of the former but is "the excluded and illegible domain that haunts the former domain as the specter of its own impossibility, the very limit to intelligibility, its constitutive outside" (xi). In other words, the normative constraints that attempt to impose their limits on the material body simultaneously also support the possibilities that can enable that same material body to transgress those very limits—thereby implying that it can occupy spaces that are both inside and outside these limits. According to Donna Haraway, it is through such possibilities that one can create "a condensed image of both imagination and material reality, the two joined centers structuring any possibility of historical transformations" (191). For Haraway, this image is the transgressive and blasphemous cyborg, a "hybrid of machine and organism, a creature of social reality as well as a creature of fiction" (191).

Haraway has argued that cyborgean identity could only have been made possible through the new global technoculture—the "informatics of domination"—which has replaced advanced capitalism with "a world of production/reproduction and communication" based on the "social relations of science and technology" (Ebert 106). And whereas before both capital and labor structured the social relations within industrial societies, it is now communication sciences and modern biologies that have "translated the world into a problem of coding, a search for a common language in which all resistance to instrumental control disappears and all assembly can be submitted to disassembly, reassembly, investment, and exchange" (Haraway 206).

In this poststructuralist context, what would be the consequences for the disabled body? Historically, the disabled body (particularly one described as severely disabled) has always been called upon to reassert its viability as an intelligible body (i.e., the body that matters) in order to claim its presence at least within a liberal politics. However, bounded by the limits of the real, these efforts on the part of the disabled subject to present his/her body as intelligible are often confounded because of the physiological and mental differences that constitute this disabled body. It is as a result of these incongruities that the disabled body has often been construed as the "monstrous body" (remember the Elephant Man), where the monster, as Haraway reminds us, has always determined the outer limits of community within western imaginations.

Further, the very viability of this disabled body is often sustained and rendered "livable" through a network of communication technologies and biotechnologies. In this ironic coupling, the very viability of the human necessitates a dependence on the nonhuman. As a result, Haraway points out in her only reference to the disabled body, in the "Manifesto for Cyborgs":

> Perhaps paraplegics and other severely handicapped people can (and sometimes do) have the most intense experiences of complex hybridization with other communicative devices. . . . [After all,] why should our bodies end at the skin or include at best other beings encapsulated by skin? (220)

One could therefore argue that the disabled subjects transgress the boundaries between human/nonhuman/machine to seek a pleasurable survival as a border-crosser in the ironic political myth of a cyborgean materiality. This cyborg world inhabited by disabled subjects might be a world of "lived social and bodily realities in which people are not afraid of their joint kinship with animals and machines, not afraid of permanently partial identities and contradictory standpoints" (qtd. in Sandoval 413). As Chela Sandoval reiterates, this invention of a cyborgean subjectivity, "being a technologized metaphorization of forms of resistance and oppositional consciousness" (410), would provide both a language and a praxis of possibility for society's most marginal populations.

However, I argue that the ease with which the disabled subject lends itself to the poststructuralist articulation of "cyborg politics" is a cause for concern. Despite their insistence that they possess "livable" bodies, people with disabilities have lived through a history of segregational practices (in schools, workplaces, residences, communities, etc.) that have constructed them on the outside limits of intelligibility. More often than not, these segregational practices have also ensured that large numbers of disabled people experience lives of abject poverty. In the United States, for example, working people with disabilities earned only 63.6 percent as much as those without disabilities, according to 1995 data. Within the working population (ages sixteen to sixty-four), 30 percent of working people with disabilities live below the poverty line. Further, among people with severe disabilities who are prevented from working at all and so are qualified to receive Medicaid or SSI, 35.8 percent have incomes below the poverty level (LaPlante, Kennedy, Kaye, and Wenger 1). Moreover, in the current context of massive cuts in public spending and the increased privatization of health care, nearly 4.1 million Americans with disabilities under the age of sixty-five lack any kind of health insurance (LaPlante, Rice, and Cyril 1).

In light of this material reality, constituting the disabled subject as cyborg actually renders as immaterial the actual struggles of disabled subjects fighting for their immediate economic survival. In fact, such reinscriptions only speak to a particular form of "lifestyle politics" which strengthens the basic ethical tenets of bourgeois individuals—"the ethical construct of capitalism where one has to be free to do what one wants, free to buy and sell, to accumulate wealth or to live in poverty, to work or not, to be healthy or to be sick" (qtd. in Doyal 36). Left unquestioned are the historical, political, and economic conditions that permit only a small minority (read white, heterosexual, bourgeois, and able-bodied male) to exercise this "material" freedom to choose. For this reason, a poststructural emancipatory vision appears plausible only to the bourgeois subject (even the bourgeois subject located at the margins) who has indeed the luxury to reinvent him/herself at the margins since his/her material needs are taken care of—a luxury that has little relevance to those whose "deviant" subjectivities have required that they struggle under the exploitative conditions of late capitalism. In fact, I later argue that it is the maintenance of these conditions in the first place that demand the necessary construction of the ideology of "deviance" and thus the construction of the "disabled" body.

By limiting their reading of the social to the present, poststructuralists refuse to recognize that this movement from "labor into robotics and word processing" and "sex into genetic engineering and reproductive technology" (Haraway 202) could not have happened except through the continued maintenance of the oppressive labor relations produced by the new international division of labor and supported by advanced capitalism. If the construction of a cyborgean reality necessitates a division of labor, then it also necessitates the existence of a class-based hierarchy. Poststructuralists often attempt to blur these hierarchies by claiming that power is not confined to particular nodes (like the economy) but is diffuse—it exists everywhere. However, we do know that everyone does not have "equal access" to this power, particularly when such access involves access to knowledges, technologies, and most important, access to the means of production. For example, those disabled people who face economic deprivation on a daily basis seldom have access to the technology that can offer their "unlivable" bodies the cyborgean possibilities that poststructuralists extol. When only the bourgeois subject can have access to such emancipatory possibilities, emancipation itself becomes a divisive force, (re)inscribing the very class divisions it seeks to dismantle and therefore renders the emancipatory project of the cyborgean space ineffective. By locating their emancipatory practices within the space of the social imaginary, as opposed to the actual materiality of economic conditions, poststructuralists continue to uphold a utopic vision of emancipation that can never be achieved because it exists within the realm of fantasy.

Rewriting History: Disability and the Political Economy of Difference

Having explored the limits of the poststructural disabled subject, in this section I utilize historical materialism to argue for the (re)theorization of disability as a historical construct within the broader context of global political economy. Unlike poststructuralist discourses that see the body as wholly constituted within language, historical materialism begins with the presupposition that labor is the central organizing force in history, because human beings do not just live but instead "produce" their lives within specific historical contexts through their relationship to labor.[7] In other words, the historical materialist framework reads the subject—its body, consciousness, and meanings—as produced by and through labor. Thus, historical materialism is able to map out the dialectical relationship of individuals to social structures as determined by their locations in the social divisions of labor emerging from the social organization of the economy in specific historical contexts.

I have found Marxist feminist theory to be most useful in producing a more comprehensive analysis of the social divisions of labor, especially as this relates to the construction of disability. Whereas the classical Marxist emphasis has been on the relations of production that directly contribute to the construction of exchange value that produces profits for the capitalist market economy, Marxist feminists have extended Marxist analyses to account also for the labor relations that are involved in the production of goods and services that have only a use value and are directed toward meeting human needs and not those of the market.[8] The domestic labor debates that Marxist feminists have been engaged in for some time have been instrumental in foregrounding the oppressive and exploitative repercussions on those individuals whose useful labor has been devalued by the market economy and has not been regarded as real labor. While Marxist feminism has focused predominantly on the sexual division of labor, I have found it useful to extend this analysis to account for the particular location of disabled people within the broader context of the social division of labor. I will also offer a historical analysis to map out how disability is instrumental in the allocation of subjects marked by gender, race, class, and caste along the social division of labor within capitalist societies.

Drawing on historical materialism, Marxist theories of disability argue that the prejudice and oppression that disabled people experience on a daily basis are not an inevitable consequences of the human condition but the products of the particular form of social development associated with western capitalism. For example, Victor Finkelstein describes how the shift from feudalism to capitalism produced a labor market that demanded efficiency and productivity from individual workers, in a move that effectively excluded disabled people from participating as wage workers and therefore rendered them dependent on the state. Bernard Farber argues that these exclusions are essential because western capitalism needs a surplus labor market to minimize costs of production and is therefore required to maintain certain levels of unemployment.

Instead of describing unemployment as a necessary component of the economy, both Michael Oliver and David Nibert argue that capitalist ideologies justify the exclusion of particular populations from the world of work by claiming that individuals who lack particular social and technical characteristics deemed desirable for the economy are therefore designated as the surplus population. This surplus population has historically included disabled people, the permanent infirm, the aged, and the illiterate, as well as the permanent racialized underclass. Deborah Stone describes how members of this surplus population, by being certified as incapable of producing for exchange value, are certified as eligible to receive monetary aid as well as social services and in return are subject to the regulatory and controlling benevolence of the welfare state. These theories explain how, by rendering the failure to succeed in the capitalist economy as a problem that lies within the individual, such ideology supports the acceptance of a human hierarchy and the corresponding inequities that they legitimate as natural phenomena.

While proposing a historical materialist reading of disability, Paul Abberley among others has suggested that since the oppression that disabled people face has its roots in capitalism, the ideology of disability may also be responsible for racist, sexist, classist, and homophobic oppression. However, beyond making this suggestion, none of these theorists has demonstrated these interconnections within the historical context of capitalism. In the final section of this essay, I argue that historically the ideology of disability as constructed by capitalism had also been used to construct, justify, and sustain the most oppressive practices associated with social difference. A complete historical analysis of this phenomenon is outside the scope of this essay, so I am going to take a particular instance in history—the transformation of Western feudalism into capitalism—and mark the ways in which "disability" got socially institutionalized as "deviant difference," its emergence connected to "the emergence of a modern society, the professionalization of medicine, the rise of medicine as a 'natural science,' the rise of science and of modern economy" (Mies 83).

The transformation from a feudal society to a capitalist economy necessitated changes in the economic and social spheres. Whereas feudalism required "divine order" and armed retainers to maintain the peasant population as subordinate to the feudal lords, the expansion of the capitalist economy engendered the ideology of free enterprise and universal rights. However, as alternative histories have recorded, this transformation from feudalism into capitalism and the construction of the modern state of Western Civilization was dependent on violence, subordination, and exploitation on a global scale exemplified in colonialism and imperialism, characterized by the appropriation of mineral resources, cash crops, and land as well as slave labor.[9] At the same time, the shift in emphasis from agriculture to industrial production displaced a large population of peasants who migrated to urban centers in search of wage employment. With the urban centers unable to manage this vast influx of migrants who lived in conditions where pauperism, violence, and crime flourished, the bourgeoisie was compelled to justify this exploitation and to devise more efficient means to control these populations.

Such conditions therefore produced contradictions that needed new ideologies to justify and thereby "naturalize" these divisions of labor in modernizing capitalist societies. It is in this context, then, that I argue that "disability" became established as a pathological condition produced amid the material vicissitudes of social upheaval in seventeenth- and eighteenth-century Europe. At the same time, it was these circumstances that initiated the construct of the welfare state with its proliferation of poor houses, hospitals, correctional facilities, asylums, and educational institutions in order to offer economic relief to those populations unable to participate in capitalism's labor force as well as to protect the bourgeoisie from any threat these conditions would pose to capitalist accumulation.[10] Thus, these institutions in each of their assigned roles constructed complex methods by which to separate those having no labor potential to sell (the deserving poor) from those refusing to sell their labor (the undeserving poor) to the capitalists.[11] The former, once identified, were relegated to a life of isolation and segregation in state institutions, while the latter were rehabilitated through the criminal justice and education systems to prepare (if possible) for their reentry into society.

With the advent of Darwin's theory of evolution and the new science of genetics, a biological basis of difference was constructed in order to justify exploitation and exclusion of particular populations from the labor force. Medical science sought to "naturalize" disability, rejecting any possibility of theorizing "disability" as a historical rather than a biological category—i.e., as a by-product of the complex divisions of labor constructed by capitalism (i.e., material conditions).

Using this same logic of "disability" as "deviant difference," medical science collaborated with the state to justify the unequal social divisions of labor even while it upheld the humanist claim of universal rights to life, liberty, and the pursuit of happiness. Thus, in order to justify why some classes (the bourgeoisie) could maintain dominance over other classes (the proletariat), the inferiority associated with the working class was attributed to "biological defects" similar to those observed in disabled individuals. Such associations of the working class with defective biologies is apparent in even modern cinematic representations like *The Elephant Man* with its eugenicist implications. Paul Darke describes this in the following passage:

> As a modern discourse the film *The Elephant Man* acts as a modern version of the warning of biological contamination. . . . All the scenes of the working class, and their environment, are shown as dirty, disgusting, loud, violent and exploitative. This contrasts with the bourgeois scenes of clean, quiet sensibility and sensitivity. Consequently in the film all that is 'good' and 'healthy' is bourgeois, and all that is 'bad' and 'diseased' is working class. The safeguard of society is thus placed in the hygienic bourgeois world and not the unhygienic working-class one. (332)

By "naturalizing" the biological inferiority of the working classes, capitalist ideologies used the construct of "disability" to justify the unequal division of labor, which was also deemed a "natural" division within capitalism.

By the same means, history witnessed the institutionalization of the sexual division of labor that organizes the allocation of labor on the basis of gender difference and at the same time devalues women's labor. Prior to capitalism, women held relative autonomy over their economic roles in household production, as artisans and as health providers in their communities, where both production and reproduction were organized almost exclusively at the household level.[12] However, with industrialization, an idealized division of labor arose in which men's work was to follow production outside the home, while women's work was to remain centered in the household, with the exception of women in working-class households as well as immigrant and racial-ethnic families, where men seldom earned a family wage and so women and children were forced into income-earning activities in and out of the home (Nakano-Glenn 4–5).

To support this division of labor, the capitalist state drew upon scientific claims of "biological deviance" to construct women as "naturally" inferior to men, as domestic by nature, and therefore incapable of participating in skilled waged labor. Further, these ideologies, by now constructing women as economically dependent on men through the process of "housewifization" (Mies 100–110) also served to reorganize the social relations in capitalism by constructing "private" social units (the heterosexual nuclear family)—with the man as breadwinner and both the women and children as his dependents. Capitalist production transformed reproductive labor (the labor required to replenish the labor force on a daily and on an intergenerational basis, and therefore essential to capitalism) as nonproductive labor and therefore unworthy of a wage. In this way, women were socialized into subordinate roles in the household on the basis of biological determinism fueled by "scientific" conceptualizations of disability.

Mies, however, points out that women did not passively give up their economic and sexual freedoms. Several women of independent means or occupations (e.g., artisans and midwives) actively resisted the control that both patriarchy and capitalism exerted over their lives. These women often became the targets of violence on account of their resistance. By assigning to these women supernatural powers in order to demonstrate the "madness" in their resistance to the dominant order, the witchhunt became a means to violently eradicate dissent and consolidate the political authority of science. Here, the logic of "deviance" not only justified the sexual division of labor and prescribed women's "natural" roles in society but also institutionalized compulsory heterosexuality in order to support capital's continued expansion.

However, it was not just women's reproductive labor that was appropriated as nonwage labor by capitalism; so was slave labor through the violent process of colonialism. And once again the ideology of disability was used to support the deterministic belief in the inferiority of all other races in comparison with Europeans. The Enlightenment's scientific conceptualization of "universal man" was constructed as a "pervasive figure of racial superiority; [he] was disciplined, constant, self responsible, of culture . . . the conduit for the ubiquitous, all defining gaze of general enlightenment" (Yolton et al. 442). In Enlightenment terms, the savage, originally meaning "man of the woods," was seen as "a wild uncivilized creature contrasted to the political animal identified as 'European citizen'" (473). Thus, as Yolton et al. explain:

> Rousseau's hypothetical reconstruction of natural man, relieved of all attributes and institutions which could only have been generated by society, such as reason, language, aggression and property, portrayed a simple creature whose indolent, solitary and nomadic existence bore striking similarity to the life of the real orang-utan of south-east Asia. (473)

This racist construction of the savage is closely related to concepts of disability, as is visible in Bogdan's *Freak Show*. Bogdan describes the world fairs organized in the late nineteenth century, which exhibited disabled people as freaks so as to depict the "non-western other" in "the exotic mode." In these instances, disabled individuals, many of them in the most blatant distortion of the exotic mode (e.g., a tall black North Carolinian from Dahomey was exhibited as a "Wild Man from Samoa") were represented as natives of a "mysterious part of the world—darkest Africa, the Wilds of Borneo, a Turkish harem, an ancient Aztec kingdom" (105). In this way, these fairs played an important role in socializing patrons into racist ideologies that sought to justify the violence inherent in colonialism and slavery by claiming that they were on a "civilizing" mission to tame this inalienable Otherness. Working in dialectical relationship with each other, the categories of both "race" and "disability," by being depicted as "different, depraved, dishonest, unloyal, and not really the same" (Povinelli 122), rendered the "savage" accessible to the rest of "civil society"—not as historical subject but as its ahistorical Other.

I have argued that the construction of disability is a material concept—essential for capitalist accumulation to take place. Instead of conceptualizing "deviant difference" as a product of "bad" attitudes or the "unstable" sign, a historical materialist perspective is able to explain how disability has been used to justify class divisions in society, which in turn are naturalized by reaffirming the ahistoricity of disability. As Teresa Ebert explains:

> Class societies naturalize the social division of labor by means of pre-given ("natural") attributes such as sex, race, age, gender. Difference in class societies is the difference of economic access, which is determined by the position of the subject in the social relations of production. Difference, in other words, is socially produced at the site of production. However, it is secured and legitimated by reference to the natural features of the workers (age, race, gender) in order to keep down the cost of labor power (the only source of value) and thus increase the level of profit. (91)

Following from the logic of Ebert's argument, I would like to advance my own: The construct of "disability," or what has otherwise been commonly understood as "deviant difference," has been historically used to justify and to regulate the ways by which the accumulation of surplus is allocated to a small yet powerful minority belonging to the capitalist class. In other words, it is this "ideology of disability" which has been used to justify the sexual division of labor that constructed gender as a political and economic concept, the production of class/caste differences that first sustained the feudal order and later capitalism, the production of racial categories generated by the imperialistic practices of slavery, colonialism, and now neocolonialism; and the upholding of compulsory heterosexuality so as to preserve "family values" in an effort to naturalize the oppressive systems that allow capitalist accumulation to take place. "Disability" or "deviant otherness" has been used as the underlying ideology to legitimate who gets what allocations, even in the face of claims to a liberal democracy.

Given this explanation, what happens to the disabled subject under the present regime of exploitative capitalism that defines productivity in terms of the generation of maximum surplus for capitalist accumulation? On account of the real physiological challenges that disabled people face, as well as the reality that very few have access to technologies that can enable them to be productive as determined by laws of extraction of maximum surplus, disabled people have been actively excluded from the economy. Their exclusion has often been justified on the grounds that they cannot meet the economy's needs for an efficient and productive workforce, which is required to meet the socially constructed consumerism initiated by the privileged bourgeoisie. But productivity is not an objectively established given. Neither is it an imaginative myth. As Ebert argues, "The productivity of labor is derived not from its concrete usefulness but from its social form, which is determined by the social relations of production. It is not labor that determines its productivity; rather, the productivity of labor is determined by its situation within the modes of production" (102). Therefore, it follows that the only space in which the disabled subject can resurrect her own subjectivity would be under conditions where labor is not commodified by imputing to it exchange value, but is instead deployed in order to produce use-values that satisfy human needs.

However, by decentering labor as a crucial category in identity formation, poststructuralist theories actually sever the significant dialectical relationship between production and consumption embedded within the relations of global capitalist production. To put it simply, I am working on the assumption that the existence of productive forces in society provides the preconditions for the possibility of consumptive practices to exist and vice versa. However, within capitalism the unequal social relations that arise from the unequal distribution of economic resources allow only a small minority to participate in consumptive practices without actually participating in any real way in production processes. By having access to the means of production and other cultural/social resources, the bourgeoisie, now exempted from participating in productive labor, can therefore invest time and energy in the construction of transgressive subjectivities that are unhampered by the presence of limits of social borders. On the other hand, for most of the working class, participation in the labor force, even amid the most exploitative conditions, becomes the precondition that will enable them to participate as consumers within the global economy rendering this dialectical relationship between production and consumption as crucial to their survival. Thus, even as Butler and Haraway argue that there exist possibilities of constructing counterhegemonic practices to subvert the dominant modes of social organization, these oppositional practices are in the final instance subject to the laws of production and consumption within capitalist societies.

At the same time, we do know that the capitalist economy needs to maintain a certain level of unemployment in order to maintain the necessary profit margins and is therefore unable to absorb all those who do not have independent economic means. In fact, capitalist markets only absorb as wage laborers those who through their labor power can in the most efficient way expedite the maximum extraction of surplus for the capitalist. Those individuals whose labor power cannot efficiently contribute to surplus accumulation are excluded from participating in the market and go to form the surplus population. They are now constructed as the clients and consumers of "special services" offered through social institutions like schools, the welfare system, the health system, etc.; labeled as "delinquent," "physically and mentally handicapped," "problem families," etc.; and bear the stigma of being unproductive as a result of their nonparticipation in the market. In this case, unlike the bourgeois consumer for whom the separation of the relationship between production and consumption works to his/her benefit, the worker, now separated from production relations and reduced to his/her singular role as consumer, is deemed parasitic and thereby experiences a debilitating subjectivity on this count. It is for this reason that Paul Abberley points out that any utopia where one's identity as a worker is crucial to social integration would continue to support unequal relations, because if disabled people are unable to work, then even though they would be adequately provided for within the system of distribution, they would continue to be excluded from the system of production.

Conclusion: Making Bodies Matter

In this essay, I have argued that poststructuralism's attempts to fragment all social analyses into incommensurable parts can only offer us the discursive possibilities of new and ironic interpretations of our social world. However, such practices, notwithstanding their temporal usefulness, continue to uphold the economic structures that have produced social difference on a global scale. On the other hand, moving beyond interpretations, I have demonstrated how a historical materialist analysis can explain how all social differences (disability, gender, race, sexuality, and class) have been systematically produced and continue to operate within regimes of economic exploitation. Moreover, I have argued that "disability" is the critical ideological category that is constructed so as to justify the exploitative relations that are implicated in the production of race, gender, class, and sexuality as well. By locating these exploitative relations within the larger context of a social totality and by understanding how global structures work to produce difference in all its complexity, we can change these same structures so that all bodies can actually matter. After all, to paraphrase Marx, isn't the whole point to change the world, rather than merely interpret it?

Notes

I wish to thank Cynthia Lewiecki-Wilson and James Wilson for their helpful editorial suggestions for this paper.

1. For example, Jeremy Rifkin's book, *The End of Work: The Decline of the Global Work Force and the Dawn of the Post-Market Era,* predicts that the global economy is undergoing a fundamental transformation in the nature of work, since the new technologies (sophisticated computers, robotics, telecommunications, etc.) are producing nearly workerless factories and virtual companies. Such transformations have also eliminated most possibilities for those otherwise unemployed (like persons with severe disabilities) from ever getting to work, forcing society to grapple with the question of what to do with the vast numbers of people whose labor is needed less or not at all.

2. See, e.g., Suzanne Pharr's attempts to draw connections between economic relations, sexism, and homophobia in her book, *Homophobia: A Weapon of Sexism,* by drawing on the "common elements of oppression" and Chantal Mouffe's essay "Feminism, Citizenship, and Radical Democratic Politics," where she argues for the construction of radical democratic formations that are based on the principle of "democratic equivalence" as opposed to the simple politics of identity groups (379).

3. There are a number of books that do just this, particularly within the genre of multiculturalism. In fact, in all these books, the term *disability* is always present, but usually exists as an afterthought. This is because at no point do the authors ever actually stop to consider how any serious engagement with disability would rearrange the theoretical terrain. See hooks, *From Margin to Center,* and Giroux, *Border Pedagogies,* as just two of several examples of theorists who treat disability in this way.

4. For a more thorough discussion of the humanist perspective, refer to Chris Weedon, *Feminist Practice and Poststructuralist Theory;* Terry Eagleton, *Literary Theory;* and Philip Rice and Patricia Waugh, *Modern Literary Theory.*

5. See, e.g., Howard Becker, *The Other Side;* Douglas Biklen and Lee Bailey, *Rudely Stamped;* Robert Bogdan and Steven Taylor, *Inside Out;* Lennard Davis, *Enforcing Normalcy;* Robert Edgerton, *Cloak of Competence;* Nancy Groce, *Everyone Here Spoke Sign Language;* Michael Oliver, *The Politics of Disablement;* Robert Scott, *The Making of Blind Men.*

6. See, e.g., Jane Campbell and Mike Oliver, *Disability Politics;* Rosemary Crossley and Anne MacDonald, *Annie's Coming Out;* Diane Driedger, Irene Feika, and Ellen Batres, *Across Borders;* Michelle Fine and Adrienne Asch, *Women with Disabilities;* Temple Grandin, *Emergence, Labeled Autistic;* David Hevey, *The Creatures Time Forgot;* Jenny Morris, *Pride Against Prejudice;* Susan Wendell, *The Rejected Body;* and Nancy Mairs, *Carnal Acts.*

7. See Maria Mies, *Patriarchy and Accumulation on a World Scale,* where she explains this in detail by quoting Marx and Engels: "All human history is characterized . . . by 'three moments,' which existed as the beginning of mankind and also exist today: 1. People must live in order to be able to make history; they must produce the means to satisfy their needs: food, clothing, shelter, etc. 2. The satisfaction of these needs leads to new needs. They develop new instruments to satisfy their needs. 3. Men who reproduce their daily life must make other men, must procreate" (49).

8. Detailed discussion of the many debates pertaining to the sexual division of labor are beyond the scope of this essay and can be gleaned from Maria Mies, *Patriarchy and Accumulation on a World Scale;* Teresa Ebert, *Ludic Feminism and After;* Bonnie Fox, ed., *Hidden in the Household: Women's Domestic Labor Under Capitalism;* Marilyn Waring, *If Women Counted: A New Feminist Economics;* Annette Kuhn and AnnMarie Wolpe, *Feminism and Materialism: Women and Modes of Production.*

9. For a detailed description of colonialism and its effects on people of color, see Walter Rodney, *How Europe Underdeveloped Africa;* Maria Mies, *Patriarchy and Accumulation on a World Scale;* and Alex Callinicos, *Race and Class.*

10. For example, see the work of Foucault, *Madness and Civilization;* James Trent Jr., *Inventing the Feeble Mind;* Diane Paul, *Controlling Human Heredity;* and Philip Safford and Elizabeth Safford, *A History of Childhood and Disability.*

11. See Deborah Stone, *The Disabled State,* for a fascinating description of how the construct of disability assisted in the origination of the welfare state.

12. Both Maria Mies's *Patriarchy and Accumulation on a World Scale* and Evelyn Nakano-Glenn's "From Servitude to Service Work" in *Signs* have described the historical shift of women's labor from the private to the public sphere during the colonial era.

Works Cited

Abberley, Paul. "The Concept of Oppression and the Development of a Social Theory of Disability." *Disability, Handicap, and Society* 2 (1987): 5–19.
———. "Work, Utopia, and Impairment." Barton 61–79.
Barton, Len, ed. *Disability and Society: Emerging Issues and Insights.* London: Orient Longman, 1996.
Becker, Howard, ed. *The Other Side: Perspectives on Deviance.* New York: Free P, 1964.
Biklen, Douglas, and Lee Bailey. *Rudely Stamp'd: Imaginal Disability and Prejudice.* Washington: UP of America, 1981.
Bogdan, Robert. *Freak Show: Presenting Human Oddities for Amusement and Profit.* Chicago: U of Chicago P, 1988.
Bogdan, Robert, and Steven Taylor. *Inside Out: The Social Meaning of Mental Retardation.* Toronto: U of Toronto P, 1982.
Butler, Judith. *Bodies That Matter: On the Discursive Limits of Sex.* New York: Routledge, 1993.

———. "Contingent Foundations." *Feminist Contentions: A Philosophical Exchange.* Ed. Nancy Fraser, Seyla Benhabib, Judith Butler, and Drucilla Cornell. 35–58.

———. *Gender Trouble: Feminism and the Subversion of Identity.* New York: Routledge, 1990.

Butler, Judith, and Joan W. Scott, eds. *Feminists Theorize the Political.* New York: Routledge, 1995.

Callinicos, Alex. *Race and Class.* Chicago: Bookmarks, 1993.

Campbell, Jane, and Mike Oliver, eds. *Disability Politics: Understanding Our Past, Changing Our Future.* New York: Routledge, 1995.

"Copenhagen Declaration on Social Development." 8–15 June 1995. *United Nations Economic and Social Development.* <URL:www.dna.affrc.go.jp.10081> 25 June 1998.

Crossley, Rosemary, and Anne MacDonald. *Annie's Coming Out.* New York: Penguin, 1980.

Darke, Paul. "*The Elephant Man* (David Lynch, EMI Films, 1980): An Analysis from a Disabled Perspective." *Disability and Society* 9 (1994): 327–42.

Davis, Lennard J. *Enforcing Normalcy: Disability, Deafness, and the Body.* New York: Verso, 1995.

Driedger, Diane, Irene Feika, and Ellen Batres. *Across Borders: Women with Disabilities Working Together.* Charlottetown, PEI, Canada: Gynergy Books, 1995.

Eagleton, Terry. *Literary Theory: An Introduction.* Minneapolis: U of Minnesota P, 1983.

Ebert, Teresa. *Ludic Feminism and After: Postmodernism, Desire, and Labor in Late Capitalism.* Ann Arbor: U of Michigan P, 1996.

Edgerton, Robert. *The Cloak of Competence: Stigma in the Lives of the Mentally Retarded.* Berkeley: U of California P, 1967.

Farber, Bernard. *Mental Retardation: Its Social Context and Social Consequences.* Boston: Houghton Mifflin, 1968.

Fine, Michelle, and Adrienne Asch, eds. *Women with Disabilities: Essays in Psychology, Culture, and Politics.* Philadelphia: Temple UP, 1988.

Finkelstein, Victor. *Attitudes and Disabled People: Issues for Discussion.* New York: World Rehabilitation Fund, 1980.

Foucault, Michel. *Madness and Civilization: A History of Insanity in the Age of Reason.* New York: Vintage Books, 1965.

Fraser, Nancy, Seyla Benhabib, Judith Butler, and Drucilla Cornell. *Feminist Contentions: A Philosophical Exchange.* New York: Routledge, 1995.

Giroux, Henry A. *Border Crossings: Cultural Workers and the Politics of Education.* New York: Routledge, 1992.

Grandin, Temple, with Margaret Scariano. *Emergence, Labeled Autistic.* Novato, CA: Arena P, 1991.

Gray, Chris Hables, ed. *The Cyborg Handbook.* New York: Routledge, 1995.

Groce, Nancy. *Everyone Here Spoke Sign Language: Hereditary Deafness on Martha's Vineyard.* Cambridge: Harvard UP, 1985.

Grosz, Elizabeth. *Volatile Bodies: Towards a Corporeal Feminism.* Bloomington: Indiana UP, 1994.

Halberstam, Judith, and Ira Livingston, eds. *Posthuman Bodies*. Bloomington: Indiana UP, 1995.

Haraway, Donna. "A Manifesto for Cyborgs: Science, Technology, and Socialist Feminism in the 1980s." Nicholson 190–233.

Hevey, David. *The Creatures Time Forgot: Photography and Disability Imagery*. New York: Routledge, 1992.

hooks, bell. *Feminist Theory: From Margin to Center*. Boston: South End, 1984.

Kuhn, Annette, and AnnMarie Wolpe, eds. *Feminism and Materialism*. London: Routledge, 1978.

LaPlante, Mitchell, Joe Kennedy, H. Stephen Kaye, and Barbara Wenger. "Disability and Employment—#11." *Disability Statistics Rehabilitation Research and Training Center, San Francisco*. <URL:http://dsc.ucsf.edu/abs/ab11.html> 15 June 1998.

LaPlante, Mitchell, Dorothy P. Rice, and Juliana K. Cyril. "Health Insurance Coverage of People with Disabilities in the U.S.—#7." *Disability Statistics Rehabilitation Research and Training Center, San Francisco*. <URL:http://dsc.ucsf.edu/abs/ab7.html> 15 June 1998.

Mairs, Nancy. *Carnal Acts*. New York: HarperCollins, 1990.

Mies, Maria. *Patriarchy and Accumulation on a World Scale: Women in the International Division of Labor*. Atlantic Highlands, NJ: Zed Books, 1986.

Morris, Jenny. *Pride Against Prejudice: Transforming Attitudes to Disability*. Philadelphia: New Society, 1991.

Mouffe, Chantal. "Feminism, Citizenship, and Radical Democratic Politics." Butler and Scott 369–84.

Nakano-Glenn, Evelyn. "From Servitude to Service Work: Historical Continuities in the Racial Division of Paid Reproductive Work." *Signs: Journal of Women in Culture and Society* 18 (1992): 1–18.

Nibert, David. "The Political Economy of Developmental Disability." *Critical Sociology* 21 (1995): 59–80.

Nicholson, Linda, ed. *Feminism/Postmodernism*. New York: Routledge, 1990.

Oliver, Michael. *The Politics of Disablement: A Sociological Approach*. New York: St. Martin's, 1990.

Paul, Diane. *Controlling Human Heredity: 1865 to the Present*. Atlantic Highlands, NJ: Humanities P, International, 1995.

Pharr, Suzanne. *Homophobia: A Weapon of Sexism*. Little Rock, AR: Chardon P, 1988.

Povinelli, Elizabeth. "Sexual Savages/Sexual Sovereignty: Australian Colonial Texts and the Postcolonial Politics of Nationalism." *Diacritics* 24 (1994): 122–50.

Rice, Philip, and Patricia Waugh. *Modern Literary Theory: A Reader*. New York: Edward Arnold, 1992.

Riley, Denise. *"Am I That Name?" Feminism and the Category of 'Women' in History*. Minneapolis: U of Minnesota P, 1990.

Rodney, Walter. *How Europe Underdeveloped Africa*. Washington: Howard UP, 1981.

Safford, Philip, and Elizabeth Safford. *A History of Childhood and Disability.* New York: Teachers College P, 1996.

Sandoval, Chela. "Cyborg Feminism and the Methodology of the Oppressed." Gray 407–22.

Scott, Robert A. *The Making of Blind Men: A Study of Adult Socialization.* New York: Russell Sage Foundation, 1969.

Stone, Deborah. *The Disabled State.* Philadelphia: Temple UP, 1984.

Trent, James Jr. *Inventing the Feeble Mind: A History of Mental Retardation in the United States.* Berkeley: U of California P, 1994.

Waring, Marilyn. *If Women Counted: A New Feminist Economics.* New York: Harper, 1990.

Weedon, Chris. *Feminist Practice and Poststructuralist Theory.* New York: Basil Blackwell, 1987.

Wendell, Susan. *The Rejected Body: Feminist Philosophical Reflections on Disability.* New York: Routledge, 1996.

Yolton, John, Roy Porter, Pat Rogers, and Barbara M. Stafford. *The Blackwell Companion to the Enlightenment.* Cambridge, MA: Basil Blackwell, 1991.

Part Two

Rhetorics of Literacy:
Education and Disability

7

Deafness, Literacy, Rhetoric: Legacies of Language and Communication
Brenda Jo Brueggemann

> Almost since its inception the education of deaf people has been marred
> by divisive controversy concerning the most appropriate modes of
> communication.
> —Margaret Winzer, *The History of Special Education*

> [A]n inability or unwillingness to deal with deaf children in terms of
> their own needs and capabilities. In 1880 this was understandable, as
> education for deaf children was in its infancy. But in the 1970s?
> —Richard Winefield, *Never the Twain Shall Meet*

> The clear contrast of excellence to equity is obvious.
> —Amatzia Weisel, *Issues Unresolved:*
> *New Perspectives on Language and Deaf Education*

"Deafness is a big country," writes Owen Wrigley in *The Politics of Deafness*, as he seeks to ethnographically document the "land," the "absent anchor," of the people who belong to the culture he writes about—the culture of the Deaf.[1] For all its nonexistence in chartable, tangible terms, the territory of "deafness" looms no less large in its absence. It is simply huge; its terrain is vastly diverse, and the possibilities for negotiating and navigating in it—or around it—abound. Maps are many. And both their multitude and their various and often conflicting representations guarantee that the going may, in fact, be made harder by using them.

The resources and richness of the land, too, are no less for its physical absence: There is precious ore to be mined here. The size of its population alone guarantees that. Depending on different accounts, on which map is consulted and what criteria are used for establishing "deafness," the count varies. One tally, for instance, tells us that there are 15 mil-

lion deaf persons worldwide—"on par with a modest size nation"—
when commitment to cultural "deafness" is the marker (Wrigley 13).
Other accounts give records at 1.7 million, or 6.5 million, or wait, 13.3
million or, no, count again, even 21 million in the United States alone,
depending on which specific terms and classifications are used to define
deafness. These are just some sets of the available figures.[2]

Despite the diversity and preciousness of its resources, there are also
dangerous mines in this country—mines long abandoned and not carefully marked, mines boarded shut, with warnings of "Danger! Keep
out!" There are explosive mines above ground as well, in a potentially
dangerous field. The promise and perils of educating deaf students have
been laid out in such possibly charged minefields. Education matters,
literacy matters—and often it matters violently (see Stuckey). Furthermore, education and matters of literacy explode (like the "stop," the
"plosive," our most articulate of speech sounds) on the figurative tongue
of deafness.

I want to discuss the rhetorical construction of deafness in our educational system, touching on (1) the history of deaf education; (2) the
terms used; (3) the people who serve in the deaf educational system; and
(4) the people who are served by this system.

In constructing this rhetorical-cultural map within the grids of literacy, I cannot avoid the problem of speaking for others; I agree with
Roof and Wiegman (97, 102) that "the neutrality of the theorizer can
no longer, can never again, be sustained, even for a moment." I would
not pretend otherwise. But still I must write and I must theorize and go
about "naming silenced lives."[3] I try to do it with sensitivity to those
silences, with respect for the ruptures that even I have surely created
within the system and upon the lives of those who work in deaf education and those, too, who try to navigate through its minefields. In some
ways I am one of each of them; in some ways, I am not.

My method then is somewhat like Cicero's in the second book of *De
Inventione*. Here Cicero relates the story of the "citizens of Croton" who
sought out a famous painter (Zeuxis of Heraclea) to paint for them "a
picture of Helen so that the portrait though silent and lifeless might
embody the surpassing beauty of womanhood."[4] Zeuxis gathered all
the city's loveliest women, then selected the five most beautiful from
among them "because he did not think all the qualities which he sought
to combine in a portrayal of beauty could be found in one person" (167).
Thus, his finished portrait was a (perhaps false, perhaps true) composite representing a (perhaps false, perhaps true) beauty, Helen.

Following this example, Cicero adopts the Zeuxian method for writing about rhetoric: "In a similar fashion when the inclination arose in
my mind to write a text-book of rhetoric, I did not set before myself some

one model which I thought necessary to reproduce in all details, of whatever sort they might be, but after collecting all the works on the subject, I excerpted what seemed the most suitable precepts from each, and so culled the flower of many minds" (*De Inventione* 169).

In similar fashion, when I decided to write about rhetorical constructions of deafness, I felt that the most gifted of speakers and writers in the classical period, Cicero, might serve well enough as my model. My portrayal here is surely neither the most true nor false (nor the most beautiful): it is a composite of excerpts from personal interviews and published materials, from collected works, and from suitable (and perhaps unsuitable) precepts.

With that composite sketch, the three sections that follow redraw, rhetorically, the territory of deafness as a disability in the nexus of literacy. First, I consider the "problem" of deafness in education from a rhetorical framework, by taking Quintilian's concept of the *vir bonus* (the "good man speaking well") as my cue. I argue, following humanities scholar Richard Lanham, that the legacy of Quintilian's ideal citizen, rhetorically educated, has shaped our educational system at large and therein has shaped the deaf educational system. Second, at the heart of my own argument about deafness, literacy, and rhetoric, I explore what I call the "literacy legacy" of viewing literate acts (reading, writing, speaking, listening, gesturing) as either language or communication. The simplistic conflation of these two kinds of literate practices, language with communication, where deafness is concerned, will be the legacy I seek to refashion, the argument I wish to remake. Theories and practices of literacy—as either product or process, oral or literate, cross-cultural or community-based, or academic or "critical"—come into consideration here, particularly as they intersect constructions of "deafness" in deaf education. Third, in an act of opening more than of closure, I turn to the subjects, turn to lend my ear to those who have been (or are being) educated in the deaf educational systems; I turn to see what signification they make, what maps they draw, of their own literate lives.

When Education Falls on Deaf Ears

As he begins book 12 of his voluminous *Institutio Oratoria*, the Roman educator and orator Quintilian ponders the *vir bonus*. Can this "good man speaking well," this Perfect Orator, be both a good person and a good speaker?

The answer to Quintilian's question, claims Richard Lanham, "has underwritten, and plagued, Western humanism from first to last," in deciding how and what citizens/students ought to be taught. Furthermore, in attempting to answer the question "in the West from the Greeks onward," Lanham posits that we have tended to offer two defenses.

"The Weak Defense argues that there are two kinds of rhetoric, good and bad. The good kind is used in good causes; the bad kind in bad. Our kind is the good kind; the bad kind is used by our opponents" (654). The second defense, far more interesting and relevant for my own argument here, is the "Strong Defense"—also perhaps now known best in many academic and philosophical circles as social constructionism—which "assumes that truth is determined by social dramas, some more formal than others but all man-made. Rhetoric in such a world is not ornamental but determinative, essentially creative. Truth once created in this way becomes referential, as in legal precedent" (Lanham 654). It is just such a "strong defense" for the goal of western education at large (and particularly since the eighteenth century, I believe, when literacy became accessible to the "common" masses) that has stood at the center of deaf education. It is no mere coincidence that deaf education and its concomitant social drama "came of age" at the point in western history when literacy became more commonplace and education was made available to more than aristocracy and clergy. It is no mere coincidence either that a tradition of educating "the good man speaking well" would come to see deafness as a puzzle at best, an ugly hole to fill at worst.

For how might a deaf person come to be taught what was good if he could not hear the wisdom of the ages? This is a concern carried forward from St. Augustine, who interpreted the Pauline dictum "Faith comes by hearing" to mean that "those who are born deaf are incapable of ever exercising the Christian faith, for they cannot hear the Word, and they Cannot read the Word" (Winzer 22).[5] If we carry this exclusion from the word of God over to exclusion from the "voice of reason" and then to exclusion from the word(s) of law and order that govern a land and its people, we see, as Lennard Davis has argued, that deaf citizens become, in their ignorance, "a threat to the ideas of nation, wholeness, moral rectitude, and good citizenship" (82).

Furthermore, in addition to their exclusion from the moral content of proper rhetorical education, deaf persons were doubly damned by their inaccessibility to learning the right "style" of speaking. "Eloquence," offered Augustine, was really a matter of imitation, and thus a matter that depended on one's "reading and hearing the eloquent," on "reading and listening to the orations of orators, and, in as far as it is possible, by imitating them" (*On Christian Doctrine* 4.4–5). A deaf student entering upon a rhetorical education, pursuing the path of the *vir bonus,* could barely be expected to master the nuances of correct pronunciation, to produce the right tones and the "exactest expressions, nicely proportioned to the degrees of his inward emotions," that Thomas Sheridan, the "champion of the elocution movement in the eighteenth century" (Bizzell and Herzberg 649), claimed was a "necessity of [the] social state to man both for the unfolding, and exerting of his nobler faculties" (Sheridan, Lecture 6, 730). Thus, even more potentially disabling when we consider the plight of a deaf student in receiving a rhetorical education—how might they become good speakers having never heard words, let alone tones and pronunciations, themselves?

If we turn to Quintilian's own definition of rhetoric, we see the potential for the disruption of deafness on the ear and order of rhetoric itself. Rhetoric, writes Quintilian,

> will be best divided, in my opinion, in such a manner that we may speak first of the *art*, next of the *artist*, and then of the *work*. The *art* will be that which ought to be attained by study, and is the *knowledge how to speak well*. The *artificer* is he who has thoroughly acquired the art, that is, the orator, whose business is *to speak well*. The *work* is what is achieved by the artificer, that is *good speaking*. (*Institutio Oratoria* 2.14)

Speaking: Quintilian's definition of rhetoric, intertwined as it is with a definition of education, repeats the central precept of speech.

By the Enlightenment, when literacy and education became more widespread, this precept sometimes fell on deaf ears. Literally. As Davis tells us, "Before the late seventeenth and early eighteenth centuries, the deaf were not constructed as a group," and furthermore, when the attention of philosophers and educators during the Enlightenment did turn to deafness, "one might conclude that deafness itself was not so much the central phenomenon as was education" (51, 52).[6] Thus, it was through and in education that deafness began to be known as a group trait, as a sociocultural category, rather than as an individual difference (as it seems to have been referenced in writing about deafness before this point— in the Old and New Testaments and in work by Aristotle, Descartes, and others).

The birth of deaf schools—or rather the separation of deaf persons from any educational "mainstream" by placing them primarily in deaf "institutions" (or "asylums," as they were often called)—began both in Europe and in the United States during the Enlightenment.[7] The management of deaf lives, particularly through their education and their language, has been tied up in the legacy of Quintilian's *vir bonus*, the "good man speaking well" who lies at the heart of our humanistic tradition. He who does not speak well must be trained, maintained, contained, restrained. In training the deaf person (who was long designated as "deaf-mute"), deaf education is like the entire humanistic tradition of education that Lanham asserts we have carried forth from that initial "Q Question": "Humanism, construed in this rhetorical way, is above all an education in politics and management" (692).

For the most part, I want to argue, those political and educational moments of "management" are mined from sources where literacy is seen often divisively as either language or communication. It is on the anvil of literacy that deafness, following the multiplicitous possibilities of my metaphor, might be hammered into precious ore or explosive danger.

Literacy for Communication, Literacy for Language

Richard Lanham claims that the matter of educating the good man speaking well, all comes down to the motives for education, and in the curricula we must always design in order to carry out those motives. I could not agree more. I only beg to differ about what those essential controlling motives are: for Lanham they are "play, game, and purpose" (691). For my argument here, those controlling motives are literacy, seen either as a matter of communication or as language. When I look to the recent explosion (both beautiful and dangerous) of research on literacy, I see its products and processes divided all too simply; as often as not, they are divided into literacy for/as communication (as a product) and literacy for/as language (as a process).[8]

I might return to Quintilian. Even in the consummate product of a lifelong process of rhetorical education—even in the *vir bonus*—I think the division potentially appears: the "good man" as one goal, and the "speaking well" as the other. The rhetorically educated "good man" uses literacy for and as language. He desires, attains, and uses literacy to convey thoughts, morals, ethics, both his own and those of the community, nation, or culture at large. Here literacy is a process, a means of exchange and change, a way of belonging to a place and people—a language.

Meanwhile, the rhetorically educated man "speaking well" stands in for literacy as communication. Here he masters the "products" of literacy, attaining and retaining skills at style, delivery, memory, pronunciation, tone, gestures, diction, etc. (Later, in the age of print, he masters further skills like punctuation, paragraphing, spelling, and penmanship.) His goal is the correctness of his language, the appearance of the product itself, and his ability to convey information "accurately."

Both the "good man" and "speaking well" are worthy goals, and both were goals for Quintilian. It is just as interesting (if not perplexing) to see the way these two have become separated in literacy education and then, even more sharply, in deaf education. Let me labor a moment, then, at mapping them in literacy education so that I might turn to some of the ways they explode—violently and sometimes with casualties, sometimes with goods gained—in the lives of deaf students.

Communicating a Product

Literacy as a means of learning to communicate (as a product) implies that literacy is a skill to be obtained and retained. Such a perspective tends to hold literacy in stasis, setting it up as an end in and of itself. Moreover, such a perspective puts literacy as an individual attribute rather than as a social achievement and also foregrounds what Deborah Brandt calls the "strong-text account of literacy" where becoming literate is becoming textlike—"logical, literal, detached and message-focused" (7–8).[9] Literacy as a communicative product means the individual is either a "have" or a "have-not." Finally, literacy as a product focuses on the consequences of either having or not, as do some fairly familiar accounts by literacy scholars and public intellectuals Jonathan Kozol, E. D. Hirsch Jr., Jack Goody and Ian Watt, Walter J. Ong, and David R. Olson, to name a few.

And what the literates have, according to Deborah Brandt in her argument against product-centered theories of literacy, is textlike qualities themselves. To be literate in the strong-text descriptions that have characterized literacy education in the United States, Brandt argues, is to "force attention away from the world and onto the text" and to "transcend dependency on social context and making meaning out of the fixed, semantic resources of language-on-its-own" (7, 8). As such, becoming literate is anything but a dynamic, interactional, involved process (i.e., it is anything but language); instead, it requires divorce from context and lack of involvement with the world and others, while wedding oneself to the text alone. And the text is, of course, a product, fixed and unchangeable, a text that "communicates," that imparts information, a text like the one in the middle of the old sender-message-receiver conduit of communications theory.

Literacy, then, becomes a matter of just "getting it right," of just getting the message the sender intended through that conduit so that the receiver understands it completely. This is literacy for communication only.

Processing a Language

When literacy is viewed as a process, students—both deaf and hearing—have a chance to become involved in language, to interact with the process of language, to change and fashion it, and to place themselves somewhere in the process. This kind of process is what happened at Gallaudet University in 1988 when deaf students, buoyed by recent linguistic legitimization of American Sign Language (ASL) and by their own growing pride in their culture and its unique language, closed the university for several days until their demands for a deaf president (among other things) were met.

When literacy for/as language stands at the center of educational and social institutions, then literacy becomes about "social identity," about power, about self-transformation, about speaking and listening to others, and about changing schooling and other social institutions by engaging students and citizens in critical literacy.[10] To teach critical literacy, as Giroux describes it, requires teaching more than just communication; it requires language—language not only for knowing things but for freedom. When, as Giroux writes, literacy is about language and its roles and shapes in society, then students engaged in such literacy learning are gaining critical skills that not only help them understand why they resist but also allow them to recognize what this society has made of them and how it must, in part, be analyzed and reconstituted so that it can generate the conditions for critical reflection and action rather than passivity and indignation ("Literacy, Ideology" 231).

In fact, what Giroux would have these students analyze and reconstitute are the very "mechanical approaches" to reading and writing that he characterizes as the "instrumental ideology" of literacy education. Within an "instrumental ideology of literacy" writing is "strip[ped] of its normative and critical dimensions and reduce[d] to the learning of skills" (212). The instrument here is communication: When literate acts are seen as being only about or for the purpose of communication, when literacy is only about or for the correct use of skills to convey a message clearly (and here the message goes one way), then the beauty, let alone the power, of what language can do is lost. And with the loss of language comes the loss of culture, of communities, of ethics, of morals.

Indeed, this sheerly skilled and singular potential for language and rhetoric as a "craft" was what so alarmed Plato in *The Phaedrus*. If the explosive and beautiful possibilities were taken away from language; if the complexity, complications, and contradictions of social and individual nuances that make up language were entirely given up in favor of "only information" and just "clear communication"; if the cultural, moral, critical, and ethical content were removed, the "good man" also potentially disappeared. Stripped of these things, there might still be communication. There might still be someone "speaking well," speaking pretty and pleasing words, clear and even "sublime" words. But the words might be false or empty or even immoral. There would be no language.

"I'm Ready to Roll Up and Pass It"

Let me now try to illustrate what follows from the separation of literacy into communication and language as it impacts the lives of deaf students. In these brief and loosely stitched stories I hope to show the range of possibilities—literacy as communication, literacy as language, and even literacy as both—in the tradition of Quintilian's *vir bonus* (which, I think it is important to remember, Quintilian claimed it took an entire lifetime to educate and create).

Let me note first, though, that as I enter into interviews and conversations I have had with deaf or hard-of-hearing students, I come to a significant interpretive difficulty over language. In some cases, even though I have medium-range skill in American Sign Language, I used an interpreter (usually when the person I was interviewing was a native signer and/or they requested an interpreter); in some cases, no interpreter was used (as with Anna, whom I have written about in *Lend Me Your Ear: Rhetorical Constructions of Deafness*) and the interview tended to proceed with any of the various forms of English-ASL "contact" languages—SimCom and Pidgin Signed English most notably among them. In either case, with or without an interpreter, I was left with the interpreter's dilemma upon transcribing the interviews and again, upon choosing to use quotations from them in my text. Because I am more than aware of the way "broken English" tends to get translated as "broken intelligence" in our culture (indeed, that is my very point), I have chosen to interpret, transliterate, and then quote what was "said" using its English equivalent. When what is quoted was a student's written text, however, I have maintained the exact and original text.

If I had to think of one central precept that might possibly hold a composite of deaf students that I have known, it would be that of "passing." In virtually every interview I conducted and in informal conversations, we turned always at some point to "passing." Even in an interview I had with a hearing person who was the assistive listening device (ALD) consultant for deaf persons at a local speech and hearing clinic, the issue of passing was not passed by: "I noticed you had a lot of questions about passing. Is that going to be a focus of your work?" she asked me toward the end of our interview (Sue 11 April 1996). Her question came, too, after she had told me at least half a dozen stories of "people who walk in the door" and their various degrees and successes with "passing" in the hearing world.

Most memorable among these stories for me were the students at the state university in town who refused to use the "services" offered to them by the university's Office of Disability Services—primarily because those services, either an interpreter or an FM audio loop system, prevented them from "passing" culturally even as forgoing the service jeopardized their passing academically. Indeed, two students I interviewed told of their experiences trying to pass in hearing colleges and also told me of their refusal to wear FM systems: Paul spoke of his discomfort with the FM system because of his effort to "be like them," and Lynne confessed, "I don't know why. I just feel that I was embarrassed or something [to

wear the FM system], because I was with hearing people . . . you know?"
(Paul 21 May 1996; Lynne 10 October 1991).

This is a painful paradox: By "passing" culturally as hearing when
they don't use an aid like the FM system in a regular hearing classroom,
these students risk not passing in the other necessary ways in the academic and communicative arenas. They risk learning to speak well; they
risk active participation—communication—in the classroom; they risk
knowledge and understanding. Two women who were part of "mainstreaming" efforts in the late 1970s and early 1980s told me stories
about the price of passing, socially or academically, when communication is the key in the literacy learning classroom. One now very successful
social worker remembers some of her struggles in the public schools:

> Among my deaf classmates, I was the brightest; among my hearing class-
> mates, I was not. I didn't understand that my deafness had a lot to do
> with that. When you're young, you don't see it that way, and you com-
> pare yourself without knowing that there's a difference between you
> and other hearing peers, so my self-esteem was not really very high. . . .
> And I can remember feeling much more inferior to my classmates in
> reading and English, because I always had to struggle with it. I had a lot
> more corrections on my papers than my hearing classmates. (Kathy 20
> June 1996)

Because of those painful experiences, Kathy now heads a community
program to help fill social voids and provide deaf role models for those
students currently in educational "mainstreaming" experiences. The program organizes a monthly social gathering for students who are mainstreamed into hearing schools; Kathy describes its inception and philosophy as follows: "So we started the program with the concept of wanting
to provide a social need to fill that void that many of them had in the
mainstreaming programs. We also wanted to give them something that
other programs for kids had been doing for years, and that is giving them
self-esteem and confidence."

The self-esteem inherent in "passing," in being able to fit in with the
dominant culture and in being able to communicate effectively in that
culture's "social grammar" (Giroux), is no small goal for many deaf
students. The other woman I interviewed who spent her life, like Kathy,
predominantly trying to "pass" in the "mainstream," once wrote me a
paper explaining the premium she placed on passing:

> When I went to a high school, I wanted to be in a regular english class
> with other hearing students. The reason why I wanted to be in it because
> I would like to take this class for a challenge. I was trying to be like them
> but my english teachers think it would be too hard for me. They decided
> to put me in a special education class. I really didn't learn much english
> in high school. (Anna 8 October 1991)

Later, she amplified that story verbally:

> I opened the book [in the "regular" English classroom] and thought,
> Whoa . . . this is hard." But I don't care if I get an F and fail. I want a
> challenge. But right away when they found out I got an F on my first
> test, they took me out and put me in a special education class again. I'm
> not going to learn anything about English. I was not happy. (30 Octo-
> ber 1991)

Anna is also the one who most exemplifies for me the importance of
literacy for communication, and for communication only, in the path
to passing that many deaf and hard-of-hearing students take. Indeed, it
is Anna who became the focus of an entire chapter in my book and who
gave me that chapter's resonant title, now five years ago: "because it's
so hard to believe that you pass," she once told me tearfully on the day
she discovered that she had finally passed the basic English course at
Gallaudet University, a course she had taken three times. That phrase
has stuck with me through all the thinking and writing and teaching I
have done about and with literacy, whether with deaf or hearing, native English or non-native English speakers.

What has stuck, too, are Anna's words about what English literacy
is and what it is for. When I once asked her to write me a short paper that
defined or explained writing, she wrote: "Writing is part of english to
have good communication. Writing have grammers in it. It can help some
people what the paper is telling when you write something on it" (12
November 1991). While the grammatical and communicative ironies
abound here, this short statement has also come to represent for me the
"literacy as communication" mode that often engages deaf students.

When literacy is about communication, grammar, usage, or vocabulary, it is about passing. Just passing. Getting by. Adapting, functioning, getting graced (with that grade). I think again of one young
Gallaudet student who told me of her two failed efforts at passing the
basic English course there. "This time," Bev said, "this time, I think I'm
ready to roll up and pass it" (Bev 5 September 1991). In failing once
again to "speak well" and carry the English idiom through, Bev rolls
up not just her colloquial sleeves but her entire self.

How fitting a metaphor I have found in Bev's missed idiom: The carpet of literacy, extended when literacy is taught as a mode and means
of communication only, can (and will) get rolled up at any moment, often
without advance warning. And as often as not, the student, having
missed the moment of communication, will get rolled up in it. What's
more, the carpet creates a mirage. The moment of perfect communication is always "out there" somewhere, always just a little beyond where
the student is right now, always there with the next level achieved, the
next test passed, the next graced grade. "I'm almost there," says one of

the students at Gallaudet that I have known for five years now as he tells me—on the eve of his college graduation, a week before he is to turn forty-five—of his literacy levels being quite near that of the what he has heard is Gallaudet's goal of eighth-grade literacy skills. "I struggle and struggle," Charlie tells me, "but I haven't quite reached that level" (Charlie 9 May 1996).

"Because English Can Express It Beautiful"

Where I think Charlie would really like to get, though, is past the mirage of literacy sheerly for communication and on to holding literacy as language. He is moving close these days, grasping, "almost there." He and several of the other older and residentially educated Gallaudet students I have known and interviewed have made it clear that while communication is good, communication is right, and communication is a worthy goal for literacy, in the end it is not enough. I have seen them sign of language as the goal of literacy—of how the person who "speaks well" must also be a "good person," a person who uses language for more than just the dress or perfection or the "getting-the-message-across" informational conduit.

To be sure, Charlie has spent more than enough of his educational time trapped in that one-way conduit. When I asked him recently what has happened to him at Gallaudet since I last interviewed him five years ago—when he was struggling through Gallaudet's infamous basic literacy course, English 50, for the third time—he told me an alarming story about the violence of literacy. I recount the story here with bracketed insertions of my own because it is worth recounting, because it signifies for itself:

> Last time we talked, in English 50 after you were with me, I passed English 50, and then I took English 102. I didn't know who the teacher was when I signed up. I went into the classroom and didn't like the teacher; it was a strange teacher. He'd be writing and writing at the blackboard, and then when he finished he'd sign exact English [a non-ASL, pidgin form] what he just wrote. Why did he repeat what he just wrote? The exact same thing. I read it, I understood it. And his structure of expressing the meaning [in ASL] wasn't accurate; conceptually, it wasn't appropriate. And so I failed 102. So I repeated 102 with a better teacher and I improved a great deal. I still had some problems, but I passed and took English 103 and failed that two times. The third time I took 103 I passed, and the teacher thought that there was something wrong with me, that I might be learning disabled and asked me if I was. I said I never knew. Who, me? Possibly, I don't know. So I thought I might need to get myself checked out. So I took English 203, and again, I failed. And I thought well, maybe I have a learning disability. I took it [English 203] again and again. Finally, after I became a junior, I passed and I had to select a ma-

jor and I chose American Sign Language. And then I took English 204 and got another lousy teacher, slow signs and difficult to understand, wasn't clear, so I withdrew from that and took it the second semester and finally passed and got a C, a 72, so that was okay. I was frustrated but satisfied. So then I applied to be an ASL major, and the person said, "Well, you've got this C in English. I have a friend who is an English teacher. Why don't you come down and get tested and see if you have a disability. Go ahead and try. So I took the evaluation, and found out that I have a reading disability. I reverse letters and words. Dyslexia. Yeah. Remember, I showed you my evaluation paper before? So they waived the C and I became an ASL major. But now I learned that I had a disability and they give me accommodations. (9 May 1996)

There are several remarkable things going on here. First, Charlie is a nontraditional student in his midforties who had a successful career as a drafting engineer, who has experience as a deaf actor, and who happens to be one of the most skilled users of his native language, American Sign Language (ASL), that I have personally known. He may not necessarily "speak well," but Charlie uses language well. The second point is his perseverance in the face of what could be only called an absolutely appalling experience with English literacy. If I add up all the attempts he made at "passing" through the four required English courses for graduation at Gallaudet, I count twelve classes in all.

Here I need to pause and outline briefly the basic English program as it was at Gallaudet in 1991. English 50 is not required for graduation at Gallaudet. It is only seen as a voluntary preparatory course for those entering Gallaudet students whose pretested language skills are not quite up to par in English on a four-part test consisting of reading comprehension, vocabulary, grammar, and writing. Most students have difficulty with the 150-word writing sample, in which they must compose a thoughtful argument, description, or narration in response to a question. The other three parts of the test are aimed at measuring literacy for communication, literacy as "functional adaptation" (Scribner) that can be tested for standardization, literacy as "instrumental" (Giroux). It is also worth noting that, although the course is declared voluntary, the pressure for students who are at risk to take it is enormous. They can keep retaking the English Language Placement (ELP) on their own each semester, without ever taking English 50, if they choose. Until they pass the ELP, they cannot be admitted to Gallaudet as full-time college students. Finally, they have four chances (four semesters) to take the ELP; if they fail four exams, they are disenrolled from the university. When I was at Gallaudet in the fall of 1991, 51 percent of students did not pass the ELP on the first try and therefore were likely to enroll in English 50. What is more, many of those enrolling in English 50 failed the course and the ELP repeatedly or they dropped out of Gallaudet.

Third, Charlie discovered late in life that he was dyslexic. He sat in twelve introductory-level English courses before someone—not an English professor but an ASL teacher—made sure he got tested for learning disabilities. Were they all so "deaf-set" on the idea that Charlie's inability to learn English, his inability to pass at basic English literacy, was surely just a function of his deafness that they could not see past their own limited expectations? What was going on here?

I don't know. But despite the limitations of literacy being taught as communication only, Charlie's passion for literacy as language was not squelched. And that, I think, is remarkable. This is what Charlie told me about his summary of "the English problem" at Gallaudet:

> One problem I feel is that for deaf students here it is difficult for us to learn English because of the teacher's signing skills. I think that is a direct relationship. The teachers, I feel, should learn two languages—learn both languages [English and ASL]. Because they work with the deaf they should learn our language. It would make teachers look good. And it would help students improve their skills It's destiny—students would be destined for success then. If they've grown up with ASL, then the translation [from ASL to English] is a lot easier. And writing [in English] is a beautiful language. It can be beautiful in English—if the teacher knows how to teach from an ASL standpoint. If they want to improve our English and they are concerned with that then they need to learn our language. (5 Dec. 1991)

Here is someone who cares not just about his language, ASL, but who respects the beauty and capabilities of any language, all languages. Here is someone who has experienced literacy learning for the sake of language—seemingly in spite of the educational system that focused mostly only on literacy learning for communication. Here then, in Charlie, is what I think Quintilian would have been proud of—a good man speaking well.

Ellen, another Gallaudet graduate and perhaps not surprisingly, another gifted user of ASL and, in fact, a noted ASL teacher herself, might illustrate the same point I have tried to make with Charlie. Despite the enormous troubles she has with English, Ellen professes a "love" for it. She has a history with "lousy grammar"—a picture of herself as a somewhat "screwed-up" user of English that she's come to internalize after all these years: "I always had a problem with writing because [like] with lip-reading, I could catch certain things, but then I would miss so much. I put things together, but it was usually screwed up" (3 June 1996). Like Charlie, she has spent more than enough educational time trying to learn just to communicate in English—time that she indicates was as fruitful as it was fruitless:

> And I was giving up my recess at the deaf school so that I could have private speech lessons one on one. I benefited, yeah, because I can com-

municate with my family better and with some people. And sometimes I
feel like I can talk and that is really nice. But really skilled sentences, no.
Little phrases I can say, short and sweet. (3 June 1996)

Maybe Ellen is not exactly what Quintilian had in mind, but I would
not be too sure. She is a skilled user of language and a "good person"
who uses language thoughtfully for making meaning in herself, her
community, her world. She is a known comedienne, storyteller, and poet
in the Deaf community; she teaches American Sign Language and Deaf
literature to both deaf and hearing students; and she teaches future
ASL teachers.

She stays connected, too, to English. She is currently enrolled in a
Ph.D. program in a state university, and it is through that program, she
tells me, that she continues to use and attempt improving her "English
reading and writing." And she does so for far more than just purely for
communication; there is a longing, too, for what language can do:

> I love English because it really broadens my horizon so much I feel like I
> want to express things and I can't through ASL always. And English helps
> me to express more, writing jokes and stories—like that. ASL is great for
> videotaping, but hearing people don't appreciate that. I want people to
> appreciate both [languages, ASL and English], so I use English for that
> and I find it a challenge to find a way to say things that will make people
> laugh in English, too. (3 June 1996)

Thus, Ellen sees literacy as more than just a matter of communicating,
as more than just achieving the functional necessities that impart information but that still keep the boundaries clear and yet contentious between the "haves" and "have-nots" in any culture and in any language.

For Ellen, I think, literacy (and the educational process it is learned
in) is not about building and maintaining "standards" and communi-
cational borders but about "broadening" oneself and one's community—about expression, laughter, challenge, and appreciation shared
across, through, within that language. As someone who is herself a product of "the system" (having once been a "deaf student"), who has taught
deaf students in the public schools, and who now teaches (both deaf and
hearing students) at Gallaudet University, Ellen knows about the boundaries established by education, the lines drawn tight by literacy. When I
ask her where all the current categories and classifications that characterize "deafness" so variously now might have come from, she responds
quickly, definitively—drawing the map with bold strokes:

> I think the boundary is made up by society, the educational system. "The
> deaf can't function in the hearing world. They're stuck and they have to
> go to a deaf residential school." [She is imitating hearing educators here.]
> I think that kind of thing has set up a boundary. . . . I wish that the deaf
> and hearing worlds were mixed from the beginning, that hearing people

could talk and sign and deaf people could talk and sign. What caused the separation? I think education, the system. (3 June 1996)

And it is a system that, for deaf students, tends to separate language from communication, emphasizing the latter over the former and in doing so leaving, by its own "audist" terms, deaf students linguistically lacking, audiologically disabled, civically crippled, culturally deprived. To be sure, this is strong rhetoric. These strong-text communicative portraits are most often drawn by what Harlan Lane disdainfully calls "the audist establishment"—a colonial mechanism that keeps the deaf "dumb," purportedly unable to communicate, never speaking (let alone writing) well enough while hearing people remain in power, victorious always through a "violence of literacy" that sets communication and language against each other and severs Quintilian's twin goals of the "good man" who also "speaks well." I call this truly a disabling rhetoric.

Notes

Reprinted with permission from *Lend Me Your Ear: Rhetorical Constructions of Deafness* (Gallaudet UP, 1999), copyright Gallaudet University Press.

1. See the opening chapter of Wrigley's *Politics of Deafness*, esp. 13.

2. These three sets of figures are represented in the following: Wrigley (13); Schein and Delk; and NICD, "Deafness: A Fact Sheet."

3. *Naming Silenced Lives* is the title of a book by McLaughlin and Tierney.

4. It is no coincidence either that my example involves a painter commissioned to portray "silent and lifeless" beauty—a portrait presented more than enough in the history of attitudes about deafness.

5. This damnable dilemma is discussed in an often-cited book on Deaf culture by sociolinguist James Woodward, *How You Going to Get to Heaven If You Can't Talk to Jesus? On Depathologizing Deafness.*

6. Davis's own double-edged argument about the construction of deafness and the "moment of deafness" that began in the Enlightenment is fascinating— and one I take up more in my book, *Lend Me Your Ear: Rhetorical Constructions of Deafness.* Davis illustrates how deafness became recognized and studied, and how deaf people became grouped together, both because of the theories of language and education at the time. But he also argues that eighteenth-century Europe became "deafened" as literacy rates rose and people engaged in the "deaf" acts of reading and writing more and the "hearing acts of speaking and listening less." I might add that this swing from speaking/listening to writing/reading is a major one in the history of rhetoric.

7. Here I have not capitalized the word *deaf* because I do not believe it was imagined as a cultural entity at this time; this belief is supported as well by Lennard Davis.

8. I want to note here that I am wary and weary of the all too traditional and reductive move—a classically rhetorical one, a classical rhetoric one—of dividing, categorizing, classifying. I might attempt to exculpate myself by not-

ing that I am only "discovering" the truth that was already there, that was created before me. But, sadly, I know that not to be the truth; I know instead that the "discoverer" of categories continues the splitting and ensures their existence, carries out their creation, by using what she claims to have "found." For now, I rest guilty as charged.

9. Sylvia Scribner distinguishes between literacy as an individual or social attribute.

10. For work on "literacy as social identity," see Gumperz, Kannapell; for literacy as power, see Foucault; for literacy as self-transformation, see Stromberg; for literacy as speaking and listening to others, see Geissler, Weis and Fine; for "critical literacy," see deCastell, Luke, and Egan; Giroux.

Works Cited

Interviews

Anna, Gallaudet student. Sept.–Dec. 1991.
Bev, Gallaudet student. 5 Sept. 1991.
Charlie, Gallaudet student. Sept.–Dec. 1991 and 9 May 1996.
Ellen, ASL teacher, Gallaudet graduate. 3 June 1996.
Kathy, social worker, Gallaudet graduate. 20 June 1996.
Lynne, Gallaudet student. 10 Oct. 1991.
Paul, Ohio State University student. 21 May 1996.
Sue, assisted listening device specialist, Columbus, Ohio. 11 Apr. 1996.

Published Works

Aristotle. *On Rhetoric.* Trans. and ed. George Kennedy. New York: Oxford UP, 1991.
Augustine. *On Christian Doctrine.* Trans. D. W. Robertson Jr. Indianapolis: Bobbs-Merrill, 1958.
Baker, C., and R. Battison, eds. *Sign Language and the Deaf Community: Essays in Honor of William Stokoe.* Washington: NAD, 1980.
Bizzell, Patricia, and Bruce Herzberg, eds. *The Rhetorical Tradition: Readings from Classical Times to the Present.* Boston: Bedford/St. Martin's P, 1990.
Brandt, Deborah. *Literacy as Involvement: The Acts of Writers, Readers, and Texts.* Carbondale: Southern Illinois UP, 1990.
———. "Literacy as Knowledge." Lunsford, Moglen, and Slevin 189–96.
Brill, Richard G., Barbara MacNeil, and Lawrence R. Newman. "Framework for Appropriate Programs for Deaf Children." *American Annals of the Deaf* Apr. 1996: 65–76.
Brueggemann, Brenda Jo. "The Coming Out of Deaf Culture and American Sign Language: An Exploration into Visual Rhetoric and Literacy." *Rhetoric Review* 13 (1995): 409–20.
———. *Lend Me Your Ear: Rhetorical Constructions of Deafness.* Washington: Gallaudet UP, 1999.

————. "Still-Life: Representations and Silences in the Participant-Observer Role." Kirsch and Mortensen 17–34.

————. "They've Got Power—They're Hearing: Case Studies of Deaf Student Writers at Gallaudet University." Geissler and Decker.

Cicero. *De Inventione. De Optimo Genere Oratorum. Topica.* Trans. H. M. Hubbell. Loeb Classical Library. Cambridge: Harvard UP, 1960.

Cook-Gumperz, Jenny, ed. *The Social Construction of Literacy.* Cambridge: Cambridge UP, 1986.

Davis, Lennard J. *Enforcing Normalcy: Disability, Deafness, and the Body.* London: Verso, 1995.

Davis, Townsend. "Hearing Aid." *New Republic* 12 Sept. 1988: 20–22.

deCastell, S., A. Luke, and Kiera Egan, eds. *Literacy, Society, and Schooling.* Cambridge: Cambridge UP, 1986.

Delpit, Lisa. *Other People's Children: Cultural Conflict in the Classroom.* New York: New P, 1995.

Foucault, Michel. *The History of Sexuality.* Trans. Robert Hurley. New York: Vintage, 1990.

————."Nietzsche, Genealogy, History." *The Foucault Reader.* Ed. Paul Rabinow. New York: Pantheon, 1984. 76–100.

Freire, Paulo. *Pedagogy of the Oppressed.* Trans. Myra Bergman Ramos. New York: Continuum, 1990.

Freire, Paulo, and Donald Macedo. *Literacy: Reading the Word and the World.* South Hadley, MA: Bergin, 1986.

Geissler, Kathleen, and Emily Decker, eds. *Situated Stories: Valuing Diversity and Composing Research.* Portsmouth, NH: Boynton/Cook, Heinemann, 1998.

General Description of the English Language Program. Gallaudet University English Department Handbook, 1990.

Giroux, Henry A. "Literacy and the Pedagogy of Political Empowerment." *Literacy: Reading the Word and the World.* Ed. Paulo Freire and Donald Macedo. 1–27.

————. "Literacy and the Politics of Difference." Lankshear and McLaren 367–77.

————. "Literacy, Ideology, and the Politics of Schooling." *Theory and Resistance in Education: A Pedagogy for the Opposition.* Ed. Henry A. Giroux. 205–32.

————. *Schooling and the Struggle for Public Life: Critical Pedagogy in the Modern Age.* Minneapolis: U of Minnesota P, 1988.

————, ed. *Theory and Resistance in Education: A Pedagogy for the Opposition.* South Hadley, MA: Bergin, 1986.

Goody, Jack. *The Interface Between the Written and the Oral.* Cambridge: Cambridge UP, 1987.

————. *Literacy in Traditional Societies.* Cambridge: Cambridge UP, 1968.

————. *The Logic of Writing and the Organization of Society.* Cambridge: Cambridge UP, 1986.

Gumperz, John J., ed. *Language and Social Identity.* New York: Cambridge UP, 1982.

Hirsch, E. D. Jr. *Cultural Literacy: What Every American Needs to Know.* Boston: Houghton Mifflin, 1987.

Kannapell, Barbara. "Inside the Deaf Community." Wilcox 21–28.

———. *Language Choice Reflects Identity Choice: A Sociolinguistic Study of Deaf College Students.* Diss., Georgetown U, 1985. Ann Arbor: UMI, 1986.

———. "Personal Awareness and Advocacy in the Deaf Community." Baker and Battison 105–16.

Kintgen, Eugene R., Barry M. Kroll, and Mike Rose, eds. *Perspectives on Literacy.* Carbondale: Southern Illinois UP, 1988.

Kirsch, Gesa, and Peter Mortensen, eds. *Ethics and Representation in Qualitative Studies of Literacy.* Urbana: NCTE, 1996.

Lane, Harlan. "Constructions of Deafness." *Disability and Society* 10 (1995): 171–89.

———. *The Mask of Benevolence: Disabling the Deaf Community.* New York: Knopf, 1992.

———. *When the Mind Hears: A History of the Deaf.* New York: Random House, 1984. Penguin, 1988.

Lanham, Richard. "The 'Q' Question." *South Atlantic Quarterly* 87 (1988): 653–700.

Lankshear, Colin, and Peter McLaren, eds. *Critical Literacy: Politics, Praxis, and the Postmodern.* Albany: SUNY P, 1993.

Lunsford, Andrea, Helene Moglen, and James Slevin, eds. *The Right to Literacy.* New York: MLA, 1990.

McLaughlin, Daniel, and William G. Tierney. Naming Silenced Lives: Personal Narratives and the Process of Educational Change. New York: Routledge, 1993.

Moores, Donald. F. *Educating the Deaf: Psychology, Principles, and Practices.* Boston: Houghton Mifflin, 1978.

National Information Center on Deafness. "Deafness: A Fact Sheet." Washington: NICD, 1989.

———. "Educating Deaf Children: An Introduction." Washington: NICD, 1987.

Oliver, Michael. *The Politics of Disablement: A Sociological Approach.* New York: St. Martin's, 1990.

———. *Understanding Disability: From Theory to Practice.* New York: St. Martin's, 1996.

Padden, Carol A. *Deaf Children and Literacy: Literacy Lessons.* Geneva: International Bureau of Education, 1990.

———. "The Deaf Community and the Culture of Deaf People." Baker and Battison 89–103.

Plato. *Phaedrus.* Trans. Alexander Nehamas and Paul Woodruff. Indianapolis: Hackett, 1995.

———. *Republic.* Trans. Paul Shorly. Cambridge: Harvard UP, 1970.

Quintilian. *The Institutio Oratoria of Quintilian.* Trans. H. E. Butler. 4 vols. Loeb Classical Library. Cambridge: Harvard UP, 1963.

Resnick, Daniel P., ed. *Literacy in Historical Perspective.* Washington: Library of Congress, 1983.

Roof, Judith, and Robyn Wiegman. *Who Can Speak? Authority and Critical Identity.* Urbana: U of Illinois P, 1995.

Schein, Jerome D., and Marcus T. Delk. *The Deaf Population of the United States.* Silver Spring, MD: NAD, 1974.

Scribner, Sylvia. "Literacy in Three Metaphors." Kintgen, Kroll, and Rose 71–81.

Sheridan, Thomas. *A Course of Lectures on Elocution.* 1796. Delmar, NY: Scholar's Facsimiles Reprints, 1991.

Stromberg, Peter. *Language and Self-Transformation.* Cambridge: Cambridge UP, 1993.

Strong, Michael. *Language Learning and Deafness.* Cambridge: Cambridge UP, 1988.

Stuckey, J. Elspeth. *The Violence of Literacy.* Portsmouth, NH: Boynton/Cook, Heinemann, 1991.

Weis, Louis and Michelle Fine, eds. *Beyond Silenced Voices: Class, Race, and Gender in U.S. Schools.* Albany: SUNY P, 1993.

Weisel, Amatzia, ed. *Issues Unresolved: New Perspectives on Language and Deaf Education.* Washington: Gallaudet UP, 1998.

Wilcox, S., ed. *American Deaf Culture: An Anthology.* Silver Spring, MD: Linstok, 1989.

Winefield, Robert. *Never the Twain Shall Meet: Bell, Gallaudet, and the Communications Debate.* Washington: Gallaudet UP, 1987.

Winzer, Margaret. *The History of Special Education: From Isolation to Integration.* Washington: Gallaudet UP, 1993.

Wrigley, Owen. *The Politics of Deafness.* Washington: Gallaudet UP, 1996.

8

Going to Class with (Going to Clash with?) the Disabled Person: Educators, Students, and Their Spoken and Unspoken Negotiations

Deshae E. Lott

When performing social roles and identities, disability—like gender, class, and race—becomes a point of confrontation and negotiation in a given contact zone. The academic setting, with its conflicting expectations that students be cooperative and passive as they examine differences (Goodburn, Leverenz, Ritchie), provides an interesting context for the dynamics of displaying disability. Whether the person with a perceivable disability is the teacher or the student, tensions emerge over the issue of author/ity. Ideally, higher education fosters the ability to move beyond "group think." Consequently, having a person with a disability in the classroom affords an excellent opportunity to explode stereotypes about such persons. But just who determines the comfort zones of the "deviant" person and the nondeviant others; or rather, how does one inform about deviance or learn about deviance without imposing on another's personal space? Further, how can those perceived as disempowered be empowered without drawing excess attention to that process; or better, how does one assist the person with unique learning needs without (further) disabling that person? As a disabled student, as a disabled college instructor, and as a college instructor of disabled students, I can furnish case studies for exploring such questions. Specific examples from each role that I have held in a "deviant" classroom reveal the interplay of stereotypes and status therein: the orchestration of confrontations and the negotiation of perceived limitations.

Negotiating Classroom Norms: When the Student Has the Disability

As a student with a visible disability, I have been in the minority in all classroom settings except one (that being the Canine Companions for Independence Team Training, where I learned to work with my service dog). Each of us recognizing that in some fundamental way I am different, my teachers, my classmates, and I have consistently tried to normalize our classroom experiences. How we each went about this, however, has varied drastically. Researchers document derogatory cultural stereotypes for the disabled (Biklen "The Culture," Bogdan, Byrd, Chevigny "Altered Selves," Gerber, Gerbner, Link, Richardson, Yuker, Zola), but I internalized this long before I discovered such scholarship. I did my best to defy limiting, unexamined definitions of how I would act because of my deviance, and I quickly learned that subversive approaches often worked better than direct confrontations. As a college student, for example, I would establish my mental acuity (by performances on examinations and contributions to class discussions) before attempting to establish a relationship with a professor. I did not want people in positions of authority thinking that I thought of myself as a victim who expected compensation and special consideration from them. As David Gerber notes, this response is common among persons with disabilities. I saw myself as quantitatively different but not qualitatively different. At the same time, I was aware that stereotypes presented me as qualitatively different in the eyes of many others.

The media, sustaining a cultural focus on fitness and materiality, continually suggest that my less physically active life is qualitatively less valuable. The presentation of scientific "facts" regarding persons with disabilities serves as one of their more subtle techniques of stereotype propagation. Although many people I know would agree with Ruth Bleier that "science as a method and body of knowledge is, as it must be, a cultural and social product" (15), many others view media summations of scientific studies on disability as neutral, detached, and objective (Namenwirth 29). I, too, have been guilty of trusting media presentations of health-related research despite repeatedly finding misinformation in media reports of all kinds. Society collectively determines normalcy and collectively yearns for understanding. No matter what scientific studies suggest (for example, "Activity Level Linked to Quality of Life"), I am not qualitatively a less valuable human being because I have a disability that affects my mobility. Likewise, I am not valuable simply because my response to my disability can inspire others. But media presentations of persons with disabilities foster such stereotypes. True, the disabled must exert extra effort to accomplish certain goals, and their efforts at times might validly be construed as arduous or valorous. Yet both ideas can too easily become mass cultural assumptions that limit the disabled person.

Positive Objectification

Academic achievement became my means of balancing scales that were not fairly calibrated originally in terms of my self-worth. As Chevigny notes is common among polio victims, the possibility that my potential might be perceived as "qualitatively less" motivated me to prove myself, to find something I could do well despite my limitations and to work toward above-average achievements in that range. For much of my life, that range was classroom scholastics.

Refusing to be limited socially by my physical limitations, in the classroom I even transgressed some of the gender lines that sociolinguist Deborah Tannen identifies. For instance, being unable to raise my hand/arm but wanting to participate in classroom discussions, I learned to take the floor without polite, feminine posturing. By doing so I assumed additional "deviant" attributes, but adopting a more typically male mannerism was the means of fostering a sense of ordinariness or normality. Moreover, in much the same way that early feminists—like Virginia Woolf in *Orlando*—advocated androgyny as a means to female empowerment, developing assertiveness became a way of announcing my self-confidence, a means of demonstrating my personal power and worth.

I further attempted to normalize myself by rebuking much well-meaning assistance. As a teacher, I now realize that teachers made special offers out of respect for my difference and in an attempt to put me on equal footing with other students. But as a student, I viewed many of their efforts as unnecessary privileging. Again, I did not perceive myself as qualitatively different, and sometimes I thought teachers' actions resulted from the assumption that I was qualitatively different. Sometimes teachers offered specific physical support—an alternative test-taking strategy, for example. Other times, as in my graduate philosophy courses, the privileging constituted a form of propaganda. The professor never asked me directly about my disability, but he asked one of my friends. And while he would not confront my difference on this level to my face, he had no compunctions against making me further stand out in the class. I was the only student the professor regularly referred to during lectures by conspicuously calling out my name (mispronounced but identifiable, which further drew attention to the persona he was creating). He also tended to be more verbally effusive in terms of public praise when he returned graded assignments to me. This happened during three courses I took with him, and by the second course colleagues were asking me if he might be highlighting my intelligence to counter stereotypes of persons with disabilities as mentally incompetent. The logic of such a conclusion might seem ill founded given that it was a graduate program, but such was the conclusion students were drawing from the professor's rhetoric. If he wanted students to associate my name and my brain with their philosophy courses, in many cases he succeeded. The students' confrontations were not so much with my mind but with the potential objectification of it. Even if a greater good motivated our professor, was it fair for him to inculcate in us the idea that "Deshae is strong, not weak"?

On the whole this philosophy professor's pedagogy ranks among those I most esteem. And I must commend him for calling attention to disability in the classroom environment. Was his method successful? Well, in many cases, I think so, for the students approached me regarding my disability in ways they did not do at any other time. But in some cases, especially with one nontraditional student, it evoked the "God bless you" response to which I am accustomed: the shaking of the head, the pat on the head or shoulder, the compliment. Given that some of my colleagues reported a sense of distaste or rage when witnessing this woman interact with me, the domino effect of this philosophy professor's method certainly raised awareness of the kinds of situations some persons with disabilities experience. And their reactions, in turn, made me more aware of the objectification I was experiencing with composure and complicity. I did not confront my professor. I complied with the process precisely because the exaggerated circumstances raised others' disability awareness.

Compensating for Deviance

Other examples abound of disability-related negotiations in the academic setting. For example, when I graduated from my undergraduate university, I was the only person that term graduating *summa cum laude,* certainly reflective of my classroom performance. Although the chancellor and I had interacted enough times for him to register that I was a wheelchair user, he still said, "Will all those graduating *summa cum laude* please stand." His minor rhetorical slip paralleled many classroom experiences such as teachers returning papers and absently holding mine out for me to grasp and suddenly recognizing I could not meet their extension, that they would have to alter their handout approach. On that graduation day, as I negotiated to the stage, I received a very lengthy standing ovation and a lavish amount of handshaking and back-slapping from the chancellor, who as the audience clapped moved from the podium and off the stage to pose for a picture with me, a picture that would outlive the memories of those in attendance and leave for posterity an unquestionable sign of his support.

If the chancellor had not been embarrassed by his inattention to my deviance, just as if my teachers had not been so obviously embarrassed by theirs, I would not have minded the oversight that situated me among the "normal" masses nearly so much. Rather I likely would have been delighted, in the way that I was delighted and full of laughter when I pointed out a problem to a friend who once procured us play tickets for the best seats in a local theater: inaccessible seats in the center of an aisle, seats that had to be exchanged. Once again I was being denied access because "normal" conceptions of access differed from my own. But this time the denied access was a victory. The circumstance arose precisely because my friend conceived of me as "normal" rather than "deviant." As a result, we both considered the pros and cons of erasing difference, and our relationship with one another and with others benefited from our negotiations.

But to greater or lesser degrees, when oversights occurred in academic settings, people responded as if the teacher had committed some taboo. In the case of my graduation, the entire attending community highlighted both the chancellor's oversight and my disability with a standing ovation begun by my professors, who ironically implied that the chancellor had committed the error. My achievement, just as any college graduate's achievement, absolutely was an achievement for my professors and the larger community that had supported me throughout my education. They deserved to celebrate with me, and I appreciated how they expressed their respect for me. Without the disability, however, the responses—the embarrassment and the praise—likely would have been much less demonstrative. But from my perspective, everyone's discomfort was more welcome than not, for it was better to be negotiating a social space for myself and other persons with disabilities than to be isolating myself from the larger community.

As in my college experiences, experiences in public elementary, junior high, and high schools built my confidence and helped me accept my abilities rather than cultivate insecurity and bitterness. Unlike other minorities' public school experiences (e.g., those depicted by Maxine Hong Kingston in *The Woman Warrior* and Simon Ortiz in "The Language We Know"), I benefited more from teachers' compassion than I suffered from their ignorance. My deviance in some ways required atypical efforts in terms of my acculturation, but my experiences were not so much a matter of the Du Boisian sense of "double-consciousness" between a dominant and nondominant culture as they were and are a matter of holding an intracultural deviant consciousness (Du Bois 8): being a minority within the dominant ethnic group. My difference was not a matter of race, class, or gender. It was not a matter of cultural literacy. It was a matter of mobility. In a very concrete, recognizable way, it was impossible for me to engage in activities involving "normal" mobility without extra, creative efforts. I could not be asked to pretend to be someone I wasn't; the laws of physics would not allow it. Teachers looked at me as an individual. But most of them associated lacks with my disability rather than with my mind and personality and, thereby, fostered favorable group responses (Langer; Nielsen 7). While teachers reached out, students often did so to an even greater degree.

This student outreach frequently occurred during field trips taken by my humanities class (a team-taught two-course period combining high school American history and American literature and offered only for the top two dozen students in the grade, which in a way made all of us in the class privileged school deviants). One time before we headed to Kate Chopin's plantation house in Natchitoches, Louisiana, one of the humanities teachers pulled me aside to inform me that there would be parts of the tour I would be unable to share with the class. Showing concern and preparing me for the way my difference soon would be highlighted, the warning was a compassionate act on my teacher's part. However, when those inaccessible parts of the outing came, without prodding or expectation, two male students toted me and my wheelchair up multiple flights and spirals of stairs. This student behavior was not unlike that which I experienced in junior high when my peers eagerly volunteered to carry my books from class to class.

Does Motive Matter?

The motivations in these situations are complicated. Was I a handy tool for prestige and other students' self-promotion? Were they attempting to acquire the good graces of the teacher, redirecting attention from me to them? When they did deflect some attentions away from me, I was grateful and became complicit in encouraging repeats with praise and thanks. If they were getting extra attention, too, extra attention seemed more "normal." Gender becomes an interesting issue in such circumstances, too. For, in some contexts, I drew upon the feminine receptivity to help, to community. Was I capable of bringing about group solidarity? Did my disability serve as a channel to disrupt and reconstruct classroom norms, to transfer power from the teacher to the students precisely because they refused to see limitations where the teacher did or because the students somewhat altered the teacher's intended focus? In high school and college, gender influenced dynamics in another way as well, a way it would take me many years to understand: Sexual attraction, which I frequently mistook as *caritas,* would encourage some males to be particularly ingratiating in physical helpfulness. My receptivity to and appreciation of their help would perpetuate the cycle. And, eventually, behavioral patterns inside the classroom would lead to confrontations outside of the classroom. My teachers, my fellow students, and I—from our different and often conflictual perspectives—all struggled to gain authority in scripting my capabilities, in normalizing my classroom experiences, and in directing my life.

Negative Objectification Continues

The mass media, on the other hand, as Douglas Biklen, Robert H. Ruffner, and Irving Kenneth Zola point out is typical of them, continued to present me as a superachiever. And here again I felt trapped between complicity (wanting others to know that disabled persons did not perceive themselves as helpless social leeches) and anger and shame (realizing that I was receiving special accolades for doing things many unsung others had done just as well and better). As a reader and a writer of stories, I understood the need to make a story—even a news story—compelling by combining differences and commonalities. Sure, I wanted to be seen as handy and as capable as the next person, and circumstances dictated that I be seen as handicapped. However, media intrusion into my classroom and academic experiences focused on how much more were my efforts based on underlying assumptions or cultural messages that there was less of me to begin with, thereby scripting me again into a lesser and deviant role rather than simply acknowledging my disability as a manifestation of the differences among us all. Or, rather than focusing on above-average achievements alone, the disability itself became the focus of the story.

The newspaper of the city where I attended undergraduate school even called attention to my disability in the least likely of places: beside my name in the list of recent graduates from the university. The area, with a community college, private college, and several university branches, had a large section of graduates listed each May. In May 1993 I was the only student given an identification of "physically disabled" beside my name. It is unlikely that I was the only disabled graduate, for I knew of at least one other—a blind man. I may have been the only disabled graduate in the area with a 4.0 or the only person with a disability to graduate *summa cum laude*. But I may not have been. I considered the announcement of my disability alongside my name highly inappropriate. Less inappropriate in my opinion was a feature article describing some of my achievements and some of my goals. But in this case, too, I was not the only *summa cum laude* graduate in the area going to graduate school; a friend of mine at the private college had also received a graduate fellowship to an out-of-state school. Where was his story? He had worked as hard for his physics degree as I had worked for my English degree; many would argue that he had worked harder. Perhaps I should have been thankful that the media was helping to shape cultural attitudes in a way that recognized the mental capabilities of the deviant. But at that point I felt martyred against my will.

Due to the amount of attention I must give my body with therapy and special routines and adaptations, I was certainly aware that I was not inseparable from it. Even if my academic achievements allowed my body to be objectified in a positive rather than a negative way, much of the author/ity I attempted to gain over my life was challenged. I thought of my academic performance as personally rewarding, a way to assure myself that I could participate well in a normal domain. I did not conceptualize my scholastic efforts as a highly political act attempting to alter social consciousness. Of course, they were. I did not prefer to be seen as a burdensome or an inspirational deviant; I wanted to be seen as a capable community member. Personal interactions allowed for the latter much better than the media's impersonal feature articles or qualifying labels beside my name, presentations that reduced me to a handicapped person doing an extraordinary thing.

Our current educational system can foster among deviants and nondeviants positive attitudes toward disability. Since personal experiences teach us in ways that theory alone cannot, the overall effectiveness of disability studies can increase when a student with a disability participates in the classroom. Such a group necessarily confronts mass cultural assumptions about disability and negotiates among acceptable ways for transgressing limiting conceptions of normalcy. Some deviants' and nondeviants' responses will be less constructive than others will, but in my experience the confrontations ultimately enhanced my abilities to be a cultural participant. In the classroom environment I was not a personified inspirational object but a human being interacting with other human beings, all of us active learners. Teachers play an important role in creating the environment where active learning becomes possible: They can establish the pattern of responding to the deviant student as an individual, and they can establish the attitude that, with some cooperation and creativity on the part of all class members, the deviant student can fully participate in the group.

Deviance in the Lectures: When the Teacher Has the Disability

As a teacher with a disability, I reflect upon potential methods that I can employ to orchestrate mutually edifying investigations and confrontations regarding my physical condition. Each class period offers an opportunity for such explorations. The atmosphere must be open and fluid for students to feel confident enough to address an issue that could jeopardize their position with an authority figure. However, classroom control must be maintained, too. A sense of structure must remain intact so that participants feel enlightened, not hopelessly confused, by the explorations. From the first day of class, I take care not to disempower myself before my students. I present opportunities to assist me as being empowering for the students: not only as a way for them to receive my compliments and sincere gratitude but also as a way for them to become more engaged in the course material and more involved in creating their learning environment. As studies of classroom dynamics suggest (Miller), my students seem to like having more control over their class and more human interaction with me, their instructor. While it is essential to develop a sense of rapport in order to facilitate any discussions and negotiations regarding deviance in the classroom, there are definite boundaries on both sides. Studies show that people respond more favorably to disabled persons when they focus on that person's capabilities rather than on the disability itself (Bowman). Moreover, as a former student, I know that resentments emerge when teachers self-disclose to what students consider an excessive degree; such teachers are seen as off task and as having ego problems that disrespect the students by taking advantage of the captive audience.

So, how can the disabled teacher facilitate discussions on deviance without counterproductively alienating his or her audience? Having a service dog provides me with a nice springboard for confrontations regarding physical differences. Although I do not fully explain my disability to the class, I do explain the role of my service dog. Then I joke about returning graded papers that I have dropped and Ulina has retrieved. As a teacher with a disability, I get to legitimize the excuse about the dog eating one's homework. While she provides an opportunity for me to admit my weakness, she also empowers me physically—by increasing my capabilities—and creates an immediate common ground with the many animal lovers in the room. I often show the class how Ulina picks things up from the floor that I cannot reach. In this nonthreatening way, I introduce the issue of difference on the first day of class. I honestly announce to students that I am weak and strong, that I need help and can offer help. This serves as one of the ways I try to facilitate an interactive community that respects individual differences, a model I hope that students also will apply beyond the classroom.

Student Responses: Silence to Straightforwardness

Students definitely are aware of my difference; they move their feet out of the way as I roll by and, without prodding, help with handouts, props, multimedia, and furniture rearrangements. But there is an amazing degree of silence regarding my deviance (at least to my face). In fact, I often receive more sexual innuendoes from male students than inquiries from either sex regarding my disability, as if the objectification is being channeled or transferred for male students at least into a better-known system of interplay. There are, however, a number of students each term who are bold enough to mention my disability directly—some during the first day or week of class, others after the term is under way; some to my face, others via E-mail, on quizzes, or in course evaluations; some with no pretext but curiosity, others with the pretext of wanting to heal me (e.g., inviting me to church retreats), learn from me (e.g., physical therapy and education majors), offer me hope (e.g., technology), or explain to a friend or a parent exactly why I use a wheelchair. A student has yet to ask a question about my physical disability that offends me. I value the spirit of curiosity and the opportunity to educate. Whatever motivates students' attentions to my dog or their general assistance to me and their inquiries about my health—whether it be a love of animals or a forced compliance with the deviant authority figure and a desire to use the deviance to their advantage—negotiations and consciousness-raising do occur: Classroom dynamics and course evaluations demonstrate that students overall perceive me as handy, capable, and handicapped.

Still, consciousness-raising remains incomplete. When I read course evaluation comments and get the invariable "amazing lady" statement that stereotypes me in a way that the mass media would, I have to wonder if I use my disability in the classroom to the advantage of myself, my students, and disability awareness in general. Similar questions arise when incidents occur such as when a student named Kay informed me that she recently had seen a film in which a woman with multiple sclerosis had a service dog. Kay related the plot: After being bitten by a vampire, the service dog bites its human teammate. As a result, the woman and dog are teammate vampires, and the woman is no longer disabled. The possibility of the woman's becoming able-bodied excited my student, who thought the storyline "so cool!" and "so neat!" While I was fascinated as usual by Kay's discourse, my own response to the story was one of horror.

The benefits of physical ability were being advanced at what price to the disabled woman transmogrified into a vampire? For the comfort of being a less obvious social deviant? So that she might move from being a "burden" on society to being a social parasite? In order for her to exchange the position of social freak for trendier social freak? Kay's report of the movie plot and her response to that plot disturbed me. After interacting for over four months, Kay assumed that I would share her enthusiasm on this subject. I could only wonder if I might have established too much common ground with my students if they would so easily project their own responses on to me. But did I integrate my questions into a classroom lecture or even into a private appointment with Kay? No. The complicated nature of the dynamics of such a discussion and the need to deal with issues more directly related to the class made it easy to choose as I did. But at what price to myself, other persons with disabilities, and my students?

Disabled educators have a unique opportunity to engage students in disability studies. They also have unique responsibilities. Education ideally enhances the life of the individual and his or her community and thereby meets private and public needs. Careful contemplation can help the teacher with a disability transform social attitudes toward disability without foregrounding a disability-rights agenda. But internal contemplations must be combined with external orchestrations. The teacher with a disability must introduce a receptivity to explorations of cultural conceptions of disability, watch for situations that naturally allow for addressing the subject, and—most important—embrace such opportunities.

Teaching Deviant Students: A Deviant Teacher's Perspective

As a teacher of students with disabilities, I deal with issues of confrontation and negotiation from two primary perspectives: as their teacher and as their comrade in Otherness. Part of my general teaching philosophy entails creating a balance between embodying the compassion and demanding the quality that I associate with the humanities. But when and how should the teacher express to the deviant student a willingness to negotiate that student's means of meeting course expectations? Should the teacher or the student instigate such exchanges? And would a student feel more or less threatened by impositions from someone whom the deviant student expects to understand, but perhaps does not, because all disabilities and ways of dealing with those disabilities differ? Wanting to give the deviant student opportunities to prove him or herself, do I impose unfair standards? Because I expect so much of myself, are my expectations higher for disabled students than for other students? Am I more sensitive when the deviant student accepts disempowered positions? How do I create opportunities for renegotiating power structures within the classroom?

In the course of encounters with "deviant" students, I have had to ask myself all of these questions. A few examples will show some of the ways disability-based conflicts have been negotiated in my classroom. Bodie, a quadriplegic, brought his notetaker to class with him every Tuesday and Thursday. She was always there and almost always attempting to do her chemistry homework during the time the State of Texas was employing her to assist Bodie with his education. The situation infuriated me, but Bodie seemed apathetic. I refrained from inquiring about his apathy toward what I considered an abusive situation, about why he would continue employing this young woman. I refrained from asking the young woman if she understood the words *responsibility, compassion,* and *ethics.* But I did my best to require Bodie to require his attendant to do her job: I called upon him regularly.

I didn't want this web of relations, intricate and sticky, to trap Bodie further. Perhaps it is not aptitude but strategy—a desire to stand out neither way—that motivates some deviant students of mine to situate the self precisely in the middle of the bunch in terms of scholastic achievement. If I insist that the disabled student take advantage of his learning opportunities as a student, am I imposing my vision on the disabled student's life? Moreover, if I insist that the disabled student develop what I think are constructive skills as an employer (skills that Bodie and I require, since we hire health care attendants), is it my place to determine what constitutes preferable personnel management skills? Having to work with personal care attendants myself, I understand that the power dynamics are extremely complicated. Whether inadvertently, unconsciously, or consciously, personal care attendants tend to explore the boundaries of vulnerability and responsibility, of strengths and weaknesses. And both parties understand that at all times some degree of physical abuse remains a viable option for an employee of the physically limited. Boundaries tend to get challenged, and abuses—major and minor—do occur. From that perspective, my direct confrontation with Bodie's employee, no matter how great my indignation and desire for justice, would have been unwise. Instead, I opted to report the employee's unethical behavior to the support services office on campus that recruited her and the state agency that paid her wage.

I would like to say that, if the situation arose again, I would challenge Bodie directly to make sure that he understood how he could exert self-control and problem-solving techniques. But I cannot honestly be certain that I would. Bodie used a speakerphone, never was alone, and had to have someone else hold the papers that he read. If I had addressed the issue, we would have had an audience. Even if I asked his employee to wait outside of a closed office door, already a taboo, I would put him in an unfair position. From his perspective, I might be trapping him as much as any other person or factor in his life. In that situation, I didn't deem explicit confrontation the wisest strategy. If I had witnessed greater abuse or if it had been a different student with a different disability, I might have responded differently.

Students with more invisible disabilities, physical and emotional, constitute an entirely different conflict zone. Just minutes before his group presentation, for instance, Jeff approached me with the information that he had panic-disorder syndrome and an excuse from his doctor for not completing the assignment. He had yet to inform his group, who were counting on him for a third of the project. There were several problems here, timing being the biggest. I denied Jeff's requests to excuse him from the class period and the day's quiz and to tell his group that he had become suddenly ill. I told him that the choices at that point were his but urged him to at least be responsible enough to inform his group members immediately that he was not prepared to make a presentation so that they had a couple of minutes to prepare an alternative approach. And, giving more input than necessary, I told him that I considered his acts (he previously had suggested both to me and his group members that he would be an active participant in the final product) duplicitous and irresponsible. Jeff chose not to attend class but did inform his group members, whom I am proud to report handled the situation with grace and maturity.

Now during my course introductions and on my syllabi I stress even more that students inform me of their individual circumstances so that we can negotiate educational strategies that will benefit them. Sometimes this strategy proves constructive, but sometimes it also invites students to impose limits on themselves that they might otherwise have challenged. For instance, would Jeff have contributed to the project at all and learned from it in the ways that he did if he had been straightforward initially? And would his group members and I have learned as much from the experience? In this sense, I disagree with Lee Brattland Nielsen's argument that "other students should be given accurate information, in advance, about the disability of a student who is being placed in their class" (9). While the disability needs to be addressed, the person with the disability needs to participate in the discussions. No individual's relationship to a deviant physical condition can be adequately rendered with a textbook definition or an instructor's mediation. This is certainly the case with descriptions of my own disability, limb-girdle muscular dystrophy. I understood Jeff's hesitancy in asking for modifications when, by emphasizing his limitations, he could negatively influence people's opinions of him. But perhaps because my own disability is not an invisible one and my lifestyle requires ongoing modifications, I was as guilty as the nondisabled person in lacking sympathy for the person whose body or adaptive devices do not broadcast his differences for him.

It is hard to find the happy medium in terms of silence. Although I write into my syllabus and stress in my introductory course lecture that students with special needs should contact me and the university's disability services immediately, hesitancies seem natural in light of the facts that audience analysis takes time and acknowledging disability is a form of personal disclosure. Then there is the issue of disclosure: The teacher's and the student's conceptions of what is an acceptable amount of disclosure regarding any given deviance are likely to differ. Take, for instance, the case of Courtney, one of my former students with an invisible disability, Crohn's disease. Unlike Jeff, who announced his inability to complete his assignment minutes before it was due, Courtney announced her inability after she learned her final course grade, which she asked that I alter with emotional appeals, "I thought *you especially* would understand." She was petitioning each of her professors, as if a grade change were the requisite consolation for her personal pain. And I, a fellow victim, her rhetoric implied, was supposed to be particularly sensitive to her plight. Courtney is perhaps the most potentially talented student with a disability that I have taught in the last eight years; she wants to publish stories, and she's likely to do so. But the teacher in me wanted her to refine her skills rather than request a grade based on her potential. As a student I had worked to show people that I was not mentally and emotionally breakable because my body was weak. I was my body, but I was more than that. I was a person who could contribute positively to society despite having a deviant body. After weighing the multiple issues, I eventually agreed to give Courtney an opportunity to earn a different grade by having extra time to do makeup work. I refused to agree to her first choice, to tell her that because she had suffered she had earned what she had not earned. Her first six weeks' performance in my class (before the flood of doctors' excuses) as well as her overall GPA for the last two years suggested that average student work was her norm. She argued that the grades were a product of instructors' insensitivity to her health this particular semester and their insensitivity to her race the semesters before. Although her argument is worthy of consideration, it also supports an ideological position that potentially traps both teacher and student in limited and limiting roles. Compromising with student requests to be excused from coursework requires less effort on a teacher's part than negotiating alternative assignments, but does this ultimately help deviant students or change social attitudes toward the disabled?

William was similar to Courtney in his approach, but his disability was an emotional one resulting from years of sexual abuse. He, like Courtney, wanted me to give him extra concessions and wanted me to be his confidante. Understanding the problems of psychological involvement with students, I suggested that he investigate the campus counseling services. He replied that he already had and that the counselor "took a job at another university right after I laid it all on the floor." William felt that it had been futile to trust someone; he felt that he had been abandoned the moment he expressed his vulnerability. Now he was turning to me. While supporting his desire to heal, I cautioned him about self-victimization and suggested potential sources he might contact for future counseling.

Students with disabilities may sometimes appear to perpetuate their own victimhood. But how much of this is caused by their unconscious complicity with cultural expectations? And if as an educator and a former student with a disability I can help them consider the differences between self-empowering and self-defeating requests for special considerations, should I? Or is such an approach unethically invasive and capable of drawing student litigation, as was the case with Colby College sociology professor Adam Weisberger, who evoked student outrage over assignments requiring students to delve into personal issues and circumstances (Shalit)?

Teacher: Teach Thyself

Tensions between me and students with disabilities constitute only part of the classroom confrontations. There are also unvoiced tensions between me and nondeviant students. For instance, I contemplate why it bothers me that some students appear not to see the disability of their classmate when it is precisely that aspect of me that I strove to downplay. On the one hand, when I perceive other students not reaching out (enough), I wonder if it reflects a poor model on my part. My experiences show that when teachers lead the way toward promoting tolerance and equity, students follow. Am I so against presentations of victimhood that I actually limit negotiations toward inclusion? On the other hand, downplaying disability is precisely what I attempt to do. When students appear not to see the disability of their classmate, shouldn't I be glad? Maybe. But in such situations I have often found myself (hypocritically?) bothered by others' insensitivity and blindness, by the lack of community and the degree of alienation in the world that such silence regarding difference represents. In the teacher role, I find myself frustrated by an institution that silences difference (Leverenz) just as in the student role I found myself frustrated by attempts to highlight difference. Although on one level student silence regarding another's disability may suggest an embracing of the Other, on another level I know that to truly embrace alternatives and differences requires carefully considering them and grappling with the interplay of embedded cultural constraints.

My experiences as a deviant teacher of deviant students can benefit nondisabled teachers by providing a dual-perspective on deviant student-teacher relations. Deviant and nondeviant teachers alike, for instance, need to be aware of the complications that emerge when teaching the disabled student who lacks privacy. Sensitivity in general needs to be cultivated concerning how a disabled student's dependence on caregivers influences his or her behaviors. Ignorance or knowledge of the disabled student's perspective, however, should not foster undue concessions in terms of course requirements. Teachers of deviant students would better serve the student and the community by creatively negotiating a deviant student's means of meeting course expectations than by necessarily altering those course expectations. In terms of being a model in and out of the classroom, the teacher can foster community awareness of deviance and, just as important, community cooperation with deviance.

Disability Studies: Respecting Individuality, Fostering Community

Tensions emerge in any deviant classroom. All of my aforementioned anecdotal incidents raise questions that, if explored, can lead to the clarification of cultural attitudes concerning the disabled. The study of disability in the classroom helps cultivate others' awareness of cultural constructions of disability and their own power to alter such constructions. Understandably, different audience members confront the tensions related to disability and negotiate rhetorical positions in dissimilar ways. Kenneth Burke suggests that "a rhetorician . . . is like one voice in a dialogue. Put several such voices together, . . . let them act upon one another in cooperative competition and you get a dialectic that . . .   can lead to views transcending the limitations of each" (qtd. in Karis 120). Classroom deviance works within but also explodes arbitrary boundaries regarding persons with disabilities and academic norms. Every person with a disability—visible or invisible—differs from every other person.

Sometimes there are benefits to creating separate schools administered by people with physical limitations similar to those of the students, such as is the case with Gallaudet University, where its deaf students demanded a deaf university president (Shapiro 5). But in systems aiming to represent each interest somewhere, systems reflecting our democratic ideals, it is imperative to address in classrooms some of the issues related to disability. E. D. Hirsch argues that multicultural education "inculcates tolerance and provides perspective on our own traditions and values. But however laudable it is, it should not be the primary focus of national education. . . . To teach the ways of one's own community has always been and still remains the essence of education of our children" (449–50). While schools certainly must disseminate culturally shared knowledge along with helping students develop their critical thinking skills and their respect for human differences, primarily teaching the ways of the community does not necessarily promote progress. Retrospection and introspection need to be coupled with vision. Only by cultivating receptivity and sensitivity to the positions of those we are less familiar with can we create a community of collective health. What is health? How can we attain it? To answer these questions, we must articulate our different perspectives and negotiate among them.

In eliminating ignorance, we cannot ignore difference; we must explore it and react to it emotionally and intellectually. But what are the methods a teacher can employ to orchestrate such investigations and confrontations in ways edifying for deviant and nondeviant students alike? And how can visible and invisible disabilities be included in the learning process? Thomas M. Stephens's comments on the language of race and ethnicity equally apply to the language of disability: "No member of an in-group or out-group can avoid being labeled, but language acts can ameliorate, change, or clarify the perceived status of the classification, depending on the linguistic context, political biases, or social situation" (144). Precisely for ameliorative, transformative, and clarification purposes regarding the issues of race, ethnicity, class, gender, and sexuality, liberal arts and social science courses at the university level often address the issues Stephens presents. However, less often explored are individual and cultural cognitive strategies relating to spirituality and disability. Jenny Franchot argues that American scholarship avoids religious topics, and she calls for such a focus in much the same way that Rosemarie Garland Thomson notes a lack of scholarship on disability and calls for more studies. To a greater degree than to religious studies, disability studies has an interdisciplinary advantage. Some science classes can approach alternate physiologies and their labeling, and business courses can address disability issues by means of the Americans with Disabilities Act. Of key importance in any discipline's presentations on disability is the treatment of aberrance. While this constitutes a form of advocacy in the classroom, lectures can propose to students the option of respecting and accepting diversity as opposed to harboring and fostering Otherness.

Teaching students to challenge the ways of the community—to ascertain past and current trends and to determine which of these to adopt and which to alter—trains students to create the future ways of their communities. If as Hirsch argues, "Literate culture . . . excludes nobody; it cuts across generations and social groups and classes; it is not usually one's first culture, but it should be everyone's second" (452), then disability studies must become a part of our cultural literacy. Like multicultural studies, disability studies can inculcate tolerance and provide perspective on community values. But hopefully disability studies will teach more than tolerance toward difference. Receptivity and creativity are essential. Together these attitudes foster supportive acts that enable persons with bodily limitations to live as independently and productively as possible. By bringing disability studies into the curriculum even in small ways, we further move toward a cultural ideology that embraces the continual negotiations advantageous to the welfare of persons with disabilities as well as to their nondisabled fellow citizens.

Works Cited

"Activity Level Linked to Quality of Life." *Morbidity and Mortality Weekly Report* 47 (1998): 134–37. <www.yahoo.com/headlines/980227/health/stories/hea9_1.html> (2 Mar. 1998).

Biklen, Douglas. "The Culture of Policy: Disability Images and Their Analogues in Public Policy." *Policy Studies Journal* 15.3 (1987): 515–35.

———. "Framed: Journalism's Treatment of Disability." *Social Policy* 16 (1986): 45–51.

Bleier, Ruth, ed. *Feminist Approaches to Science.* New York: Pergamon, 1986. 1–17.

Bogdan, Robert, Douglas Bilken, Arthur Shapiro, and David Spelkoman. "The Disabled: Media's Monster." Nagler 138–42.

Bowman, James T. "Attitudes Toward Disabled Persons: Social Distance and Work Competence." *Journal of Rehabilitation* 53 (1987): 41–44.

Byrd, E. Keith, and Timothy R. Elliott. "Media and Disability: A Discussion of Research." *Attitudes Toward Persons with Disabilities.* Ed. Harold E. Yuker. New York: Springer, 1988. 82–95.

Chevigny, Bell Gale. "Altered Selves." *Nation* 30 Mar. 1998: 32–34.

Dijk, Teun A. van, ed. *Discourse and Communication: New Approaches to the Analysis of Mass Media Discourse and Communication.* Research in Text Theory 10. New York: Walter de Gruyter, 1985.

———. "Forgotten but Not Gone." *Nation* 6 Oct. 1997: 39–44.

Du Bois, W. E. B. *The Souls of Black Folk.* New York: Vintage–Library of America, 1990.

Franchot, Jenny. "Invisible Domain: Religion and American Literary Studies." *American Literature* 67.4 (1995): 833–42.

Gerber, David. "Anger and Affability: The Rise and Representation of a Repertory of Self-Presentation Skills in a World War II Disabled Veteran." *Journal of Social History* 27 (1993): 5–27.

Gerbner, George. "Mass Media Discourse: Message System Analysis as a Component of Cultural Indicators." Teun A. van Dijk 13–25.

Goodburn, Amy, and Beth Ina. "Collaboration, Critical Pedagogy, and Struggles over Difference." *Journal of Advanced Composition* 14.1 (1994): 131–48.

Greenberg, Ruth B., and Joseph J. Comprone, eds. *Contexts and Communities: Rhetorical Approaches to Reading, Writing, and Research.* New York: Macmillan, 1994.

Hirsch, Edward Donald, Jr. "Literacy and Cultural Literacy." *Investigating Arguments: Reading for College Writing.* Ed. Jeffrey Walker and Glen McClish. Boston: Houghton Mifflin, 1991. 437–63.

Karis, Bill. "Conflict in Collaboration: A Burkean Perspective." *Rhetoric Review* 8 (1989): 113–26.

Kingston, Maxine Hong. *The Woman Warrior: Memoirs of a Girlhood Among Ghosts.* New York: Vintage Books–Random House, 1989.

Langer, Ellen J., Richard S. Bashner, and Benzion Chanowitz. "Decreasing Prejudice by Increasing Discrimination." *Journal of Personality and Social Psychology* 49.1 (1985): 113–20.

Leverenz, Carrie Shively. "Peer Response in the Multicultural Composition Classroom: Dissensus—A Dream (Deferred)." *Composition Theory for the Postmodern Classroom.* Albany: SUNY P, 1994. 254–73.

Link, Bruce G., Francis T. Cullen, James Frank, and John F. Wozniak. "The Social Rejection of Former Mental Patients: Understanding Why Labels Matter." Nagler 212–37.

Miller, Judith, John Trimbur, and John Wilkes. "Group Dynamics: Understanding Group Success and Failure in Collaborative Learning." *New Directions for Teaching and Learning* 39 (1994): 33–44.

Nagler, Mark, ed. *Perspectives on Disability.* Palo Alto, CA: Health Markets Research, 1991.

Namenwirth, Marion. "Science Seen Through a Feminist Prism." Bleier 18–41.

Nielsen, Lee Brattland. *The Exceptional Child in the Regular Classroom: An Educator's Guide.* Thousand Oaks, CA: Corwin, 1997.

Ortiz, Simon J. "The Language We Know." Greenberg and Comprone 267–74.

Richardson, Willie, and Gwenevere Daye Richardson. "How the Media Manipulate Us with Code Words." *Editor and Publisher* 24 Apr. 1993: 128+.

Ritchie, Joy. "Beginning Writers: Diverse Voices and Individual Identity." *College Composition and Communication* 40 (1989): 152–73.

Ruffner, Robert H. "The Invisible Issue: Disability in the Media." Nagler 143–46.

Shalit, Ruth. "The Man Who Knew Too Much: A Professor's Probing Teaching Methods Put His Career in Jeopardy (and His School in Court)." *Lingua Franca* Feb. 1998: 31–40.

Shapiro, Joseph P. "Ten Years Ago, the World Listened." *U.S. News and World Report* 23 Mar. 1998: 5.

Stephens, Thomas M. "Research Report: The Language of Ethnicity and Self-Identity in American Spanish and Brazilian Portuguese." *Ethnic and Racial Studies* 12.1 (1989): 138–45.

Tannen, Deborah. *Gender and Conversation Interaction.* Oxford Studies in Sociolinguistics. New York: Oxford UP, 1993.

———. *Gender and Discourse.* New York: Oxford UP, 1994.

———. *You Just Don't Understand: Women and Men in Conversation.* New York: Ballantine, 1990.

Thomson, Rosemarie Garland. *Extraordinary Bodies: Figuring Physical Disability in American Culture and Literature.* New York: Columbia UP, 1997.

Woolf, Virginia. 1928. *Orlando: A Biography.* Orlando, FL: Harvest–Harcourt Brace, 1956.

Yuker, Harold E. "Labels Can Hurt People with Disabilities." *Et cetera* 44 (1987): 16–22.

Zola, Irving Kenneth. "Depictions of Disability—Metaphor, Message, and Medium in the Media: A Research and Political Agenda." *Social Science Journal* 22 (1985): 5–17.

9

Signs of Resistance: Deaf Perspectives on Linguistic Conflict in a Nineteenth-Century Southern Family

Hannah Joyner

During the late nineteenth century, American schools for the Deaf dramatically changed their educational philosophies and methods. In antebellum America, most teachers of the Deaf used sign language in their classrooms. After the Civil War, however, increasing numbers of teachers prohibited the use of sign language and instead trained students to speak and lip-read. In *Forbidden Signs,* Douglas Baynton argues that the debate about communication methods had little to do with either teaching methods or the wants and needs of Deaf people. The change from manualism to oralism highlights the large cultural shift occurring in the United States at the end of the century from a rural society rooted in paternalism, Christian religion, and respect for the natural world to an urban industrial society connected to ideals of progress, increasing faith in science, and a climate of nativism (see Baynton, esp. 1–11).

During the antebellum period, Americans worried that Deaf people were separated from the Christian community by their inability to hear the word of God. Teachers of the Deaf felt that manualism remedied this separation from religion. Using sign language, the reformers could teach Christian principles to Deaf people. By the end of the nineteenth century, American reformers were less interested in Deaf people's isolation from Christianity. Instead, the post–Civil War emphasis on nationalism led reformers to fear the Deaf community's separation from the larger English-speaking community. Differing from mainstream America was not tolerated. Only through the use of speech could the Deaf prove that they were part of the nation, not a threat to its unity (Baynton, 15–35).

In the early nineteenth century, creationism was in vogue. Americans believed that God created humans as pristine beings who continually fall from perfection. Because many Americans believed early humans used gesture rather than speech, signed language was deemed closer to God than spoken language. This belief encouraged the use of manualism in schools for the Deaf. Evolutionary theory swept the nation in the late nineteenth century; humans were now seen as continuously improving, each generation superior to the previous. The ability to speak was now the evolutionary marker between humans and beasts. Therefore, oralists claimed the use of sign language and gesture doomed the Deaf to a sub-human status. Only speech could restore them to their humanity (Baynton, 36–55).

Before the Civil War, most teachers of the Deaf were men. Using sign language, male professors taught students deemed old enough to care for themselves. During the postbellum period, as was true throughout American education, the teaching force became increasingly female. Baynton argues that the shift from manualism to oralism further encouraged this trend in schools for the Deaf. Speech training required a lower teacher-student ratio. To avoid higher educational expenses, women were hired because they could not demand the high salaries men received. In addition, oral education was thought to be effective only for very young children. Only women were seen as appropriate surrogate mothers for these youngsters (Baynton, 56–82).

In the early nineteenth century, manualists believed sign language to be universal. It was seen as the "direct expression of nature itself." The natural language of signs was contrasted with the artificial, culturally created spoken languages. By the end of the century, however, oralists redefined sign language as unnatural. Anything that diverged from the mainstream was seen as abnormal and undesirable. Respect for sign language was exchanged for respect only for speech (Baynton, 108–48).

Baynton concludes that both manualists and oralists were unable to treat signing Deaf people as equals. Manualists understood that the Deaf were different from the hearing in both language and culture, but they could not accept Deaf people in positions of authority. On the other hand, oralists advocated equality for Deaf people, but they could not allow sign language because it represented a difference between hearing people and Deaf people. Neither manualists nor oralists could accept both equality and difference (Baynton, 149–63).

Baynton does not explore the Deaf community's perspective in this book, stating that his work is predominantly a study of hearing people and their attitudes toward the Deaf community and their language. He does, however, suggest that Deaf people themselves knew manualism, since it was in their interest to know it, despite the discrimination of hearing proponents. Deaf people supported sign language because it allowed them a space to construct oppositional meanings of their lives—meanings that constructed deafness as both normal and positive (Baynton, 10–11, 149).

Baynton's excellent study joins a large literature analyzing the shift from manualism to oralism. Like Baynton, other scholars in Deaf history have not explored the topic from the perspective of Deaf people themselves. Nor have historians considered why hearing parents, rather than hearing administrators, made the decision to abandon sign language education in favor of the recently developed oral schools (see Benderly; Fisher and Lane; Gannon; Higgins; Higgins and Nash; Lane; Lane, Hoffmeister, and Bahan; Padden and Humphries; Sacks; Schein; Van Cleve; Van Cleve and Crouch).

This essay is an attempt to pay attention to the perspectives of Deaf people and their developmental experiences within hearing families. The time has come for the cultural and intellectual studies of Deaf history to be joined by the insights of social history. The time has come to address Simi Linton's complaint that "disabled people's voices are almost completely absent" in scholarly studies of disability and must be considered before scholars will ever have a more complete and balanced picture of the historical lives of people deemed disabled (Linton 37). This essay explores the experiences of the Lawrences, a Louisiana family, during the middle of the nineteenth century. As I will explain, what Towny Lawrence's story seems to tell us is that while his perspective should be heeded, his voice should never be heard.

In nineteenth-century America, the diagnosis of a child's deafness was usually a great disappointment for hearing parents. Because of social and familial fears about deafness, Deaf children were often dragged to doctors for experimental treatments and to a variety of schools for new kinds of educational therapies. In the long run, these searches merely served to pathologize the children's condition. This essay addresses how one young man understood his own deafness. Unlike most hearing Americans, Deaf individuals typically did not see deafness as deserving of pity or in need of cure. Instead, they saw their struggle as one primarily of self-determination.

Shaped by cash-crop agriculture (that is, crops grown to sell rather than to eat) and an oppressive system of racial slavery, the South differed from the industrializing North. In an effort to maintain a separate culture from the rest of America and to protect the institution of slavery, powerful white Southern leaders encouraged the South to secede from the Union and form its own alliance of states. In 1861 the new Confederacy went to war with the rest of the United States. The story of Towny Lawrence's resistance is set during that tumultuous time.

The Lawrence family grieved when they realized that their children could not hear. As soon as they made the discovery, Henry and Fanny Lawrence began to search for a cure. After months of experimental treatment, Henry's hopes turned sour. To Fanny he reported, "I hoped ere this that I should have had some good account to give thee about our little boys, but as yet I cannot see any change." The doctor suggested that the reason for his failure to cure the children was Henry's doubts. Henry explained that the doctor had "no doubt I have no faith at all but live on hope. But my fears are stronger than my faith." Although Henry felt that the doctor used "fairly rational means" and "ought to make them hear if there is anything to hear with," he could not let go of his suspicions: "I fear to say what I think of him." He decided to continue with the children's treatments. Although his belief in the treatments was failing, he did not yet abandon his dream: "I am sad but I hope on" (Brashear-Lawrence Family Papers [BLFP] 6 Mar. 1853). After years of research, the Lawrences finally recognized that their efforts were not likely to be successful and that their hopes for what they considered normal children must come to an end.

As the Lawrences debated how best to respond to their children's permanent deafness, they tried to form bonds of communication. The earliest book on deafness published in the United States, John Burnet's *Tales of the Deaf and Dumb* (1835), claimed, "Nature . . . has not proved herself such a cruel stepmother as to throw these children of misfortune upon the world without a language." The Deaf had the language of signs. Burnet argued that the language of signs was "a universal language" that all people who "observed nature and her operations" could use (16). Many advocates for Deaf children argued that hearing parents, especially mothers, already knew the language of signs, whether or not they realized it. As one said, mothers knew "*two* languages, one for the *ear,* and the other for the *eye.*" She could "talk with her eyes" by "looks and gestures" that both Deaf and hearing children could understand. Through her natural behavior, thought many people, mothers "daily and hourly, held intelligible conversation" with their children (Burnet 12–13). Advocates for the Deaf argued that women were uniquely qualified for their role. Following the gender norms of the antebellum South, mothers usually took primary responsibility for the daily welfare of young children. They were, said society, less tied than men to the world of abstraction and the spoken word. The community believed that women were, "if any are," more "capable of becoming *ears to the deaf and a tongue to the dumb*" (Burnet 17).

In order to improve their communication with Deaf children, Burnet suggested that mothers "endeavor . . . to forget *words* and think only of *things,* become for the time dumb." When they could not use words, mothers would be forced to turn to the physical language of the body—of facial expressions, gestures, and mimicry—to communicate. Precise imitation would require close observation of the "spontaneous expressions of the feelings and passions in the countenance" and "those gestures which nature prompts us to make." In addition, mothers should look for "clear and well defined ideas of the forms, qualities, and uses" of household objects and "the characteristic circumstances" of actions so they could "cultivate the faculty of IMITATION" in their signs (17–18). After a family initiated the use of a sign, the Deaf child would learn its meaning quickly and adopt those signs (*Biennial Report* 20).

The "home sign" used by families was often started not by mothers but by Deaf children themselves as they tried to express basic needs to their parents. For example, if the child was thirsty, he or she might imitate action of drinking out of a cup. When hungry, the child might "move his mouth as if chewing" (*Biennial Report* 20). As the child became more aware of the world and its processes, the signs could become more elaborate. For example, when the child saw a cow being milked, or water being drawn from a well, perhaps he or she might mime those actions to distinguish between milk and water (Burnet 19).[1]

Signs to represent specific family members and friends were also quickly developed. As Fanny Lawrence wrote to Hannah Lawrence, when she showed her Deaf son Bob a handkerchief belonging to his aunt, he "immediately made his sign" for her (BLFP 3 July 1853). Having name signs for family members connected Deaf children, at least to a degree, to their parents and siblings. Their name signs were usually determined by the individual's physical characteristics. Often the chosen characteristic was "a dimple, a scar, a mole" or some other physical marker. The sign might refer to unusual clothing or typical behavior (*Biennial Report* 20). Even when the concrete reference no longer applied (for example, when a funny hat was removed), name signs already established by the child generally remained (Burnet 20).

Clearly the communication that children were "born knowing" was not American Sign Language, complex and well developed, used by the Deaf community in the United States.[2] The informal communication between hearing parents and Deaf children was, in fact, rarely more than a collection of gestures, mimicry, and a few agreed-upon signs to describe basic ideas. Home sign had great limits. Parents typically had more difficulty conveying information than their Deaf children did. They often could not easily explain abstract thoughts or unexpected events to their Deaf children. Using their family's home sign, children often found it difficult to understand "every thing beyond their immediate vision" and were often unable to perceive "the causes of phenomena of much that they see and feel" ("Sermon" 11) because their parents could not explain them. For example, when one boy's father traveled away from home, the child was confused. When his father's "cup was taken out at breakfast for Sister," the young boy "made signs" insisting that it was not her cup, explaining that his father always "drank . . . coffee out of it," by repeatedly pointing to his father's usual breakfast seat. He had witnessed his father's departure, and he "gave an account" of the departure to his family "very clearly by his signs." The boy walked to the window and pointed "to the river, moving his fingers along in the direction the boat went." When the family still did not explain what had happened, he "gave the account of your going away . . . again," starting "with your going out the front door and getting into the carriage." The little boy was frustrated, and "expressed much feeling on the subject." But his family could not explain to him why his father had left them (NPTFP, Virginia Trist to Nicholas Trist, 5 Dec. 1834).

Increasingly, the Lawrences and their children felt frustrated in their communications with each other, especially as their children matured and could not share their developing thoughts with their parents. Because of their frustration, the parents began to explore educational plans available for their Deaf children. Six months later, the Lawrences were still undecided about the appropriate action for their Deaf children. Henry's sister Lydia inquired of a teacher of the Deaf what he recommended as "the best way to manage and educate" Deaf youngsters. He responded that "decidedly the best course" was to hire a young woman "in the house until they are eleven or twelve years of age." Under the tutelage of a live-in teacher, "they will learn more and better in that way than any other." She could "get the children on in their studies much faster" than in a residential school, where "the younger ones are generally overlooked for the older and more advanced ones" (BLFP, Lydia Lawrence to Frances Lawrence, 4 Dec. 1855).

Although the Lawrence family probably did not yet know it, the addition of a young Deaf woman would expose the children to sign language that would connect them to Deaf society. She would share more than just a language with the children. She could, like the children, understand how the hearing society around them treated the Deaf. In addition to sharing the discriminations of being Deaf in a society constructed for the hearing, a young tutor could show the children the possibilities for advanced education, self-sufficiency, and community bonding with other Deaf people.

At the institution near Lydia's home, she reported to Fanny, that there were "very many excellent young women" who were completing their education and "would be very glad to get a good home" with a family such as the Lawrences (BLFP, 4 Dec. 1855). Unmarried Deaf women did not have many employment alternatives after graduation. The financial support, intellectual challenge, and emotional connection with Deaf children that went along with home tutorship probably made the job quite sought after. There were also disadvantages, however: Working in a particular family's home would remove the Deaf women from the society they had developed at the state school for the Deaf.

The chosen tutor, Lydia wrote, "would go for $150 or $200 a year"— less than one child's tuition at many residential schools. In addition to educating the children in "something that may be useful to them in after-life," one relative thought that having the children taught could be "such a relief" for Fanny. She hoped that the educated Deaf children could become "a source of comfort to their parents" rather than giving their mother "a life of trial" (BLFP, 4 Dec. 1855). Unfortunately, no family letters have been preserved that discuss the experiences during the several years when the tutor lived with the Lawrences.

By 1860, Walter and two of his younger brothers, Towny and Buddie, were students at the residential Louisiana school for the Deaf, as evidenced by Fanny's letter of 28 Dec. 1860 to her sons there. Although this institution was always in a precarious financial position, educators sought to teach pupils basic academic subjects (particularly written English), moral and religious topics, and vocational skills. All of these were taught at the Louisiana school by means of American Sign Language. Social activities were also central. For example, young Towny Lawrence wrote a letter about the weekly "tableaux"—similar to staged skits—which the students proclaimed "splendid" and "fine" (BLFP, Towny Lawrence to Hannah Lawrence, 15 [illegible] 1861). Deaf faculty and staff at the school often took charge of extracurricular entertainment. Activities such as these allowed Deaf students and faculty to spend time with each other and to establish a long tradition in the Deaf community of storytelling.

In the early 1860s, the Civil War broke out, disrupting almost every southern institution for the Deaf. The Louisiana school closed, and Towny and his brothers returned to the family. The Lawrences again hired a young woman to teach the boys and their younger children: "Miss Robinson is here teaching the children. All are home and learning well," reported Henry to his sister (BLFP, 2 July 1861). Not only was a Deaf adult in the Lawrence family home with the younger Deaf children, but the older children, already exposed to the language and culture of the state institution, were in the home with their younger Deaf siblings. The youngsters could grow up with a large number of people with whom they could communicate easily. Growing up Deaf in the Lawrence household became a normal way of life.

The Lawrences knew that the Civil War was "a terrible contest between friends and brothers," as Henry wrote to Fanny (BLFP, 10 Dec.

1862), and that it would change their lives profoundly. When a massive comet passed overhead, Henry felt it to be a sign: "It must have something to do with the extraordinary times we live in" (BLFP, Henry Lawrence to sister, 2 July 1861). As the years of war went by, there were more hardships and more pessimism. As Henry wrote to his wife, "People are tired of the war and crying for peace" (BLFP, 10 Dec. 1862). The disruption of the children's educational experiences at the residential school was one part of the Lawrence's wartime frustration. The parents felt that the young tutor was unable to provide any significant academic experiences. The children complained that they missed the daily contact with their Deaf friends. The Lawrences began to look for alternatives. Soon the children were enrolled at the New York School for the Deaf, a prestigious Northern residential school.

When the war came to an end, the Lawrence family lost much of its fortune as a result of the end of slavery and the destruction of agricultural land by warring armies. Soon Henry began to believe that the financial promise of the South was no longer in plantation agriculture but in the developing businesses and industry. He opened a lumber yard. He began to fear that his Deaf children would be unable to fill his shoes. Before the Civil War, he had imagined that they could become farmers and live with other hearing family members on the Lawrence plantation. But Henry thought his children would never be able to communicate with business clients. His Deaf children could not speak, and many of the clients in this poor rural area were illiterate and could not communicate by reading or writing. Henry promised his Deaf children that "a good home will be made for you always," and he knew they could help him "attend to my Business"—but he felt that they would not be able to continue the work after he died. He feared they would become helpless (BLFP, Henry Lawrence to Robert Lawrence, 30 Dec. 1865). He decided to bring the older boys home to apprentice in the business with him rather than continue their academic education. Although this arrangement did not answer his concerns, he could think of no alternative.

By the early 1870s, the Lawrence family discovered that alternative. They enrolled Towny and his young sister Maggie in the new Whipple School in Connecticut. It was an oral school, promising to teach the pupils to speak and read lips. Henry Lawrence felt that the years of searching for a cure for deafness was now finally answered—not by medicine but by education. The children, he felt, would essentially no longer be Deaf. They would be able to communicate with him (always a great difficulty) and with clients. He was ecstatic. He felt his Deaf children "ought and must learn to talk and read the lips" in order to take charge of his business. Their ability to speak, he wrote in a letter to Fanny, "would enable me to give up all things to my sons and they could go on and manage as well as I could and to know and hear them speak and Read the Lips understandingly, I would be willing and ready to die and feel I had done my Duty to them." He felt that the ability to speak was "worth years of practice to be able and feel able to stand upon man's platform of equality, usefulness, and intelligence" (BLFP, 7 May 1875).

Towny and Maggie were not so happy with their situation, however. They soon complained about the teaching methods at the school. These were different from what they had experienced in the sign language–based schools of Louisiana and New York. At the new oralist school, Zerah Whipple tried to teach Towny and Maggie to contort their mouths and throats to produce sounds. To accomplish his goal, Whipple touched the students' faces and expected them to touch him. Raised with strict southern standards of appropriate and inappropriate physical contact between men and women, Maggie especially hated being touched by an old man. Her father sought to reassure her: "Do all you can to oblige Mr. Whipple. He would not ask you to do anything which was not proper and you must make an effort to talk" (BLFP, 18 June 1874).

Henry was enthusiastic about his children's oralist training. "I feel so much interest in the instruction of the deaf to talk," he told Maggie (BLFP, 18 June 1874). But Fanny was less sure. She could communicate effectively with her children in sign language, and she wrote to them often. She knew their concerns.

In order to keep the pupils, Whipple frequently sent word of "the pleasing intelligence" or the children's "continuing improvement" (BLFP, Frances Lawrence to Maggie Lawrence, 22 June 1874). His words spread throughout the extended family. One cousin, Lizzie Lawrence, passed along to Nannie, a hearing sister, "Mr. Whipple's account of Towny's great improvement" (BLFP, Lizzie Lawrence to Nannie Lawrence, 22 Nov. 1874). She was sure that he would "with time be able to understand perfectly and make himself understood" in spoken English. She continued, echoing other hearing members of the Lawrence family, "What a great thing it would be for him and how fortunate to have the one talent which has for years been withheld brought at last into use," the talent of speech (BLFP, Lizzie Lawrence to Maggie Lawrence, 14 Dec. 1874). Nannie then wrote to Maggie, "Mr. Whipple says Towny will make a fine talker. . . . [He] speaks very highly of you, says you and Towny are doing splendidly." She continued that Whipple was "astonished . . . the way Towny was learning so very fast and we were *very, very* delighted to hear of it" (BLFP, 29 Dec. 1874).

The hearing family's great desire to have their Deaf children learn to speak made Towny and Maggie feel it was their duty to submit to the oralism training. Although they continued to complain, Fanny hoped that the two would "try to have patience and bear all the little unpleasant things—till you can learn to talk" (BLFP, Frances Lawrence to Maggie Lawrence, 24 Feb. 1875). She advised Maggie, "Learn all you can—talk all the time" (BLFP, 10 Apr. 1875). She missed her children terribly, she admitted, and "the only thing that reconciles me to the absence of my children" was "the thought they are being benefitted in some way, doing better than they could by remaining home with us" (BLFP, Frances Lawrence to Maggie Lawrence, 22 Mar. 1875).

The Lawrences were so pleased with what Whipple said about their children's progress, and so desperate to have their older brothers Walter and Robert learn to speak, that they considered sending the young men to the Whipple School to learn his written alphabet (designed to guide students in their productions of sound) and the "first sounds." They also considered hiring a graduating student of the Whipple School, a young woman who was probably hard-of-hearing, to tutor the boys in Louisiana. Fanny wrote to her daughter to see if the young woman might be qualified to teach not only the beginners but the more advanced Towny and Maggie. She stated her concern: "I expect Towny knows as well how to pronounce as she does." Her request for information about the proposed tutor would, she was afraid, offend Whipple as it would threaten to remove two of his paying pupils. She advised Maggie: "Better burn this up, as Whipple would not like it perhaps" (BLFP, 24 Feb. 1875).

Whipple had already had disagreements with the Lawrences. When Henry visited the Whipple School, he had almost removed his children when Whipple demanded that he pay their tuition in advance. He "was afraid he would be cheated out of his money." Henry was offended by Whipple's distrust of him. His first desire was to remove his children right then, but the desire was tempered by his goals for the children: "He was so anxious for you to learn to talk well," Fanny wrote to Maggie, "that he determined to send him some money in advance" (BLFP, 24 Feb. 1875).

At this time, Towny staged a protest significant enough that it left his parents confused, disappointed, and frustrated. He left the Whipple School, refusing to continue his oralist education, and he refused to speak ever again.

As Towny reported to Maggie, still at the Whipple School, he "would not go back to [Connecticut] at all. I have told Mother I would never learn to talk, give it up wholly. I don't believe in articulation for Deaf Mutes." He was frustrated with his efforts at the Whipple School, and had been convinced by some of the leaders of the New York manual school of the "incapacity of Mutes of ever learning to talk and read lip language" (BLFP, 6 May 1875). Towny, as his mother wrote to Maggie, "prefers to talk on his hands." Despite all her pleading, she could not "induce him to read [aloud] or talk" (BLFP, 10 Apr. 1875).

Towny was tired of the practice of learning to speak, saying he was "perfectly disgusted with it, as I look ugly when I talk (the motion of the lips, I mean)." He was also frustrated with the difficulty of speech reading. He warned his sister: "I bet that you will not be able to read every invisible word spoken by certain strangers." Speech and speech reading did not seem like practical skills, compared with the academic and vocational training he had received at the Louisiana and New York schools. Rather than seeming practical, oralist training seemed only for show. The boy was sick of being an object of fascination and display. When his aunt and her friends asked Towny "to speak for them for curiosity," he refused, angering his aunt. As he explained to Maggie, "It seemed to me that she did not like me for giving up the attempt" (BLFP, 6 May 1875).

Towny attacked the motives of hearing oralist teachers. He felt that "Whipple only wants to make money," knowing that many hearing parents were desperate to have speaking children and would try anything to accomplish that goal. Whipple was not alone in his pecuniary motivations. Towny wrote to Maggie that oralist teachers were "too lazy to be hard workers for their living by being farmers" (BLFP, 6 May 1875).

At the heart of Towny's anger was his parents' refusal to acknowledge and accept their Deaf children fully. His parents would not admit the importance of his charge. As Towny's mother reported to Maggie, "Towny is mad with me about something of no importance—some trifle—an unintentional affront. I suppose he told you about it. He says your Father and I care nothing about our mute children." Fanny responded to him that his father wanted the children to learn to speak so he could talk with them. Henry could barely communicate by signs, unlike Fanny, who was a relatively proficient signer. Henry wanted to talk to Towny, as he said, "like I can to anyone else." Not mentioning that the father did not bother to learn sign language, Fanny noted that his desire to communicate with Towny at all was a sign of his affection. She reported to Maggie, "Father was anxious to have you all taught to speak so he could have the pleasure of talking to you. That did not seem much as if he did not care for" his Deaf children (BLFP, 10 Apr. 1875).

Fanny worried that her other Deaf children might believe that their parents did not care for them, but she hoped they did "not think the same as [Towny] does in that respect." Although there is no evidence in the historical record to suggest that any of Towny's brothers and sisters shared in his protest, there is some evidence that they agreed with these particular charges. Fanny wrote to Maggie, "All of you say Nannie," the one hearing Lawrence child, "is more indulged than the others." However, she refused to believe there was any truth in their claim: "I am sure I don't see where it is" (BLFP, 10 Apr. 1875).

Towny's passionate letters to his Deaf siblings give the historian some idea of what made his resistance possible. Certainly, because he had access to clear communication with his Deaf siblings while he was coming of age, the young man grew up self-confident, with cultural knowledge about the Deaf community. Because his first language (learned from his older brothers, Deaf tutors, and later in residential schools) was American Sign Language, spoken English seemed especially frustrating for him; he knew how easily he could communicate with a visual language.

Why was Towny the only one in his family to refuse to speak? His older brothers worked with their nonsigning father in a business with many illiterate hearing customers. The Deaf boys' difficulty communicating with them may have made the attempt to learn to speak seem more reasonable. This attitude was strengthened by their father, who felt that no one who could not speak could run a business. Like his older brothers, Towny's much younger sister did not fiercely resist oralism. But she may have accepted oralist training because she never received the strong foundation in sign-based education that Towny and the older boys did. Her brothers were away at school or working for much of her childhood. And she lived in a society with very strict gender roles that did not allow women independence. Towny had the unique combination of support, self-esteem, age, gender, and ASL fluency to allow his protest.

The story of Towny Lawrence offers historians a lens into the perspectives of Deaf people facing the switch from manualism to oralism during the late nineteenth century. From the analysis of private lives and individual stories of the Deaf, scholars will begin to create a more complex portrait of oralism. Clearly, scholars' portrayal of the damaging effects of oralism on Deaf pupils is accurate. But the pedagogical move away from sign language did not mean cultural and linguistic genocide for Deaf people. Being Deaf often led to hearing discrimination. On the other hand, a strong Deaf identity could also lead to everyday acts of resistance, to fights for rights and for respect, and to the continuation of a culture and a set of values that Towny Lawrence and his peers held dear.

Notes

Items from the Nicholas Philip Trist Family Papers and from the Brashear-Lawrence Family Papers are quoted courtesy of the Southern Historical Collection, Wilson Library, the University of North Carolina at Chapel Hill.

1. The ASL sign for milk looks like hands milking a cow, even though most American children today have never seen milking. Home sign depends on a concrete connection between act and the sign, but ASL does not. ASL vocabulary often has historical connections to concrete behavior, but the signs are now arbitrary—that is, their connection to the concrete is no longer important.

2. Almost certainly, however, home sign affected the development of ASL and continues to shape it.

Works Cited

Baynton, Douglas C. *Forbidden Signs: American Culture and the Campaign Against Sign Language.* Chicago: U of Chicago P, 1996.

Benderly, Beryl Lieff. *Dancing Without Music: Deafness in America.* Garden City, NY: Anchor-Doubleday, 1980.

Biennial Report of the Board of Trustees of the Tennessee Deaf and Dumb School. Nashville: S. C. Mercer, 1852.

Brashear-Lawrence Family Papers (BLFP). Southern Historical Collection, Wilson Library. U of North Carolina, Chapel Hill.

Burnet, John R. *Tales of the Deaf and Dumb; with Miscellaneous Poems.* Newark: B. Olds, 1835.

Fischer, Renate, and Harlan Lane, eds. *Looking Back: A Reader on the History of Deaf Communities and Their Sign Languages.* Hamburg: Signum Press, 1993.

Gannon, Jack. *Deaf Heritage: A Narrative History of Deaf America.* Silver Spring, MD: National Association of the Deaf, 1981.

Higgins, Paul C. *Outsiders in a Hearing World: A Sociology of Deafness.* Beverly Hills: Sage, 1980.

Higgins, Paul, and Jeffrey E. Nash, eds. *Understanding Deafness Socially.* Springfield, IL: Charles C. Thomas, 1987.

Lane, Harlan. *The Deaf Experience: Classics in Language and Education.* Cambridge: Harvard UP, 1984.

———. *When the Mind Hears: A History of the Deaf.* New York: Random House, 1984.

Lane, Harlan, Robert Hoffmeister, and Ben Bahan. *A Journey into the DEAF-WORLD.* San Diego: DawnSign P, 1996.

Linton, Simi. *Claiming Disability: Knowledge and Identity.* New York: New York UP, 1998.

Nicholas Philip Trist Family Papers (NPTFP). Southern Historical Collection. U of North Carolina, Chapel Hill.

Padden, Carol, and Tom Humphries. *Deaf in America: Voices from a Culture.* Cambridge: Harvard UP, 1988.

Sacks, Oliver. *Seeing Voices: A Journey into the World of the Deaf.* Berkeley: U of California P, 1989.

Schein, Jerome D. *At Home Among Strangers: Exploring the Deaf Community in the United States.* Washington: Gallaudet UP, 1989.

"A Sermon, Preached in Christ Church, Staunton, on Christmas Night, December 25, 1842, by the Rev. Joseph D. Tyler." *Annual Report of the Board of Visitors of the Virginia Institution for the Education of the Deaf and Dumb and of the Blind.* Richmond: Ritchies and Dunnavat, 1843.

Van Cleve, John V., ed. *Deaf History Unveiled: Interpretations from the New Scholarship.* Washington: Gallaudet UP, 1993.

Van Cleve, John V., and Barry A. Crouch. *A Place of Their Own: Creating the Deaf Community in America.* Washington: Gallaudet UP, 1989.

Part Three

Cultural and Spatial Rhetorics of Disability

10

Textual Practices of Erasure: Representations of Disability and the Founding of the United Way

Ellen L. Barton

Disability often is defined solely as an individual's physical and/or mental impairments, treated, if possible, through medical care and addressed, again if possible, through education and services aimed at achieving independent and productive life in contemporary society. Insofar as disability is thought of socially, culturally, or historically, it is usually represented in terms of improvement: After all, people with disabilities are no longer warehoused in large institutions, children with disabilities are being mainstreamed in schools, the Americans with Disabilities Act was passed in 1990, and Americans in general are thought to be growing ever more sensitive to the justice and importance of including citizens with disabilities in the multicultural melting pot. But I would argue that disability also must be defined as a more complex social construct, one which reflects not a benign evolution of acceptance but a dynamic set of representations that are deeply embedded in historical and cultural contexts. These representations are in part created and reflected by what I call discourses of disability—stretches of language as short as a conversational exchange or as long as the literature of an academic discipline. One especially prominent discourse of disability emerges from the context of charitable organizations. Since many members of the general public interact with disability primarily in the context of fund-raising, advertising texts produced by charities play a crucial role in establishing cultural understandings of disability in America. This essay examines one particularly influential configuration of texts, textual practices, and the discourse of charitable organizations at a particularly interesting historical moment—the founding years of the

United Way in the early 1950s, an era of charity advertising that put into place some of the enduring stereotypes of disability in American culture.

Background, Framework, Materials, and Argument

The background of this essay is a larger project exploring the ways that uses of language and discourse socially construct the experience and understanding of disability in the United States (Barton). The interrelations of language and disability have been seen in the negative connotations of such terms as "cripple," "retard," "spastic," and "handicapped" (Zola; Phillips, "What"; Hillyer; Brueggemann). Terminology, however, while crucial, is just one aspect of language that contributes to the social construction of disability. Many other complex and interacting discourses—medical, legal, educational, and charitable—contribute to the social construction of disability, with charitable organizations constructing a textualization of disability that has long been influential in the American public.

The theoretical framework for this project comes from recent work in disability studies, an interdisciplinary field emerging out of work in medical anthropology and sociology, public policy, feminist studies, and activist criticism (L. Davis; Fine and Asch; Goffman; Hevey; Hillyer; Ingstad and Whyte; Longmore; Morris; Nagler; Shapiro; Shaw). The central insight of the disability studies research is that disability is not solely a medical condition but a complex social experience, one centered around the physical realities of the minority of individuals with disabilities but one constructed as an experience of difference by the majority of individuals without disabilities. Activist critic Carol Gill articulates the ultimate goal of disability studies: "[I]n the ideal world . . . differences, though noted, would not be devalued. . . . Society would accept [the experience of] 'disability culture,' which would in turn be accepted as part of 'human diversity.' . . . In such a world, no one would mind being called Disabled" (45). In the real world, however, being labeled disabled is to be labeled as different, designated as the Other, fitting Erving Goffman's classic definition of stigma: "an individual who is disqualified from full social acceptance" (*Stigma* n.p.). The experience of disability is thus more often one of segregation and prejudice than one of integration and welcome, and the representation of difference and separation in charity advertising is one of the most prominent places where such stereotypes are presented and perpetuated.

To turn the attention of rhetorical analysis to the textual practices by which such representations of disability are presented to the American public through the discourse of charitable organizations, this essay reports on an archival study of the founding of one particularly prominent charitable organization, the United Way, which began in 1949, in

Detroit, Michigan, as an umbrella organization that collected funds from workplace campaigns and distributed them to member charities such as the United Cerebral Palsy Association and the Epilepsy Foundation. The United Way archives consist of two collections in the Walter P. Reuther Archives of Labor and Urban Affairs at Wayne State University: the papers of Walter Laidlaw, executive director of the United Way from 1949 to 1968, and an ongoing collection of materials from United Way campaigns, primarily what the agency calls collateral, which includes posters, brochures, collection plans for workplaces and neighborhoods, press releases, and other fund-raising campaign materials. The selection process for the materials that were analyzed in this particular study followed two directions. From the collateral collection, I examined thirty-two posters and advertisements used between 1949 and 1964. From the Laidlaw collection, I selected Laidlaw's launch addresses for United Way campaigns, some pamphlets and plan booklets used in corporate and neighborhood campaigns during the 1950s, and press releases.

Together, these materials provide what historian Michael Hill, following Erving Goffman, calls the basic materials of an archival investigation—front-stage representations contextualized by back-stage information. In *The Presentation of Self in Everyday Life*, Goffman defines front-stage representations as those crafted for public consumption (e.g., ads). Hill defines back-stage information as the complex institutional and sociocultural contexts that generate and support front-stage representations. The operations of the United Way, its growth and development in the 1950s, and its prominence as a charitable organization create the back-stage contexts for its front-stage representations of disability. This context is reflected in the United Way's internal memoranda, planning documents, and public relations materials. This combination of front-stage representations and back-stage information holds the potential to deliver what Hill sees as the promise of an archival study—"the power to confirm as well as to disturb our collective legitimations" (6).

Beginning in 1949, United Way ads appeared in newspapers, magazines, workplace posters, and other public settings. They thus represent a particularly influential site of the front-stage representation of disability for the American public. The general argument of this essay contextualizes these front-stage textual practices in terms of the central contradictions of the American 1950s: Underlying the celebration of American goodness expressed in charity was profound uneasiness about the presence of disabled Others who were different from the American mainstream, unease that is allayed by erasure. The American 1950s were ostensibly optimistic. The success of American government and industry in the victory of World War II was recent, American businesses were growing, and the middle class was multiplying. David Halberstam notes that "in that era of general good will and expanding affluence, few Americans doubted the essential goodness of their society" (x). Beneath what Halberstam calls this "placid surface" (ix), however, lurked lingering fears from the war and growing worries about personal well-being. The postwar peace brought the anxieties of the McCarthy era at home as well as the dread of the cold war and the fear of the Third World abroad. The postwar boom brought renewed hope, conformity, and materialism. But as Kathryn Black notes,

> Into this buoyant postwar era came a fearsome disease to haunt lives. . . . Polio was a crack in the fantasy. . . . Polio created an epidemic of fear unlike any other in modern times. . . . The disease attacked everyone's sense of fairness and muddied [everyone's] notion of justice. . . . In polio epidemics, rewards and punishments were dispensed with a random, devastating hand. . . . The disease stood as an ominous reminder that Americans were still vulnerable to the forces of nature, that scientists couldn't put everything right. (Black 47–48)

As sociologist Fred Davis said about getting polio, "In short, it was un-American" (41).

I will argue that charity fund-raising of this era constructed simplistic and stereotypical representations of disability primarily by erasing the complex experience of individuals, particularly adults, with disabilities. The following sections show how this erasure is accomplished in three textual practices of United Way fund-raising in the 1950s: a move to using children rather than adults in advertising campaigns that rely on pity and fear, a growing use of extraordinary rather than ordinary individuals in campaigns that emphasize achievement and success, and a new focus on the charitable organization itself in campaigns extolling the United Way as a model American business. In each section, the analysis first describes the front-stage representations constructed by these textual practices and then contextualizes them in terms of the back-stage operations of the United Way and the sociocultural milieu of the American 1950s. In my conclusion, I argue that these textual practices of erasure contribute significantly to (mis)representations of disability that have endured as cultural stereotypes of dependence, transcendence, and difference.

Pity and Fear in United Way Fund-Raising

Charities of the 1950s actively exploited fear of disability and pity for its victims in fund-raising. As Black notes of the National Foundation for Infantile Paralysis (NFIP), "No plea for contributions was too maudlin" (105). The United Way fund-raising materials contain many examples of representations of disability that depend on familiar themes of pity and fear, quasi-religious themes that have historically pervaded charity fund-raising (Hevey). The United Way came to center most of their ads around children, a textual practice with multiple effects: Not only does it effectively erase the complex experience of disability by adults whose legitimate interests in independence and autonomy are therefore never represented; it also definitively establishes a binary distinction between the able-bodied and the disabled, separating and distancing the disabled from the abled.

One print advertisement from 1949 appeared in Detroit newspapers and was probably also used in posters, pamphlets, and other materials (fig. 10.1). It explains how one donation to the United Way would then be distributed to multiple agencies. The ad itself focused on disability and included a montage of photos illustrating the services of agencies that receive United Way funds, an approach the United Way still uses.

The most prominent photo shows a little boy standing in arm crutches. Although the agency providing services to this particular disabled child is not specified, four smaller photos show agency services actually being delivered, with two photos devoted to adult clients and two to children. One photo shows a nurse examining the hands of two adult women with the caption, "Arthritis and Rheumatism cripple more people than any other disease." These crippling conditions are seen as an acquired disability devaluing formerly productive adults: "These diseases keep thousands of people from working thus resulting in loss of income." The answer to such a loss of productivity is presented in terms of recovery and prevention: Donations to the United Way will fund research leading to "an effective treatment and cure." A second photo and its text also carry a message about productivity as a key aspect of an adult life. The photo shows an adult man being led by a dog; the caption reads, "A Leader Dog helps guide a blind person to a new world of independence. It gives the sightless an opportunity to work, play, and be a normal human being." Productivity here is presented as part of a balanced life, but the agency in the achievement of such an independent life with its balance of work and play is not the adult man; it is the leader dog. Without the service provided by the charitable agency, the sightless man presumably lives a life of dependence and perhaps despair over his inability to be normal because of his disability. The other two photos in this ad feature children being helped by charitable funds. In one, a nurse holds a baby to her chest and glances soulfully upward; in the other, a doctor examines a baby in front of its mother, easily identified by her house dress, her maternal grasp of the baby's hand, and her admiring gaze at the doctor. The captions for these photos use the presence or absence of a mother to make a distinction between worthy families who still need help in order to receive hospital/clinical/institutional care for their children, and "sick, dependent, and neglected children" who will now receive "a second chance at growing up" because of hospital/clinical care provided by agencies operating with United Way funds.

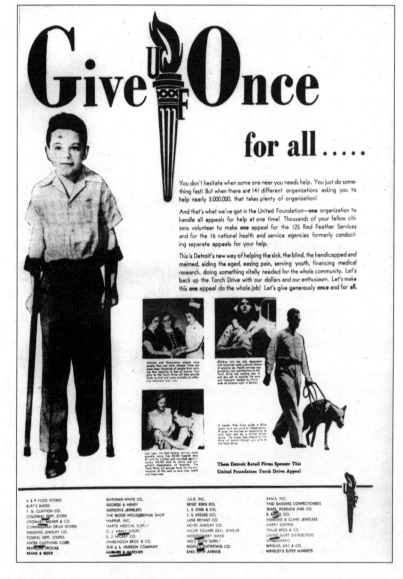

Fig. 10.1. Detroit United Foundation ad, October 1949. Walter P. Reuther Library, Wayne State University.

The general text in this ad again reinforces the separateness of disabled children and dependent adults, using generic and categorical noun phrases: "helping the sick, the blind, the handicapped and maimed, aiding the aged, easing pain, serving youth, financing medical research, doing something vitally needed for the whole community." The final phrase in this ad makes an inclusive gesture, mentioning the whole community ("Let's give generously once and for all"), but the Otherness of the disabled has already been clearly delineated. The whole community here once again is the independent able-bodied community responding appropriately to the Others in their midst (actually, at the edges) by extending the helping services of charity.

This ad from the initial campaign of the United Way falls squarely into the tradition of representing people with disabilities as pitiful cases, dependent adults and handicapped children lumped together into a class which has to make progress toward being "normal" solely through the enabling services of charities. The ads also represent able-bodied readers as compassionate donors, ones who are eager to help the progress of others toward normalcy. More subtly, however, the ads allow, even encourage, a binary opposition identifying a separate group in society— the less than human Others—diseased, disfigured, or disabled—subject to "our" voyeuristic gaze. Pity is the fulcrum in these ads, the result of the peek at misfortune and the basis for any charitable donation.

Sometimes the invitation to gaze in charity ads approaches the egregious (fig. 10.2). In one ad from the 1950s, the headline focuses attention on two success stories: "Your Torch Drive Dollars made Arthur and Pamela well again." Arthur is shown as an emaciated child in his underwear with a vacant expression on his face, sitting on what could be a medical examining table. The child's abnormal physical features are emphasized: His arms are drawn away from his sides, and his misshapen hands are pressed knuckles down on the table; similarly, his misshapen legs with their grotesquely swollen knees are drawn apart and hanging down from the table. The text invites readers to examine his specific abnormalities: "Arthritis crippled Arthur when he was five years old . . . take a *good* look at his hands and knees." The second photo, of course, restores Arthur to normalcy: Dressed in play clothes with pants covering his leg braces and a football obscuring his hands, Arthur stands, smiling and alert. The text celebrates the cured Arthur: "ARTHUR TO-DAY—all set for a fast game of football with his buddies. Now, he can romp and roughhouse just like other kids his age." Arthur's body, now normal, is no longer available for viewing, and the vacant expression is gone as well. He has made the transition from subhuman cripple to all-American boy. Pamela's photo is not quite as dramatic as Arthur's, although it raises similar contradictions. Posed like a model with her left hand tucked artificially under her chin, Pamela gives the camera a charming smile while hooked up to what looks like a portable EEG machine with multiple electrodes and dangling wires attached to her pretty hair. The incongruity of the pose and the electrodes denies Pamela the status of a model child, although once her cure ends the need for the ugly technology, she could very well become a model. The ad identifies the helping agencies, the Arthritis and Rheumatism Foundation for Arthur and the Michigan Epilepsy Center for Pamela. It reassures the reader, "To-

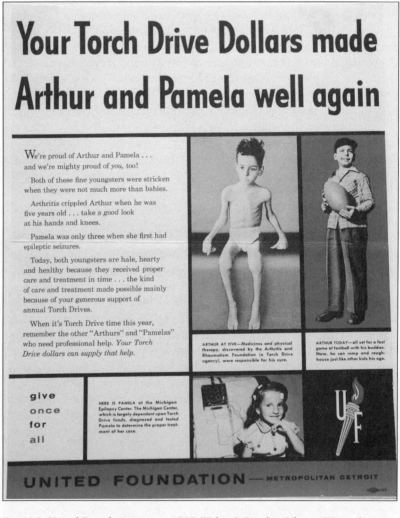

Fig. 10.2. United Foundation poster, 1955. Walter P. Reuther Library, Wayne State University.

day, both youngsters are hale, hearty and healthy because they received proper care and treatment in time." The reader is constructed as being directly responsible for this happy ending and is urged to continue this pattern of gazing with pity and giving to charity as an appropriate response: "When it's Torch Drive time this year, remember the other 'Arthurs' and 'Pamelas' who need professional help. *Your Torch Drive dollars can supply that help.*"

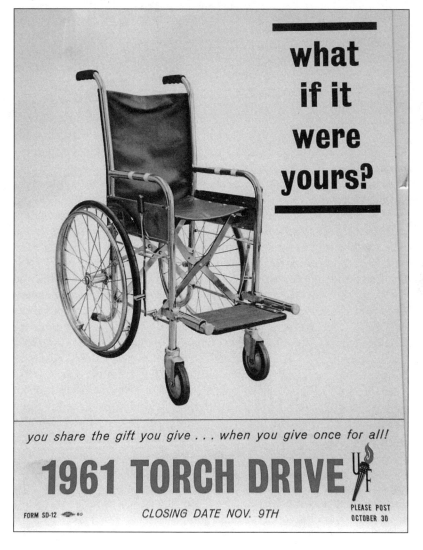

Fig. 10.3. Torch Drive poster, 1961. Walter P. Reuther Library, Wayne State University.

Pity was the dominant theme of United Way fund-raising in the 1950s, but occasionally the theme shifted from pity to fear, directly constructing the reader as vulnerable to disability. One large print ad, for example, consists of a picture of an empty wheelchair and the question, "What if it were yours?" (fig. 10.3). Unlike the usual United Way ads, which were heavy with details, this ad only reminds readers, "You share the gift you give . . . when you give once for all!" The starkness of the photo and text is presumably intended to represent the unpleasant realities of living in a wheelchair, and the reader is expected to need no more prompting to respond appropriately to the solicitation. Donations to the United Way thus assume the status of talisman against disaster. Other ads appeal to fear of disability as a caregiving burden. One ad notes, "The toughest handicap for a retarded child is that he becomes a retarded adult" (fig. 10.4). The text, however, shifts the burden of lifelong caregiving from the reader to charitable institutions: "Through the United Foundation Torch Drive, we can all give the retarded adult a chance to live a life of dignity. Your contribution helps the Metropolitan Agency for Retarded Children and its six affiliates provide educational and vocational training and residential care facilities for retarded individuals." Donations thus ensure that readers and other able-bodied adults need not be oppressed by the burden of disability once removed.

The textual practices of charity fund-raising erased the complex experience of people with disabilities. The chief means by which the United Way fund-raising of the 1950s accomplished this was to reduce the experience of disability to the figure of a child. Although the 1949 ads featured both adults and children, the ads for the next decade all showed services being provided to children. In the thirty-two ads created between 1949 and 1964, twenty-one featured children, with able-bodied adults as parents, caregivers, or volunteers. One 1949 ad depicted a poverty-stricken woman, three concerned United Way support for servicemen through the USO, and three others centered on able-bodied adults as conscientious caregivers or generous donors. For example, one included a small photo of an adult volunteer at the door of an elderly shut-in, and another featured head shots of smiling adults, presumably able-bodied, who had already made their donations to the United Foundation, with a small blank spot ready for the reader's picture (fig. 10.5).

Only two ads from this set actually focused on adults with disabilities. One features a young woman with a leader dog (fig. 10.6). The text reads, "You can see for yourself, and so can I, for now I have Pat, the smartest leader dog a girl ever had! Pat not only sees for me, but she sits by me when I'm alone. And sometimes she must be lonely, too, for she slips her warm paw into my hand, and I tingle all over just to have such a good friend." Although the nameless girl in the ad emphasizes her normalcy through the agency of her dog, the text portrays a life of separation and isolation: Pat may help this young woman to see, but she nevertheless spends her time alone, with only a dog for a friend. Just one ad in this collection portrays an adult with a disability working (fig. 10.7). In a large print ad probably from the mid-1950s, a man in a heavy factory shirt works on a large engine; there is a wrench in his right hand, while in place of his left hand is a prosthetic device holding another tool.

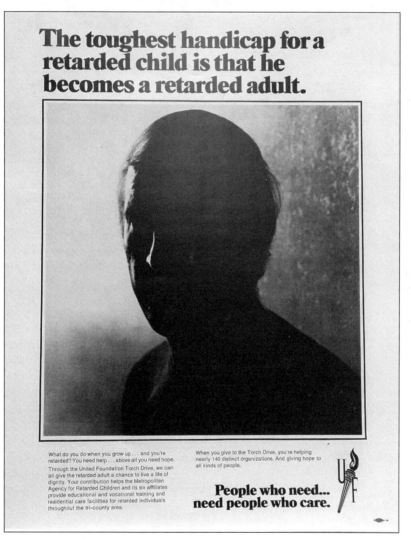

The toughest handicap for a retarded child is that he becomes a retarded adult.

What do you do when you grow up . . . and you're retarded? You need help . . . above all you need hope. Through the United Foundation Torch Drive, we can all give the retarded adult a chance to live a life of dignity. Your contribution helps the Metropolitan Agency for Retarded Children and its six affiliates provide educational and vocational training and residential care facilities for retarded individuals throughout the tri-county area.

When you give to the Torch Drive, you're helping nearly 140 distinct organizations. And giving hope to all kinds of people.

People who need... need people who care.

Fig. 10.4. Torch Drive poster, 1975. Walter P. Reuther Library, Wayne State University.

The prosthesis is almost indistinguishable from the large industrial engine the man is working on. The text of the ad, however, places the credit for this man's employment not within him or his actions but within the actions of agencies.

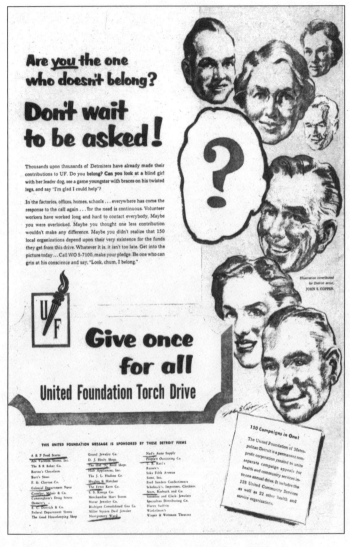

Fig. 10.5. United Way poster, October 1952. Walter P. Reuther Library, Wayne State University.

None of the ads in this study portrayed a person with a disability as
an autonomous adult, one who works or lives with some (in fact, any)
degree of independence. Adults in the ads remain dependent, even the
special category workers hired as "the handicapped" or especially nice

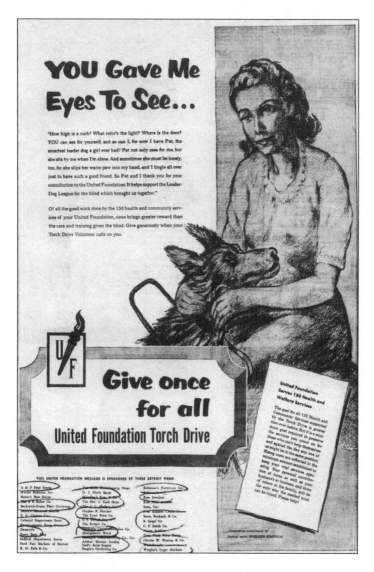

Fig. 10.6. United Way poster, October 1952. Walter P. Reuther Library,
Wayne State University.

people assisted toward "normal human life" with aids such as leader dogs, cases to be admired primarily for their willingness to overcome the assumed tragedy of disability and notable for their obvious gratitude to the agencies, charities, and donors who make their progression toward normalcy possible. Children in the ads are dependent cases as well, presented as pitiful reminders of the tragedies of life. In these front-stage representations of the United Way, neither children nor adults give voice to any complication of this representation as a grateful recipient of char-

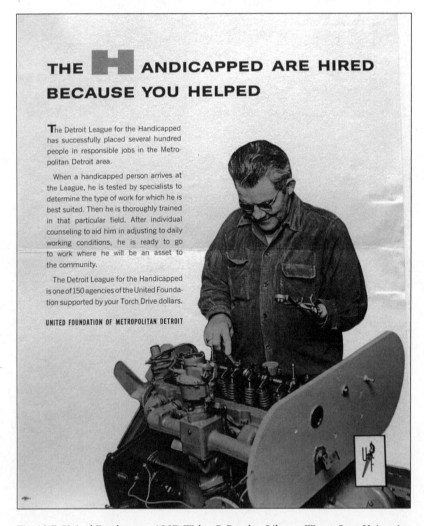

Fig. 10.7. United Fund poster, 1957. Walter P. Reuther Library, Wayne State University.

ity, one who fulfills the expectation that "victims" want nothing more than a "normal human life" as defined by agencies and charities. Nor do handicapped children or dependent adults challenge the binary construction of the disabled as completely separate from the able-bodied, especially able-bodied adults who might read the ads.

The back-stage operations of the United Way also moved to support the growing use of children and childlike adults as front-stage representations of disability. During the late 1940s and early 1950s, the United Way was an organization in flux, establishing ties with older charity organizations in Detroit. Charity traditionally had been divided into two related umbrella organizations, the War Chest and the Community Chest, both of which were directed in the 1940s by Walter Laidlaw. The War Chest grew out of the Detroit Patriotic Fund of the 1920s and 1930s and was an extremely successful World War II fund-raiser. The Detroit Community Chest evolved from the Detroit Community Fund of the 1920s and 1930s. Neither Fund had been successful, however. Laidlaw blamed the Depression and "the growing deterioration of existing fundraising machinery" for lackluster fund drives. Yet he realized that the future of organized charity lay in developing the community organization, a difficult task because the theme of wartime patriotism was no longer available in 1950 to fuel donations and the theme of community giving was, in his own view, a failure.

Under Laidlaw's direction, however, the United Way made this transition, in part by turning away from wartime soldiers and toward peacetime families and by moving its central themes away from patriotism and toward pity and fear. Perhaps the best example of this transition is in the choice of the person who lit the Torch of the United Way at the kick-off rally for the annual Torch Drive. The Torchlighter was the personification of the front-stage representations of the campaign, appearing on posters and in other publicity. In 1949 and 1950, Torchlighters were war heroes whom Laidlaw knew from his years at the War Chest. In 1951, however, the Torchlighter was a child from a local agency supported by the United Way, and by 1959 the United Way could state in its newsletter: "It is traditional that a child who has been in some way victimized by an illness or handicap, and who has shown courage and forbearance through this ordeal, be named to serve as the Torchlighter." In sum, the United Way personalized its front-stage representations in the form of a child who could evoke sufficient pity and fear to fuel donations from America's families.

This practice reflected not only the back-stage context of United Way but also the sociocultural context of the American 1950s. At the height of the baby boom, Americans celebrated children as never before. Essayist Mary Gordon argues that the 1950s were the culmination of twentieth-century ideas about the innocence of childhood and the importance of protecting children from the evils of the adult world: "The barriers protecting this zone were most effective in the years between World War II and the 1960s—a time of prosperity, of a burning desire for normalcy and peace, and of a belief in the goodness of the private world, represented by the nuclear family" (440). Both the celebration and the separation of children were important to United Way fund-raising: The presence of disabled children at the party of American childhood was a sure-fire technique to arouse pity, but it was pity aroused in able-bodied adults who were carefully constructed as separate from the experience. The use of other people's children thus distanced disability and erased a fuller version of the complexities of its experience.

Brought into prominence during the early campaigns, the representation of disability via the figure of a child remains an enduring practice in United Way fund-raising, allowing this charitable organization to continue the binary representation of the disabled as objects of pity or fear and of donors as compassionate members of the able-bodied community offering help to those Others who wish to progress toward normalcy. Some textual practices have grown more subtle over time; shock photos of crippled children in their underwear no longer appear. But the language establishing groups of excluded categories continues: "the aged and handicapped, the diseased, the destitute, the lonely and the many others in need" is from a 1950 ad, but the 1995 United Way pamphlet identifies readers as compassionate donors who have "the power to lift those who have fallen, to comfort those who are troubled and to guide those who are lost." The use of children continues as well. The contemporary pamphlet contains vignettes of families helped by United Way agencies, the "happy parents of 3-year-old Gabrielle" and "Denzel's devoted parents." "Your contribution today will give families like these hope for a brighter tomorrow," notes the ad, constructing exactly the same categories, albeit in family rather than individual terms. Now families with the special problems of children with disabilities receive our compassionate gaze and our generous donations. The textual practices of erasing the complexity of disability in favor of the evocation of pity and fear brought forth from a gaze at a disabled child have endured for more than fifty years of United Way fund-raising.

Achievement and Success in United Way Fund-Raising

An important part of the historical background for the understanding of disability in the American 1950s was laid in the 1930s and 1940s during the presidency of Franklin Delano Roosevelt. Biographer Hugh Gallagher begins *FDR's Splendid Deception* by noting that "Franklin Delano Roosevelt was the only person in the recorded history of mankind who was chosen as a leader by his people even though he could not walk or stand without help" (xiii). But this choice was not based on an open acceptance of disability as part of an accomplished life; instead, it was based on a near-total erasure of FDR's disability. Until the last months of his life, Roosevelt was never seen in public in a wheelchair, his braces were painted black to blend into his socks and shoes, and his sons and Secret Service agents developed excellent strategies to move him in the semblance of walking. Roosevelt's public life was that of an able-bodied man.

Roosevelt was the quintessential American "supercrip," to use a term coined by disability activists. According to Jenny Morris, a supercrip is a person with a disability who lives out the popular representation of disability as adversity to be overcome. Supercrips stories are American success stories, Horatio Alger with a disability (F. Davis; Phillips, "Damaged"; Wilson). Although extraordinary supercrips are the people with disabilities who climb mountains and jog across countries, ordinary supercrips are those who struggle, sometimes mightily, to wear the appellation "no one considers *you* handicapped." Supercrips abound in popular representations of disability. Autobiographies such as Christy Brown's *My Left Foot,* which Brown himself called "my plucky little cripple story" (qtd. in Morris 95), and family memoirs such as Marie Killilea's *Karen* present individuals with disabilities and their caregivers as contemporary heroes and heroines, valiantly struggling to achieve normalcy.[1]

Not surprisingly, charitable organizations have made avid use of the supercrip representation. Supercrips are comfortable representations, not challenging prevailing assumptions about normalcy too deeply. Supercrips also allow the use of seemingly independent adults as front-stage representations in charity fund-raising. In the earlier United Way campaigns, supercrips were presented in the "ordinary" version—that is, adults with disabilities were presented as striving after a "normal human life" as described, for example, in the 1950s ads featuring blind adults with leader dogs (figs. 10.1 and 10.6). Extraordinary supercrip representations have become more common in recent charity campaigns, perhaps reflecting the ever-increasing emphasis on individual achievement that culminated in decades like the American 1980s.

In a poster for the 1981 campaign of the United Cerebral Palsy Association (a United Way agency), for instance, there is a picture of a glider in midair under the headline "What does a glider plane have to do with Cerebral Palsy?" The answer is provided in the text of the ad: "Kathleen Barrett, that's what. She's the pilot of the glider team pictured at right. Although she has Cerebral Palsy, she and others like her are living proof that, more and more, people with this disability can live productive, full lives . . . thanks to United Cerebral Palsy." Another 1980s ad shows a picture of a woman on arm crutches wearing a runner's bib and standing in front of the Brooklyn Bridge. The text below the picture describes another feat: "The real winner of the New York City Marathon came in last. Long after Alberto Salazar and Grete Waitz had won their titles, Linda Down crossed the finish line, a winner in the true sense of the word. Linda has Cerebral Palsy. She saw the marathon as a chance to make a positive statement about disability not getting in the way of ability." Supercrips do not achieve solely in sports, however. In another poster, a sober-faced, blue-suited young man with arm crutches exemplifies a headline reading, "Just because you can't stand on your own two feet doesn't mean you won't go far." A small label near the photo introduces "James C. Stearns; Attorney; McKenna, Connor & Cuneo," and the text confirms our impression of a 1980s corporate superstar: "James Stearns still can't walk across a room without crutches. But he can run circles around his opponents in a courtroom."

Considerable progress seems to have been made, from the cripple hoping for a "normal human life" in 1949 to the brave sports heroes and super achieving corporate executives of the 1980s. But each of the supercrips has still achieved his or her extraordinary feats "thanks to United Cerebral Palsy," a textual line that retains the status of these adults as dependent upon the services of charitable agencies. And the basic distinction separating the disabled from the abled also remains: In a 1980s ad headlined "Strange as it sounds, there never was a better time to have cerebral palsy," the last line of the text hasn't changed substantially since the 1950s: "Remember: When you give, you help people live like human beings." The word *normal* may be gone, but its implications remain.

In some ways, then, the use of supercrip representations appears to be a move toward more complex understandings of people with disabilities, especially adults, although this move is compromised by contradictory textual practices in these front-stage representations. The back-stage contextualization of these representations, however, seemed not to change at all. In the early 1950s, there was a representational match between the front-stage and back-stage representations of adults with disabilities as dependent cases. Internal documents of the United Way matched the words and pictures of front-stage representations by routinely describing adults with disabilities as pitiful cases with no hope of leading normal, productive lives. For example, in the 1949 launch materials (the executive director's launch address and its supporting documents), the clients served by United Way agencies are described with phrases like epileptics with "wrecked lives," arthritis sufferers stricken by "this terrible crippler," polio "victims of this dread disease," and multiple sclerosis victims of "a creeping paralysis that attacks young adults." By the 1980s, however, front-stage and back-stage representations seem to have moved together toward more complex representations of adults with disabilities as achievers and even super achievers. For example, in a set of suggested captions for publicity photographs, a set of adults with developmental disabilities are no longer described as victims who cannot work but as clients of social service agencies that provide "job placement, career counseling, and rehabilitative services to individuals with psychological difficulties, mental impairment, and a history of psychiatric treatment or hospitalization" (note the person-first language). But in advisory materials for promoting 1980s campaigns, even these potentially achieving or super achieving adults remain dependent cases linked with appealing children in the stereotyped representation of disability in terms of pity and praise. In a flyer distributed to United Cerebral Palsy Associations nationwide in the 1980s, public relations officers are urged to use "Photos and Fillers—poignant pictures of children and adults." In this back-stage contextualization, adults with disabilities, even supercrips, are again constructed as dependent children, poignant reminders to able-bodied readers who are constructed as separate from such misfortune.

Supercrip representations reflect the historical context of their era. Adults striving for normalcy in the 1950s reflect the era's emphasis on conformity; sports stars and corporate movers and shakers in the 1980s reflect that era's emphasis on achievement. Like representations of children, though, supercrip representations ultimately erase the complex experience of living with a disability in American society. Supercrips can be extraordinary success stories—Franklin Delano Roosevelt as president of the United States—or ordinary successful Americans—James Stearns running rings around his courtroom opponents. But neither extraordinary nor ordinary supercrips represent any complexities of living and/or working with a disability. The conspiracy of silence that aided Roosevelt and the cascade of praise that surrounds contemporary overachievers limit the social identities that people with disabilities can lay claim to and allows society to simplify its thinking about disability, using stereotypes rather than individuals and assuming a single, able-bodied perspective on normalcy rather than thinking about multiple normalcies. Like children, supercrips can coexist comfortably with society's designations of cases that are worthy of pity, praise, and charitable support.

Supercrip representations based on achievement and success are intimately connected with representations based on pity and fear. Both are based on the concept of people with disabilities as stigmatized Others. After giving able-bodied readers their peek, pity and fear representations leave the disabled Others in their segregated places, never addressing difficult issues of independence or integration. Achievement and success representations seem to welcome disabled Others into public life, but this welcome is highly constrained. Still under the guidance and control of agencies, only those disabled willing to represent themselves as able-bodied, preferably with extraordinary abilities, are presented as candidates for inclusion. Whether individuals are segregated or integrated, however, whether their disabilities are presented as tragedies or adversities, the textual practices establishing these representations draw upon and maintain the powerful stereotype of the able-bodied that disabled bodies and disabled individuals are separate, Others in body and therefore in life. The experience of living in a disabled body, the experience of living in an able-bodied society, the normalcy of a life, particularly an adult life, with a disability—all of these complexities are erased.

The United Way as American Business

The representations of disability described above utilize long-standing cultural stereotypes. Pity and praise representations are common not only in charity but also in popular culture, fiction, and personal experience. A representation that is historically unique to the founding of the United Way, however, is that of charity as business. Since 1949, the United Way has consistently represented itself as a responsible business operation, and it has represented donors as making sensible business decisions about their charitable dollars. This shift toward the representation of a relationship between donors and disabled that is mediated by business may be the most effective of all means of erasure of the experience of people with disabilities. These particular textual practices put them completely out of the loop. It is at the same time an effective means of erasing the need for more complex reflection about the experience of disability on the part of the readers of the ads—the textual practices of erasure allow, even encourage, the erasure of reflection about pernicious stereotypes of disability, especially the stereotype that people with disabilities are unemployable as an explanation for the absence of people with disabilities in the workplace.

The self-representations of the United Way as a business organization are best summed up by its slogans—"Give Once for All" and "Fair Share." These slogans were crucial to the success of the concept of a single workplace campaign that would raise sufficient funds for a large number of community charities. In workplace campaigns, the United Way combined campaign is explained as a sound business idea: "Now, with one generous gift to the Torch Drive, Detroiters can give once for all. This is a new idea in giving, but it is an idea born of good business methods." In order to ensure that these gifts were generous, the United Way began using another slogan in its workplace campaigns—"Fair

Share." This slogan addressed a tricky problem: A single donation to a consolidated campaign had to be significantly larger than any individual donation. The United Way used this slogan to explicitly teach workers how to donate according to its own standard of giving: "How much should you contribute to the Torch Drive? In most businesses, firms, [and] factories . . . your Torch Drive workers have figured out a 'fair share' as a minimum to guide you in answering this question."

The good business methods referred to in workplace campaigns were realized specifically in two practices. Companies became United Way chapters by making a corporate donation and by running a Torch Drive. Workers then donated through the practice of payroll deductions. Donations via payroll deductions were the *quid pro quo* between charity and business: In return for their support of an in-house campaign and the administration of a payroll deduction operation, businesses were promised that the United Way campaign would be the only charitable campaign they would have to support. From 1949 on, these practices were represented as a solid business relationship. In its very first poster directed toward business leaders in 1949 (fig. 10.8), the United Way established its common identity with business: "It's just plain good

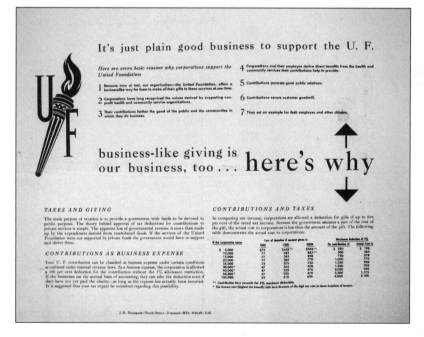

Fig. 10.8. Ad soliciting business support of the United Foundation, 1949. Walter P. Reuther Library, Wayne State University.

business to support the [United Foundation]. Business-like giving is our business, too."

The United Way was blunt in its front-stage representation of its business orientation as an improved means of charitable fund-raising. In a pamphlet distributed jointly in 1954 by the United Way and the CIO, the United Way is presented as a sensible solution to the "problem" of charity in the workplace:

> With the end of World War II, Detroiters, like Americans everywhere, were besieged by a constantly increasing number of fund-raising drives seeking money to support the organizations which fight most of the ailments common to man. At least 50 annual, personal solicitations plagued the man on the street and in the shop, and employers received as many as 134 separate requests for in-plant solicitations or corporation gifts, or as was true in many cases, both. . . . Rumblings of a plan to consolidate giving began in Michigan in 1948 when top leaders from Labor and Management throughout the state met to find an answer to the costly duplication of campaigns.

The umbrella organization of the United Way is represented as extraordinarily good business sense in response to this situation, where charity is presented as an annoying interference to "real" work. The United Way thus is able to represent itself as a model of efficient business administration:

> [T]he "Give Once for All" payroll deduction plan is becoming increasingly popular each year as the practical, sane method of eliminating duplication, time, effort and money to raise funds for the many worthwhile organizations so essential to our well-being in time of need.

This representation of the United Way as an administrative center, mediating between generous donors and a potential clamor for their funds, is one of the enduring United Way self-representations in fund-raising, repeated constantly in materials distributed to businesses in order to persuade them to become United Way chapter organizations (fig. 10.9). Chapter Plan posters, booklets, and brochures throughout the 1950s urged businesses to join the United Way in order to "eliminate the time-consuming disruption and annoyance caused by numerous charitable appeals."

The United Way's biggest innovation leading to its unparalleled success in fund-raising was that it cornered the market on workplace contributions to charity. As argued above, central to this effort was the United Way's self-representation as a business, its construction of itself as an efficient business operation, and its construction of donors as efficient business decision makers who make the prudent decision to give their "Fair Share" to the campaign that allows them to "Give Once for All." Also central to this representational effort was the United Way's need to offer evidence in support of its claims to be following tough-minded business strategies, and for this purpose, the United Way turned to details of its internal operations and relations with its member agencies. Every Torch Drive campaign has emphasized the large number of member agencies supported by United Way funds. In 1949 ads, participating agencies were identified: "125 Red Feather Services [and] 16 national health and service agencies." The same kind of list of agencies has

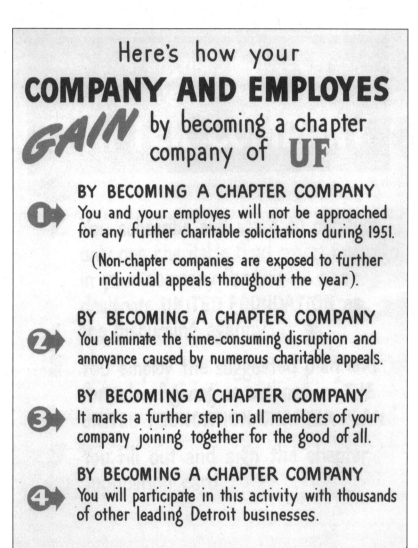

Fig. 10.9. Page from a chart book used by United Foundation corporate solicitors, 1950. Walter P. Reuther Library, Wayne State University.

appeared in United Way fund-raising ever since. In 1950, the number
was 143; in 1951, it was 150; in 1960, 195; and by 1995 the agencies
were too numerous to list individually.

Beginning in the 1950s, however, the United Way did more than simply list participating agencies and their good works. It ran campaigns
that highlighted its tough business operations with respect to these agencies, praising its own expertise in its rigorous vetting of agencies and their
fiscal operations. For example, one undated workplace poster is quite
specific about the way that the business of charity operates (fig. 10.10):
A headline reads, "Torch Drive dollars making their way to those in
need." The ad follows the flow of money from employees signing their
pledge cards in step 1 for automatic payroll donations in step 3. Then
the rigorous United Way scrutiny of agencies applying for funds begins:
step 4 describes United Way site visits to agencies; steps 7 and 8 describe
the meeting of the Allocations Committee of the United Way, which
"makes a critical review of the agency fund request taking into account
established priorities and needs assessment." Even the Allocation Committee's decisions are scrutinized: in step 10, the Central Allocations
Committee "reviews, revises or approves the panel's recommendation";
before step 11, "the agency receives its dollar allocation and services

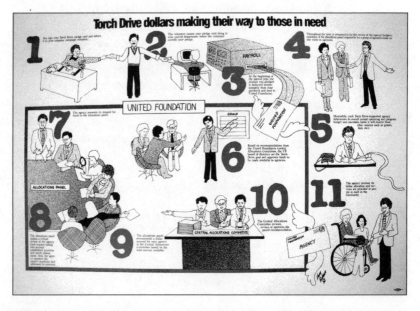

Fig. 10.10. United Foundation poster, 1988. Walter P. Reuther Library, Wayne State
University.

are provided to people in need in the community." Careful business operations thus prevail during every step in the dispersal of funds.

The promotion of the United Way as the sole charitable organization in the workplace was so successful that the American media took notice of its groundbreaking ideas and business techniques. An article in *Look* magazine, for instance, described "Charity on the Assembly Line" (Koether). Predictably, the one photo features a child with a disability, but this child in her heavy arm crutches is surrounded by powerful white male executives, including the presidents of Chrysler and General Motors, the general managers of Ford and Cadillac, and the leaders of the AFL and the CIO. The focus of the article is upon the United Way's concept of unified giving—"Give Once for All"—and on the success of the business operations. Not only does "each agency participating in the Torch Drive [receive] more money than it ever did before," but "the cost of raising that money has sunk to a record low of 4.5 per cent." The history of the United Way is presented as the success of big business: the chaotic and annoying problem of charity before the United Way "was crying for management skill and enthusiastic labor support to solve it." The article praises the United Way by using business metaphors without irony: "[The] Torch Drive is a tribute to [Detroit's] genius for doing the difficult rapidly, and to the persistence of business and labor leaders co-operating in a common cause. Working together, they literally put fund-raising on an assembly line. This time, the mass-produced product is dollars, the profit is community welfare, and the production secret is management-labor co-operation with top talent serving, without pay, at every level." In sum, "what makes the Torch Drive tick is the caliber of business and promotional brains behind it, the seriousness with which both business and labor leaders work at it, and the good will which all its participants bear to each other." The United Way is thus not only an exemplary business operation but a praiseworthy moral organization as well, one that espouses the values of big business to generate significant revenues in the service of charity.

Since its founding, then, the United Way has consistently represented itself as a business success and its donors as savvy business decision makers, and the initiation of this particular fund-raising strategy is closely connected to its historical context of the American 1950s and even to its local context of postwar Detroit. The 1950s saw phenomenal business growth as America made the transition from a war machine to a goods and services economy. Telling tales of McDonald's, Holiday Inn, Korvette's, and other businesses that became American icons, David Halberstam notes that the "era of abundance" (131) created not only prosperous businesses but affluent consumers. In the 1950s, Detroit was one of the premier sites of American business development. Flushed with the success of their role in the industrial buildup of World War II, the automobile companies and their well-paid industrial workers looked like they would dominate an ever more affluent market indefinitely. The 1950s was even a decade of relative labor peace, and all of these factors combined to spur the development of efficient corporate citizenship, at least as defined by the cooperative venture between the United Way and the leading businesses of the area and the time. The United Way and American business appeared to make a successful match; as George Koether noted in *Life,* "The whole campaign is conceived, planned and executed with the careful calculation employed in manufacturing and selling a new-model automobile. . . . Detroiters see it as the efficient way to get a job done." The United Way and American workers appeared to make a good match as well. The prosperous 1950s were a time of redefinition for American workers as consumers, and Halberstam observes that advertising was crucial in the new combination of roles: "The head of the family had worked hard and selflessly, and he had earned the right to bestow these hard-earned fruits upon his loyal family. . . . America, it appeared, was slowly but surely learning to live with affluence, convincing itself that it had earned the right to its new appliances and cars" (507).

United Way advertising capitalized on these feelings of personal success and affluence, too, by constructing prosperous donors not only as generous enough to support the less fortunate but also as savvy enough to support a businesslike charitable campaign. In sum, the workplace campaigns of the United Way were situated squarely within mainstream America, its successful businesses, and its prosperous worker/consumers.

The self-representations of the United Way during its founding years thus created a triangle of representations with the donors and the health and welfare agencies as the two base points, and the United Way as the apex of the triangle, drawing in and dispensing millions of dollars. Except for the ubiquitous handicapped child in a picture or two, the workplace campaigns of the United Way devote no attention to individuals with disabilities. Instead, the agents of interest in these campaigns are the reader, carefully constructed as a compassionate able-bodied worker ready to give his "Fair Share"; the agencies, rigorously vetted by the United Way; and the United Way itself, that paragon of business operations and moral virtue. When this representation of charity is present in the workplace, however, what is absent is people with disabilities, as workers or even as individuals who participate in agency programs (and who therefore might have some useful contributions to make to agency operations and policy). People with disabilities are simply erased, kept absent by the textual practices representing an efficient operation which has turned charity into a once-a-year signature, a signature which allows the donor to remain happily within the world of the able-bodied worker in industrial and corporate America.

These textual practices of erasure also erase the need for able-bodied American workers to think any further about disability and its complex experience, especially in the workplace. Representationally, it is akin to a vicious cycle of absence. If materials issued from the authority of the predominant charity in the workplace do not represent individuals with disabilities in the workplace, then the reader has no responsibility to think in that direction either. If these materials argue overtly that business should go on as usual, with disability represented as one small interruption once a year, then workplaces and workers need not concern themselves in more substantive ways with disability and the absence of individuals with disabilities in the workplace. When charity is abstracted as simple good business, then there is no necessity or motivation to think beyond that level, to think about the specifics of working with a disability or of working with a person who has a disability. Again, disability and the experience of individuals with disabilities remain erased. Further, the need for those without disabilities to think about the possible complexities of disability in the workplace is erased as well, eliminating the need to challenge and change attitudes and stereotypes about disability.

Conclusion: Dependence, Transcendence, Difference

From an instrumental perspective, the textual practices of the United Way have been resoundingly successful. Since its inception, the United Way has been one of the most successful fund-raising organizations in America. Its front-stage representation of individuals with disabilities as the pitied, feared, praised, and erased Other creates a powerful and persuasive rhetoric of benevolence, one that the American public is familiar with and responds to. The rhetorical appeals of these ads to pity and fear, to admiration, and to efficiency were targeted to evoke readers' feelings of good fortune, their suppressed fears of vulnerability, and their pride in American values and institutions. But this rhetoric, despite its success, regularly diminishes the experience of people with disabilities and ultimately diminishes the understanding of disability by society at large. From a critical perspective, the three sets of textual practices described in this analysis have contributed significantly to the continuation of pernicious stereotypes of disability in American culture, reducing and ignoring the complex experience of individuals with disabilities who are living in this same culture. Reducing disability to the figure of a child or childlike adult reinforces the stereotype of disability as lifelong dependence. Presenting disability in the figure of a supercrip reinforces the stereotype of disability as adversity requiring transcendence. Ignoring individuals with disabilities completely in order to transform charity into a business operation reinforces the stereotype of disability as difference. Together these practices maintain the stereotype that people with disabilities are the Other, not integrated into ordinary life, not allowed to define independence and dependence in their own ways, not allowed to be different in spite of their differences.

The implications of the reduction of disability to a figure of dependence are lasting and profound, maintaining the stereotype of all people with disabilities, including adults of any ability, as childlike, needy, and dependent, relying solely on charity and not on themselves. Evan Kemp, head of the Equal Employment Opportunity Commission during the Bush administration, criticizes these representations of the perpetual child. He says that society sees disabled people as "childlike, helpless, hopeless, nonfunctioning, and noncontributing members of society." These prejudices "create vast frustration and anger" among disabled Americans (Johnson 120).

The perpetual child representation and its widespread dissemination, especially through charity fund-raising, contributes significantly to the social oppression of people with disabilities. It is the enduring paternalistic stereotype that political activists have to contend with in their efforts to shift the context of disability from pitiful children to functioning adults whose lives are made more difficult by active prejudice in employment and housing and passive prejudice in access and indifference.

Similarly, the implications of the representation of disability in terms of a supercrip who has transcended adversity are limiting and damaging. The accomplishments of glider pilots, marathon runners, and courtroom litigators are presented as success stories, but any difficult details in those stories are suppressed and erased. The glider pilot does not show how she is a functioning member of the team rather than a figurehead; the courtroom litigator does not discuss the accommodations he may have needed to take the bar exam. Successful adults may be a step above pitiful children, but the representation still lacks the complexity of the experience of disability in America and contributes to a different oppressive stereotype about minority groups—the assumption that society need make no systematic accommodation for people in different circumstances such as disability, suggesting that successful individuals will rise to the top without making annoying demands, and unsuccessful people will fail not because of social conditions but because of character deficits.

Finally, the implications of ignoring disability completely in workplace fund-raising maintains the most insidious stereotype of all—the idea that the disabled are different, separate from the abled, especially in the workplace, not sharing the centrality of work in an adult life. In the United Way's zeal to present itself as a successful business organization, it ignores people with disabilities completely and represents charity solely as a workplace annoyance. This is a stereotype with devastating repercussions. Another continuity has been the 70 percent unemployment rate of people with disabilities (Shapiro 37).

Taken together, these stereotypes establish and maintain the cultural position of individuals with disabilities as the Other, segregated from the workplace and erased from much of the rest of social life as well. In the discourse of charitable organizations, people with disabilities are consistently separated by erasure. In 1950, for example, only one year after its founding, the United Way began another textual tradition—that of celebrating itself. Walter Laidlaw's launch message to the Detroit fundraising community notes the "intangible" benefits that go beyond the millions going to charity: "Who can measure adequately the values of a cooperative effort where the entire community is bent upon a common purpose? Here, and only here, have Catholic, Jew and Protestant, labor and management, rich and poor alike shared in a common venture. This common effort has exalted this community in spirit. What began as a mere mechanism has become an expression of this city at its best."

It is notable, however, that people with disabilities are not included in this celebration of community. Those who receive the benefits of the United Way are still the Other, their lives and experiences completely erased from representations created and maintained by those who putatively support their efforts toward independence and integration, by those who define such efforts as progress toward living like "normal human beings."

Note

1. For a reasoned discussion of the strengths and weaknesses of supercrip family memoirs, see Helen Featherstone's *A Difference in the Family*.

Works Cited

Barton, Ellen L. "Informational and Interactional Functions of Slogans and Sayings in the Discourse of a Support Group." *Discourse and Society* 10.4 (1999): 461–86.

———. "Literacy in (Inter)Action." *College English* 59 (1997): 408–37.

———. "Negotiating Expertise in Discourses of Disability." *TEXT* 16 (1996): 299–322.

———. "The Presence of Interlocutors vs. the Sites of the Internet: The Restricted Range of Disability Narratives." *Works and Days*, special issue: *The Future of Narrative: Internet Constructs of Literacy and Identity*. Eds. Gian Pagnucci and Nick Maurielo. 33/34, 35/36 (2000): 85–115.

———. "Sanctioned and Non-Sanctioned Narratives in Institutional Discourse." *Narrative Inquiry*, forthcoming.

———. "The Social Work of Diagnosis: Evidence for Judgments of Competence and Incompetence." *Constructing (In)Competence: Disabling Evaluations in Clinical and Social Interaction*. Ed. Judy Duchan, Dana Kovarsky, and Madeleine Maxwell. Hillsdale, NJ: Lawrence Erlbaum, 1999. 257–90.

Black, Kathryn. *In the Shadow of Polio: A Personal and Social History*. Reading, MA: Addison-Wesley, 1996.

Blaska, Joan. "The Power of Language: Speak and Write Using "Person First." Nagler 25–32.

Brown, Christy. *My Left Foot*. New York: Simon and Schuster, 1955.

Brueggemann, Brenda Jo. "Still-Life: Representations and Silences in the Participant-Observer Role." Mortensen and Kirsch 17–39.

Davis, Fred. *Passage Through Crisis: Polio Victims and Their Families*. Indianapolis: Bobbs-Merrill, 1963.

Davis, Lennard J. *Enforcing Normalcy: Disability, Deafness, and the Body*. London: Verso, 1995.

Featherstone, Helen. *A Difference in the Family: Living with a Disabled Child*. London: Penguin, 1980.

Fine, Michelle, and Adrienne Asch, eds. *Women with Disabilities: Essays in Psychology, Culture, and Politics*. Philadelphia: Temple UP, 1988.

Gallagher, Hugh. *FDR's Splendid Deception*. Rev. ed. Arlington, VA: Vandamere Press, 1994.

Gill, Carol. "Questioning Continuum." Shaw 42–49.

Glennon, Linnea, ed. *Our Times: The Illustrated History of the Twentieth Century*. Atlanta: Turner, 1995.

Goffman, Erving. *The Presentation of Self in Everyday Life*. Rev. ed. New York: Anchor Books, 1959.

———. *Stigma: Notes on the Management of Spoiled Identity*. Englewood Cliffs, NJ: Prentice Hall, 1963.

Gordon, Mary. "Age of Innocents: The Cult of the Child." Glennon 440–44.

Halberstam, David. *The Fifties*. New York: Fawcett Columbine, 1993.

Hevey, David. *The Creatures Time Forgot: Photography and Disability Imagery*. London: Routledge, 1992.

Hill, Michael. *Archival Strategies and Techniques*. Qualitative Research Methods Series 31. Newbury Park, CA: Sage, 1993.

Hillyer, Barbara. *Feminism and Disability*. Norman: U of Oklahoma P, 1995.

Ingstad, Benedicte, and Susan Whyte, eds. *Disability and Culture*. Berkeley: U of California P, 1995.

Johnson, Mary. "A Test of Wills: Jerry Lewis, Jerry's Orphans, and the Telethon." Shaw 120–30.

Killilea, Marie. *Karen*. New York: Dell, 1952.

Koether, George. "Charity on the Assembly Line." *Look* 19 Oct. 1954.

Longmore, Paul. "Uncovering the Hidden History of People with Disabilities. *Reviews in American History* 15 (1987): 355–64.

Morris, Jenny. *Pride Against Prejudice: Transforming Attitudes to Disability*. Philadelphia: New Society, 1991.

Mortensen, Peter, and Gesa Kirsch, eds. *Ethics and Representation in Qualitative Studies of Literacy*. Urbana, IL: NCTE, 1996.

Nagler, Mark, ed. *Perspectives on Disability.* 2nd ed. Palo Alto, CA: Health Markets Research, 1993.

Phillips, Marilyn. "Damaged Goods: Oral Narratives of the Experience of Disability in American Culture." *Social Science and Medicine* 30 (1990): 849–57.

———. "What We Call Ourselves: Self-referential Naming among the Disabled." Paper presented to the Seventh Annual Ethnography in Research Forum, Philadelphia, Apr. 1986.

Shapiro, Joseph. *No Pity: People with Disabilities Forging a New Civil Rights Movement.* New York: Times Books, 1993.

Shaw, Barratt, ed. *The Ragged Edge: The Disability Experience from the Pages of the First Fifteen Years of* The Disability Rag. Louisville, KY: Advocado Press, 1994.

Wade, Cheryl. "Disability Culture Rap." Shaw 15–18.

Wilson, David. "Covenants of Work and Grace: Themes of Recovery and Redemption in Polio Narratives." *Literature and Medicine* 13.1 (1994): 22–41.

Zola, Irving. "Self, Identity, and the Naming Question: Reflections on the Language of Disability." Nagler 15–24.

11

Putting Disability in Its Place: It's Not a Joking Matter

Rod Michalko and Tanya Titchkosky

> The story reveals the meaning of what otherwise would remain an unbearable sequence of sheer happenings.
> —Hannah Arendt, *Men in Dark Times*

> The common and the ordinary must remain our primary concern, the daily food of our thought—if only because it is from them that the uncommon and the extraordinary emerge, and not from matters that are difficult and sophisticated.
> —Hannah Arendt, "Action and the Pursuit of Happiness"

An Unbearable Happening

My partner Tanya and I, along with my guide dog, Smokie, and her dog, Cassis, were walking down the street of the small university town to which we had recently moved. Tanya had just begun teaching at the university, and I would begin my teaching in the following term. Smokie, of course, was in his harness, and so was Cassis. Although Tanya is not blind, she trained Cassis to work in harness. Occasionally, the four of us would walk together—Smokie in his harness and Cassis in hers marked with a sign "In Training." On this occasion, we chanced to meet a faculty member from the university.

Immediately, he introduced himself to me by saying, "You'll recognize me the next time you hear my voice." He told me his name was Harry and that Tanya had told him that I would be teaching next term. I replied that I was looking forward to it.

Harry told me that he taught at the university and that he was very interested in making the university accessible to "handicapped students." I responded by saying that I was glad to hear that, since the university was very inaccessible to "disabled people." Harry said, "We try to discourage handicapped students from coming here." Thinking he was joking, Tanya and I laughed.

Harry, however, was not joking. This was certainly a meeting of rival interpretations regarding disability. He explained that another university in the province was "totally accessible" and "equipped to handle handicapped students." Tanya and I stopped laughing.

Harry then told us that he had recently met a blind student in an elevator on campus. He said that the elevators on campus do not have braille markings and that the student was trying to "figure out the floors." Harry asked me whether I thought braille markings were necessary for blind people. "For some," I replied. I suggested that the elevators on campus should also have sound indicators so that blind persons would be able to distinguish the floors. This was unnecessary, according to Harry. He said that the blind student on the elevator could tell the numbers of the floors on the elevator pad since they were slightly embossed. Sound indicators, he thought, were too expensive.

Harry explained, "Retrofitting of all the buildings is too expensive. It's just not pragmatic." He then reminded us of the university designed especially to accommodate "handicapped students."

I suggested that encouraging disabled students to attend the university that was "totally accessible" and discouraging them from attending any other university would eliminate any choice they had in the matter. Harry said that this was true for able-bodied students as well. He suggested that if a student wanted to enter a specific program of study, such as "Jesuit studies," his/her choice too would be limited to a specific university. I pointed out that being limited by a program of study and being limited by a disability were two different issues. Harry disagreed.

I then asked whether he thought that restricting the employment of nondisabled professors to a specific university was agreeable. Harry said that this was already the case. "There are no teaching positions anyway," he said. "Universities get three hundred applications for one position. So what choice is there?" Again, I suggested that this was a different issue. This time he agreed.

Immediately after agreeing with me, however, Harry said that he was a "pragmatist" and that "handicapped students should go to one university and then they would have everything they need." At this point, Tanya asked Harry what he would recommend to those faculty in his university who might acquire a disability. Harry did not respond to her question. For the next minute or so, Harry continued to speak of the merits of a university that was designed to accommodate disabled students. He then explained that he was on his way to a medical appointment. We said our farewells and went on our separate ways.

Later that day, a bank teller, seeing my guide dog, assisted me in conducting my banking; as I was about to step off a curb, a pedestrian told me that the traffic light was in my favor; a clerk at a supermarket helped me find the items I wished to purchase. These happenings may certainly be described as common and ordinary. Banking, shopping, and having a quick conversation on the street are certainly things that happen to most of us, and in this sense they are common and ordinary happenings. But for each of us, something may occur that would make these ordinary happenings not so ordinary. We might meet someone on the street whom we have not seen for months, or a bank teller may make a mistake and tell us that there is no money in our account. We might accidentally knock something over in the supermarket. Such occurrences would certainly add a measure of extraordinariness to otherwise ordinary happenings.

There is always a sense of the uncommon with me even in the most commonplace happenings. My blindness is constantly with me. It goes wherever I do. I am always "with it" and "in it" (*Mystery of the Eye* 141–57). My blindness is always "with me" and "in me." Moreover, my blindness is always "marked" in public. Smokie is always with me. He is in his harness and, for most, this signifies me as blind *(The Two-in-One)*. This is one way in which I am extraordinary in ordinary places and uncommon in common ones. Appearing in public is something I have in common with everyone who does so. One feature of appearing in public is that we make an appearance in ordinary and common places. Still, in the midst of this ordinariness each person is unique and is set off from each other person. Even though we are all different, not all differences are noticed. Seeing different individuals on a busy street or in a bank is one thing; noticing their individual differences is another. In fact, the unnoteworthy character of individuals in the public realm is what makes this realm public and distinguishes it from the private.

As one method of achieving the public realm, individuals typically keep their private experiences to themselves. Announcing that we are not feeling well or are extremely happy or depressed is not something we typically do while walking down the street or while shopping in a supermarket. We may "give off" signs of such states of mind, but we do not typically announce them. Behavior in public places, as Goffman notes, is oriented to achieving and sustaining these places as public, as places common to all and thus as ordinary.

There are, however, individual features which are noticed in public. Persons who are attired in a manner uncommon to a particular setting are typically noticed, and so are those who stumble on seemingly nothing while walking on a sidewalk. These are relatively mundane features which, when noticed, are forgotten just as quickly as they were noticed.

These features become part of the "stuff" of which the commonplace and ordinary are made.

But there are other features that, when noticed in public, are not forgotten so quickly. Their noticeability does not spring from the same source as the noticeable but mundane features mentioned earlier. Uncommon attire or stumbling are features that, while noticeable, do not typically influence or change the ordinary character of the public settings in which they appear. But there are features that do influence public settings;[1] disability is one such feature. It is relatively common, for example, to see wheelchair ramps in public places as well as modifications to curbs which enable persons in wheelchairs to negotiate them. Some elevators bear braille markings and sound indicators, which enable visually disabled persons to use them. There are also spaces in parking lots that are designated for use only by those who are disabled. Thus, ordinary streets, elevators, and parking lots take on features that are not so ordinary.

While "accommodations" such as wheelchair ramps are often noticeable, what is not as noticeable is what the presence of these accommodations points to: a "public" interested in accommodating itself to those who are disabled. (This "interest" may often be motivated by law.) These accommodations also point to an essential feature of public places. Until quite recently, wheelchair ramps and other accommodations were not features of public places. These accommodations are "afterthoughts." As such, they point to an essential orientation of the public realm, namely, that it is oriented to persons within the understanding of the ordinary and the commonplace. Ordinary and common public places are oriented to ordinary and common people.

This meeting of the ordinary and the extraordinary marks the beginning of a story that may reveal the meaning embedded in the happening I described above. Our conversation with Harry was both ordinary and extraordinary. It was an ordinary conversation on an ordinary street. But the topic of this ordinary conversation was extraordinary; it was about disability. Moreover, even though the interlocutors were all ordinary people, one was blind—thus extraordinary—and another was accompanied by a guide dog "in training," giving her an air of extraordinariness as well. This conversation was a "meeting" of the ordinary and the extraordinary in the commonplace setting of a public street.

I will now recount this conversation by telling one story that lies buried in it. I will attempt to unpack the narrative of this ordinary conversation, thus revealing its meaning as well as revealing what is extraordinary about the commonplace. Instead of treating this conversation as yet one more unbearable happening in a sequence of happenings, I will orient to it as the "rich stuff" of which stories and meaning are made.

The Place of Disability

Our conversation on the street was about disability. It was a conversation about education and disability. It was not a conversation about whether disabled persons should receive an education. Instead, it was about where this education should take place.

Conversations regarding where disabled persons should attend university make implicit reference to the place of disability in our society. Where does disability fit? What is the relationship between disability and the ways in which our society is organized? What is the place of disability in our society? The conversation Tanya and I had with Harry may be interpreted as answers to these questions, which were tacitly asked and answered that day.

Our conversation raised the question of the place of disability in our society strictly in terms of physical accessibility. Can disabled students enter university buildings, enter classrooms, use the bathrooms, use the elevators? Can disabled students physically move about the university? Given this version of accessibility, we asked whether or not this particular university was a place for disabled students. The answer we gave was twofold: From Harry, "No, it isn't." From Tanya and me, "It should be."

Whether or not a place is accessible to disabled persons or whether places should be accessible turns on human understandings of "space." We find ourselves in the midst of a physical and material world that is spatially organized (Jenks 144). One understanding of this material world springs from the human imposition of distinction. Even though, like the rest of the material world, we (humans) take up space, we make a distinction between the "natural" world and the "social" world (Wolfe 4). This distinction turns on the organization of space. Nature organizes the space of the natural world, while humans organize the space of the social world. The place of the natural world is naturally given, whereas the place of humanity is a creation of humans.

The human creation of a place in the world depends upon the human distinction between humanity and nature. Human society, community, culture are the result of humans collectively making a place for themselves in the natural world. The "space-of-nature" is thus manipulated so as to "make a place" for humanity through the construction of a human artifice (Arendt, *The Human Condition* 175–247). This modern distinction between nature and society understands the place of nature as "naturally given" and conceives of the "place of humanity" as requiring making through human intervention.

This Marxist sense of the human as *homo faber* generates further distinctions. These distinctions spring from the resulting social organization of human creation and artifice and become as natural as the distinction between humanity and nature. There are, for example, the human distinctions of gender, race, ethnicity, etc., and their place in human society is often conceived of as being as naturally given as is the place of nature. For example, men and women are differentially placed in society and so placed often without regard for the "social fact" of the social construction of their distinction. In fact, one reading of the feminist movement is that feminism recognizes the socially organized character of place and thus is involved in "making a place" for women in society. Resistance to the feminist movement can, in turn, be read as resisting a collective's making a place for itself when such a place is "ready-made" (Cormack 87) and naturally given.

This sense of a "ready-made place" may be the grounds for the distinction between able-bodiedness and disability in our society. In his work on the historical and philosophical development of the "self," Taylor begins with the notion of a ready-made place framed within a spatial construct:

> My self-definition is understood as an answer to the question Who I am. And this question finds its original sense in the interchange of speakers. I define who I am by defining where I speak from, in the family tree, in social space, in the geography of social statuses and functions, in my intimate relations to the ones I love, and also crucially in the space of moral and spiritual orientation within which my most important defining relations are lived out. (35)

Who we are, our self-definition, is a matter that is inexorably tied to our orientation to the place in which we find ourselves—to our orientation to the place we find ready-made for us. We are, according to Taylor, speakers living with and among other speakers. Who we are is defined by our place in this community. Self-definition is delineated by spatial terms, by "where we speak from." "Who" we are is located in "where" we are.

The question of "where we speak from" is thus fundamental to the question of self-definition. In Taylor's terms, "we take as basic that the human agent exists in a space of questions" (29). This "space of questions" exists in the place that is ready-made for us but does not refer directly to the "ready-made" character of family and intimacy, status and function, and the rest. Instead, "the space of questions" refers to the development of an orientation to this ready-made place. It is the self-defining orientation of defining our place. Or, in Taylor's words,

> To know who you are is to be oriented in moral space, a space in which questions arise about what is good or bad, what is worth doing and what not, what has meaning and importance for you, and what is trivial and secondary. (28)

These questions arise only when we orient to our ready-made places as "moral space." As ready-made, our places give us answers to such questions without us posing them. Questions of what is good or bad and of what is important do not arise when we orient to our places as ready-made, since the places in which we find ourselves present themselves to us as solutions to problems and as answers to questions. The problem of how a place is defined and how a self defines itself in relation to that place are always-already taken care of before the immersion of a self into a place. The idea of the "ready-made" implies not only that any making of a place is no longer necessary but also that the making of an identity in relation to a place will be taken care of by the place into which the self is immersed. Thus, who we are is defined wholly by the "self" which our place has "made ready" for us to step into.

Questions of self and of identity are framed not only within the spatial terms of where one stands but also within the moral space of where one ought to stand. Even though Taylor speaks of self-definition as grounded in a community of speakers and as raising the question of where we speak from defined as speaking from our family tree, social space, status, etc., the questions of where we ought to speak from and where we belong are not raised but presupposed. It is presupposed that we belong where we find ourselves and that we ought to speak from that space. Good or not, important or not, our space is our home and that is where we speak from. As Taylor suggests, we speak from within a community of speakers and through this exchange we enter the process of self-definition. But when our home and when our community of speakers is problematized, so is our process of self-definition. When the question of "belonging" is raised, so too is the question of identity.

Speaking from an environment to which one belongs and with which one identifies oneself raises the problem of Otherness. This is one of the problems that was implicitly and explicitly raised in the conversation Harry, Tanya, and I had on the street. "Where do disabled students belong?" was the question our conversation addressed and did so by posing it in relation to those whose "belonging-to" remained unquestionable and thus certain. Our question was, "Where does disability belong in relation to the steadfast certainty of able-bodiedness?"

The Misfortune and Injustice of Place

"Disability can be viewed as a relationship between a person with a physical or mental impairment and the social and physical environment around him or her" (Gadacz 5). While this view of disability is undoubtedly true, it is just as true for persons who are not disabled. Every person has a relationship with a social and physical environment. This does not distinguish disabled persons from able-bodied persons. The distinc-

tion between the two resides not so much in the form of the relationship as it does in the content.

The environment with which a disabled person has a relationship is
described by Gadacz as being "around" him or her. While this may be
said for persons without disabilities as well, it cannot be said with the
same significance. The environment that nondisabled persons find
around them is also their environment: They perceive it with "naturally"
working senses, travel it with "naturally" working legs, understand it
with a "naturally" working intelligence. Their environment is "just
there" for them to sense, travel, and understand. What is "around them"
is their environment.

Physical and mental impairments do present persons with difficulties
in sensing, perceiving, and/or understanding the physical and social
environment. We (disabled persons) often experience difficulty in moving through the environment. In the vernacular of the day, these difficulties do present us with "challenges." Be it physical or social, the architecture of social life is often experienced by disabled persons as a
barrier, and thus what is "around" disabled persons is the environment
as barrier.

Still, an inaccessible environment does not necessarily represent the
essential distinction between disability and able-bodiedness. Even though
the environment is in general accessible to able-bodied persons, there
are some particular environments which are not. Everyone is subject to
restriction, and we accept this as "just the way things are." But there
are other instances of inaccessibility that cannot so easily be subsumed
under the rubric of "just the way things are." Restricting access on the
basis of such qualities as gender or race, for example, is conceived of as
sexist or racist. The latter formulations are certainly open to interpretation and debate, but this debate is not typically carried on within the
framework of "just the way things are," since the debate itself springs
from the understanding that "things should be otherwise." We should
not be excluded from the environment solely on the basis of our gender
or race. That such exclusion is illegal bears witness to the strength of
the argument against such injustice. But that this legality exists and is
often debated bears witness to the strength of the injustice itself (Razack
23–28). Nonetheless, these debates center on the understanding that
qualities such as gender and race do not in themselves restrict accessibility to an environment.

The conceptions of misfortune and inability are the bases for both
explaining and justifying the inaccessibility of environments to disabled
persons. The idea of "just the way things are" is a depiction of the "normal and natural" working condition of the body—able-bodiedness. Any
injustice to this "natural body" is framed within the conception of mis-

fortune—but for the misfortune of disease, accident, flawed genetics, the able-body is the normal and natural body. It is "natural" for everyone to have a natural body—"that's just the way things are"—but sometimes people don't and, unfortunate as this is, "that's just the way things go." This is the "misfortune of disability."

Unlike gender or race, the interpretation of disability as "misfortune" allows for the understanding that inaccessibility too is a misfortune and not necessarily an injustice. Everyone belongs to (is) a race, and the same holds for gender.[2] This cannot be said of disability. People belong to (are) disability only because of some misfortune. Disability is not framed within the idea of the "natural" in the same way that gender, race, and able-bodiedness are. Disability is typically a sign of the "natural-gone-wrong."

This paradigm allows for Harry's remarks to be heard as reasonable. That his university is inaccessible to disabled persons is unfortunate, but only unfortunate—that's the way things go. This sort of reasoning originates in the concept of disability as misfortune and leads to the understanding that although disabled persons may be excluded from the environment, this treatment is unfortunate and not unjust.

Judith Shklar reminds us, however, that "we must recognize that the line of separation between injustice and misfortune is a political choice, not a simple rule that can be taken as a given" (5). Thus, the reasonableness of Harry's comments lies in the abstract separation of misfortune and injustice and requires the invocation of the "simple rule" of nature "taken as a given." This rule is implicitly given when disability is conceived of as misfortune.

When inaccessibility is conceived of as a "political choice," disability is removed from the realm of nature and placed squarely into the realm of human achievement. Any inaccessible environment would now be responsible for its inaccessible character. Inaccessibility would necessarily be framed within the idea of political (human) choice and not simply within the "rule of nature" taken as a given. But the environment which surrounds disabled people and with which they have a relationship is still socially constructed from the building blocks of a concept of nature. Otherness to disability is the body-able—the natural body. Even though it may be the case that culture is "inscribed on the body," it is inscribed on a natural one. As Susan Bordo explains:

> Throughout my discussion, it will be assumed that the body, far from being some fundamentally stable, acultural constant to which we must contrast all culturally relative and institutional forms, is constantly "in the grip," as Foucault puts it, of cultural practices . . . there is no "natural" body. Cultural practices . . . are already and always inscribed, as Foucault has emphasized, "on our bodies and their materiality, their

forces, energies, sensations, and pleasures" [*The History of Sexuality* 15].
Our bodies, no less than anything else that is human, are constituted by
culture. (142)

As much as the notion of the "natural body" is an inscription of culture, it still presupposes a body upon which culture may write and be
written. Able-bodiedness is constituted by culture and serves as a method
for distinguishing between "natural" relations to an environment and
"unnatural" ones. "Gripping" (understanding) a body as disabled requires
both the script of culture and the *tabula rasa* upon which culture writes.
As much as culture constitutes this "blank slate," it requires it to write
the script of disability. The cultural idea of misfortune absolutely requires
a "natural body" even though, as Bordo says, "there is no natural body."
Relations to an environment are always-already constituted through a
concept of a human body perceiving and moving through an environment. The distinction between disability and able-bodiedness is thus
scripted by a culture that is gripped by an understanding of ability written in the language of the "natural body."

When disability is conceived of as the unfortunate condition of impairment, the "problem" of disability becomes that of developing an
adaptive relationship to misfortune. This view recommends that disabled
persons make a place in the environment by adapting themselves so that
they are "able" to "fit into" the environment that surrounds them, unnatural as it may be. With adaptive technologies and practices, disability can be shaped so that it can "fit" into the place that the environment
has ready-made for it. "Making a place" is a foreign idea to those who
understand that the only possibility open to them is that of adaptation.
Adopting an adaptive identity is one way for disabled persons to develop
the "ability" to "fit into" the environment that surrounds them.

Even though adaptation is sometimes seen as a necessary and even
as a sufficient orientation for those suffering an injustice to adopt, it is
never seen as the "highest good" attainable, as it is for those suffering
a misfortune. In fact, adapting to injustice may be seen as misfortune.
An unfortunate outcome of unjust treatment is that victims sometimes
adapt. Disability is typically conceived as misfortune, and the concept of misfortune is extended to interpret social treatments such as lack
of access to public buildings. Like disability itself, therefore, inaccessibility may be viewed as misfortune.

Despite recent legislative initiatives that define lack of access to disabled persons as illegal and thus unjust, inaccessibility is still a salient
feature in the lives of disabled persons. Legislation itself insists on accessibility, but only if accommodations are reasonable.[3] Accessibility for
disabled persons to public buildings and services such as universities is
legislatively provided unless, of course, it is unreasonable to do so. The

legislative notion of "undue hardship" offers reasonable grounds for not providing accessibility. Unfortunately, the social and physical environments remain a barrier to disabled persons, since the "social construction" of barrier-free environments is "unduly hard" to achieve.

Although the contemporary (especially legislative) concept of disability includes the idea of injustice, it still tends toward misfortune as its primary interpretative category. Shklar's notion of "political choice" is still not firmly attached to contemporary interpretations of disability. One account of society's exclusion of disabled persons is "cost"—it simply costs too much to make a society accessible to us. Society—a version of a physical and social environment—is by "nature" inaccessible to disabled persons. Wheelchair ramps, talking elevators, braille markings are "extras"—and costly ones at that—to the creation of an environment. But it is unreasonable to expect a society to bear the costs of adding such "unnatural" features to its "natural" environment. This is viewed as simply the misfortune of disability.

Shklar reminds us that in society's self-creation and perpetuation it "chooses" to exclude disabled persons. Understanding inaccessibility from this perspective removes it from the realm of misfortune and places it into the realm of injustice and requires that disabled persons be treated as members of society. The essentially paradoxical rationale of a society that excludes the very social identity it requires (membership) in order to create and perpetuate itself, once again, raises the idea of choice (Zola 244). Such exclusion makes reference to the idea that certain members are excluded despite their membership, and this returns us to the question of social identity, the place within which it is created and perpetuated and the place to which it belongs.

Identity Politics and Disability

"Disability" can be viewed as persons with physical or mental impairments who are surrounded by identity politics much in the same way they are surrounded by a social and physical environment. While the environment around disabled persons may not be theirs, the identity of the politics surrounding them certainly is. The exclusion of disabled persons from society marked by instances of inaccessibility does suggest that disability exists on the margins of society. From the margins, this liminal existence, as Murphy et al. point out, does influence the self-definition of disabled persons and does recommend a "marginal identity" (235–42).

The process of marginalization brings to the fore the collective and thus political character of self-definition and identity-formation. Disability brings people face-to-face with the environment as a barrier and provides us with a glimpse of how instances of inaccessibility depict a lack of access to taken-for-granted ways of moving in and through an environment. The ability to move in an environment is couched, both explicitly and implicitly, within the ideology of a "naturally working body." Thus, disability places people "outside of" not only the environment but also the dominant ideology of able-bodiedness. Disabled persons struggle for access to both; we fight for our "right to access" to the environment, and we sometimes struggle to gain access to the dominant ideology of able-bodiedness by emphasizing our membership in the modern ideology of "personhood." These two struggles are connected insofar as the latter justifies the former. The claim is that "we are persons first and disabled second." Or, "we happen to be disabled, we are persons with disabilities."

This struggle for the "right of access" originates from, and takes place in, the margins. In fact, such a struggle identifies one as existing on the margins. It is a struggle not only for entry into a social and physical environment marked by able-bodiedness as an essential ideology; it is also a struggle to persuade the dominant ideology to adapt its environment to disability and to change its view of disability by adopting the ideology of personhood as primary to all people and thus to understanding disability as a secondary, unessential feature. Thus, "adaptation" remains the fundamental orientation to both the environment and to the dominant ideology of able-bodiedness.

This adaptive orientation in the fight for access can be understood as the struggle for belonging expressed in the political struggle for the place of disability in society. It is to advocate for society itself as the "rightful place" of disability—disabled persons belong in society. To this end, the adaptive orientation demands that society adapt itself to disability by making itself accessible thus accommodating disabled persons. The ideas of adaptation and accommodation advocate for personhood as the essential identity of disability. Since all persons belong in society and since "persons with disabilities" are essentially persons, they too belong. This reasoning holds that disability is essentially a "happenstance," and like the happenstance of any person, disability ought to be adapted to and accommodated in order to preserve the essential belonging-ness of disability in society. The suggestion here is that there is nothing essential about disability and whatever negative effects it brings can be accepted, adjusted to, and accommodated. The possibility that disability is an essential feature of a person and of a society does not enter the realm of the adaptive orientation. This orientation privileges personhood as the only thing that may be essential and relegates disability to the inessential domain of conditionality requiring only adaptation.

Thus, underlying this adaptive orientation is the conception of disability as a condition and a negative one at that. Disability is understood as a condition, typically of the body, and is therefore made sense of under the interpretative schema of medicine. This is why disability is usually approached programmatically and why our society establishes prevention of disability as well as curative programs. Disciplines such as rehabilitation and special education are socially organized to address those "cases" of unpreventable and incurable conditions which cause the condition of disability. These disciplines are programmatically designed to show people how to adapt and adjust in order to live with a disability.

Rehabilitation and special education are political to the extent that they introduce choice into a person's life. For example, disabled persons can choose technologies and techniques that will permit them to do "the normal things" of everyday life such as read despite blindness, be mobile despite quadriplegia, and so on. Still, these practices do not guarantee access to a social and physical environment, nor do they guarantee the conceptual transformation of inaccessibility from an instance of misfortune to an act of injustice. And while adaptive technologies and techniques may make it possible for disabled persons to "function" in some segments of society, they do not guarantee that disability will be conceived as belonging in and to society. Thus, the identity of disability and disabled persons is still wrapped in the cloak of the "ability" to adapt and adjust.

If disability can be spoken of as a "challenge" at all, it is the challenge of the development of social identity and the self-definition in relation, as Gadacz says, to a social and physical environment—in relation to place.

> It's the longing to belong, a deep, visceral need that most linguistically conscious animals who transact with an environment (that's us) participate in. And then there is a profound desire for protection, for security, for safety, for surety. And so, in talking about identity, we have to begin to look at the various ways in which human beings have constructed their desire for recognition, association and protection over time and in space, and always under circumstances not of their own choosing. (West 16)

Whether or not disabled persons participate in an environment depends, of course, upon access to it. Accessible environments or not, however, disabled persons do participate in the longing to belong of which West speaks. We participate also in the desire for recognition, protection, security, and the rest. But we often construct this desire in terms of accessibility and inaccessibility to an environment.

West allows for a fleshing out of the content of the relationship between disabled persons and the environment. This relationship can be understood as one of "transaction" or "negotiation." In transacting with an environment by negotiating access to it, disabled persons are reflexively socially organizing their place as essentially outside the environment and, in that negotiation, are reflexively constructing their social identity as "marginal." Thus, the "challenge of disability" is twofold in character: First, there is the challenge of transacting with an environment through the "adaptive" process whereby disabled persons find technologies and techniques that allow us to engage in the activities of everyday life. Then there is the challenge of negotiating with an environment—a negotiation which takes place from the place and standpoint of marginality. The identity politics of disability are played out within the social space of these challenges and in the moral space where disability and able-bodiedness transact and negotiate with a social and physical environment in which each is understood as essentially Other. The reflexive character of disability resides in the negotiation of an identity. This negotiation must strive for the privileging of disability as essential—we are not people who happen to be, we are people who *are*. We speak from the place of disability, a place which must be made and remade into an essential feature of society.

When Disability Shows Up

> How can the conflict of rival interpretations be arbitrated? . . . Is it not once again *within language* itself that we must seek the indication that understanding is a mode of being?"
> —Ricoeur, *The Conflict of Interpretations*

As we can see from above, there is much to learn from everyday life, and this allows us to engage our most familiar and taken-for-granted experiences. For example, I (Tanya) am a dyslexic woman and my partner (Rod) is a blind man. Responding to discrimination on the basis of disability with laughter, anger, argument is part of my everyday routine. These responses allow me to move through such events while clarifying my view of disability and my world. However, invoking the principle that there is much to be learned from everyday life permits me to ask, "What can be learned from my lived experience of rival interpretations regarding disability?" I will now examine the conversation that Harry, Rod, and I had on the street as an attempt to contribute to the understanding of the relationship between the environment and disabled persons, thus raising the question of the relation between "how things are" and "how they ought to be."

First Encounters of a Shocking Kind

An initial meeting between an able-bodied person and a disabled person is often experienced as a first encounter of a special kind. However, "first encounter" does not necessarily mean that this is the first time that someone has met a disabled person (even though this may be empirically true). All of us possess some idea of disability provided to us by how our society collectively represents it (Michalko; Davis; Fries; Higgins; Thomson; Ingstad and White; Scott; Goffman). Whether we have met a disabled person or not, we have met disability through our common-sense understandings. Thus "first encounter" occurs on every occasion that we meet a particular person with a particular disability. We bring our general understandings (common stock of knowledge) regarding disability to these particular meetings. For example, meeting Rod, Harry said, "Oh, your partner has been telling me about you. I've been wanting to meet you. I have a special interest in the handicapped." Harry is greeting Rod with his understanding of disability, a "special interest in the handicapped" in general. His general interest in the "handicapped" is expressed in his specific interest in meeting Rod; Harry is particularly interested in meeting Rod insofar as he (Harry) is generally interested in the "handicapped."

Recall that Harry told Rod and me that his university discouraged "handicapped" students from attending. My concept of the social representation of disability as the "right" to accessibility and as a morality of belonging in the world led me to hear Harry's comment as nothing but a joke. By saying that disabled students are discouraged from attending the university, Harry is suggesting that "their type" and therefore disabled persons themselves do not belong. Without conceiving of disabled persons as belonging "anywhere in the world" and without assuming Harry held the same concept, I would have interpreted his comment as an act of discrimination and exclusion and therefore not funny at all. Recall that Harry said he had a "special interest in the handicapped." Unless I assumed that Harry has a special interest in telling disabled persons that they are unwelcome, I could hear his subsequent comment only as a joke. In a world in which I assume disability to be an essential feature, even though that world builds barriers to disability and often treats it as inessential, I must understand Harry as joking. Thus, interpreting the comment as a joke is premised upon Harry and me living in the same world and sharing similar concepts of disability. Assuming this, I could hear Harry as joking.

This assumption also generated my experience of shock. I was shocked that Harry was not joking. There are, of course, many ways in which the meeting between able-bodiedness and disability can be shocking. For example, one day Rod and I were working our dogs along a street that borders the campus. As is often the case, Cassis and I had fallen far behind Smokie and Rod. I was, however, still within range to witness the following: A car was leaving campus. It came down a side road that intersected the sidewalk we were walking on. Its driver, looking only for oncoming traffic from the left, did not notice Rod and

Smokie crossing the street from the right. As the driver pulled out and turned right, she caught sight of Rod and Smokie, who abruptly stopped to avoid the collision. The driver then greeted them with a wave.

When Cassis and I caught up to Rod and Smokie, I told Rod that it was Professor Helen who had pulled out in front of him without looking. Rod said, "You'd think that since I have met Helen many times, and she knows about me and other blind people on campus, she would be a little more careful." I remarked, "That's not all. Helen waved at you." We both laughed. This shock, on par with able-bodied persons opening doors for a blind person in absolute silence and then watching while the blind person gropes for the door, stems from an able-bodied person's unworkable concept of disability, an inability or unwillingness to address a person as a disabled person. Silently opening doors for blind people does display the collective representation of blindness as a sign of a "need for help." But this "need" remains alienated from who may need help. In silently opening the door for a blind person, the "helpful" person only opens his/herself to his/her ironic understanding of blindness as a "helpless sighted person." A blind person approaches a door. A sighted person, "knowing" that the blind person will have "trouble" opening the door, opens it. The sighted person does not indicate that the door is open. The blind person "should see" that the door is open. But not seeing this, the blind person tries to open it. The sighted person is surprised. Both stand groping. The door to the building remains open, but the door to any interactional development of what it means to be blind remains closed tighter than ever.

These apparent closures to disability are shocking. It is shocking that Harry would advocate the discouraging of disabled students attending his university, especially when he does so in front of a disabled person who is at his university. It is shocking that Helen waves at Rod. It is shocking that people silently hold doors open for blind people. Shocking as these interactions are, they are also humorous in their irony.

Given the unique character of human interaction and interpretation, Arendt correctly asserts that the only thing that humans can assuredly expect from each other is the "unexpected" (*The Human Condition* 178). What I did not expect was that Harry could say, "We don't encourage the handicapped to come here," and say this in a serious way. Harry did not expect us to laugh, for he was, as he explained, acting reasonably and pragmatically. We can assuredly expect that these unexpected responses to the phenomenon of disability point to the unique interpretations of the meaning of disability in everyday life. The three of us are engaged in an encounter with what disability means and who disabled people are. Rod and I and, we hope, Harry came face-to-face with rival interpretations of, and conflicting relations with, disability.

This raises an epistemological question: What concepts of disability are being employed throughout this encounter? In order to bring to the fore the conflict of rival interpretations, I turn to an analysis of Harry's concept of who disabled persons are and the standpoint from which this concept is derived.

Disability as a Depiction of Environment

Harry framed his first meeting with Rod with a special interest in Rod's experience of the university environment. Initially, this interest was represented in the discussion regarding blind persons' use of elevators. Harry went on to tell us about many other disabled persons he has met. He depicted each disabled person in relation to the university environment and the difficulties this environment imposes on them. For example, Harry told us of a student, new to campus, who uses a wheelchair. Harry told us of the difficulty he and other professors were having "figuring out" how this student could participate in the chapel program. "Right now," said Harry, "some bigger guys are hoisting him up the stairs to the chapel and down the stairs once inside the chapel."

All of Harry's encounters with disabled persons were framed by his sense of the difficulties a disabled student will meet within the university environment. Who disabled persons are is constructed in relation to the fact that they are moving and living in an environment that in various ways is not "set up" for them.

Harry addresses the relation between disabled persons and the environment from an epistemological position which holds that environment brings out who disabled people are and disabilities bring out what an environment is. For example, meeting a blind person on the elevator is framed by Harry's special interest in evaluating the university environment. Meeting a disabled person means, for Harry, addressing the structure and function of an environment constructed to accommodate certain types of people (able-bodied), while making movement potentially difficult for other types (disabled). Harry mentioned how cheaply and easily braille could be added to the elevator. He rejected the installation of chimes to announce floors or speaking elevators as too expensive and difficult to accomplish. Doing things to the environment for disabled persons is a part of Harry's interest in disabled persons, provided these accommodations are inexpensive and can be accomplished with ease. Whoever disabled people are, they are people whose inclusion in an environment can be addressed in a partial way, since addressing them also means addressing expense and ease. Thus, disabled persons are those who require accommodation while the environment is a collective entity willing to do so if it is not too expensive or difficult.

This suggests the "intentionality" of an environment. Harry implies that his university environment is intended to accommodate able-bodied people. Any environment intended for an able-bodied population will certainly show its intentions when the "unintended" (disabled people) show up. Except for inexpensive and easy accommodations, the university environment need not alter its intention for disabled students. After all, disabled students can attend the "totally accessible" university—an environment intended for them. Harry's university was not constructed with disabled students in mind.

Arendt notwithstanding, environments do not expect the unexpected. Harry's "special interest in the handicapped" is a special interest in how each disability, and each disabled person, draws out the intentions of an environment. This environment never intended disabled students to be part of the "able-student-body." Harry encounters disability as a living depiction of the intentions of an environment. Within the context of this encounter on the street, wanting to meet Rod as a "handicapped person" and to ask him about inexpensive elevator accommodations serves as a reaffirmation of the intentions of Harry's environment.

Social theorists such as Bordo, Liggett, and Foucault understand the environment as inscribing itself on individuals and their bodies. These theorists suggest that these inscriptions present particular and serious limits to disabled people. Harry also understands the seriousness of these limits. But what is particular to Harry is his concept of what constitutes a serious relation to the intentional character of an environment as shown by the limits it inscribes on the lives and bodies of disabled people.

A serious relation toward disability is, for Harry, a pragmatic one. For him the presence of disability represents an opportunity to change his environment but only in easy and inexpensive ways while reconfirming the intention of that environment. Disabled persons represent the collective's need to regard an environment's intentions pragmatically—to show that slight changes to an environment can pragmatically preserve its intention.

A pragmatic understanding of the relation between disability and environment can result in a community treating disabled persons' interests, aims, and goals as self-evident. Thus, the need for libraries with books shelved no higher than four feet—an example Harry raised of an accommodation that is too expensive. While pragmatism cannot explain why exclusions or inclusions occur, it does allow for action oriented to making the physical and social environment accessible to disabled persons. Harry's pragmatism, however, does not result in the "self-evident character" of the interests of disabled persons or in the subsequent need for accommodation. Instead, his pragmatic relation is oriented to the intentions and interests established by his institution. Intended as it is for "able-bodied" students, Harry's university did not expect disabled students to show up. For Harry, this "Unexpected Minority," as Gliedman and Roth call it, is even more unexpected given that there is another university whose intention it is to accommodate disabled students.

Harry's pragmatism is held together by the following assumptions: First, the intentions of the institution should be recognized as given and primary; that is, they should be seen as both obvious and reasonable. Second, Harry assumes that it is equally obvious that his institution "never intended" to be "set up" for disabled persons. This intention is reaffirmed on each and every occasion of noticing a disabled person in the university environment. Finally, this obvious organizational feature of the environment should be treated as reasonable given the bureaucratic reasonableness ascribed to the institution. This form of pragmatism is grounded in the assumption that institutional organization is obviously rational and undoubtedly reasonable within the context of its intentionality. This assumption helps to constitute what Bauman calls the "collective fiction" of any bureaucracy (78–84, 131–37). Just as a bureaucracy establishes the fiction that any task or office can be reduced to a singularly clear aim, so too can the people within a bureaucracy be regarded as a singular type with a singular goal.

But disability cannot be framed within the bureaucratic version of a "singular type" or, for that matter, singular goal. There are a variety of types of disabilities as well as a variety of types within a specific disability. Such differences cannot be taken into account when disability is an unintended and thus unexpected feature of an organization. The construction and preservation of a bureaucracy's collective fiction of a "singular type" depend on disability being "seen" as an unintended participant.

The standpoint of pragmatism constructs the reasonable and rational character of its intended exclusions in equally reasonable and rational ways. Exclusion is made a reasonable feature of Harry's university, in part, by establishing the belief[4] that there is some other institution that is pragmatically "all set up for" disabled persons. Exclusion is also rationalized on the basis of the bureaucratic logic which insists that critiquing an institution for something it never intended to include is not a pragmatically oriented evaluation and, thus, should only be regarded as a spurious and unreasonable "complaint." A pragmatic position cannot understand environmental intentions, inscribed upon the lives of disabled persons in the form of limits, as a reflection of "historical oversights" derived from cultural conceptions of the "normal (able-bodied) type." Exclusion is not an "oversight" since Harry's university did not have disabled persons "in-sight" in the first place. Thus, "we don't encourage the handicapped to come here." Exclusion is also made reasonable on the basis of the pragmatist's ability to quantify human experience. As Harry said, "It's ridiculous to fix this and that, and spend all that money, for just a few students." The strength and weakness of pragmatism begins and ends in its ability to engage its people as quantifiable things. These "things" are measured in relation to the costs and benefits they present to an institution which is conditioned by its finite resources and is governed by preestablished and rationalized intentions.

Nonetheless, it is pragmatically necessary for every institution to deal with unintended and unexpected participants—if they happen to show up. Institutions do not expect the unexpected, but the intended participants of an institution cannot escape from noticing and dealing with unexpected participants who happen to come along. There are no moral or even legal grounds for preventing the unexpected from showing up or for asking them to leave when they do so. What the pragmatist faces when he or she meets a disabled person is a challenge—the challenge of what to do in the presence of the unexpected. I now turn to an explication of the challenge disability presents.

Disability as a Challenge to Pragmatism

The presence of disabled students at a university represents, for some, the requirement of additional expense and organization.[5] There is the expense of accommodations such as wheelchair ramps, elevators, braille signage, interpreters for those who use sign language, and so on. Faculty may be required to reorganize their teaching methods to accommodate disabled students. Traditional methods of administering examinations, for example, may not work with dyslexic students. This sort of reorganization and additional expense, as well as many others like them, are understood by some as a drain upon university resources.

The challenge that disability presents to the pragmatist is the need to develop a justification for such additional expenditures. This is not to say that Harry's university is not challenged by those expenditures required by their intended (able-bodied) students. Fund-raising is an integral part of any university's life. But the raising of funds in order to construct a new building, upgrade computer systems, and the like is a justifiable activity for the pragmatist insofar as these expenditures are required in order to serve an intended student body. However, the raising of funds for wheelchair ramps, elevators, etc., in order to serve students who are not conceived of as part of the intended student body, is understood as an additional expense and as a drain on university resources.

Harry insists that his university was not constructed or organized with the intention of serving disabled students. Thus any reconstruction or reorganization is as unexpected and unintended as is the presence of disabled students themselves. Of course, any unexpected expense is always met with the need for justification and rationalization. This is part of the challenge Harry faces when he meets disabled students. He frames this challenge within a cost/benefit paradigm. What possible benefit could disabled persons present that can be tallied against their cost to the university? Harry's challenge is to "balance the books" on disability.

Harry has, however, found a way to develop such accounting procedures by transforming the lives of disabled persons into "living depictions of environmental intentions." This is the benefit of having disabled persons around. Harry sees a benefit in disability because it brings to the fore and clarifies the intentions of his university. For Harry, this is the only pragmatic justification for the presence of disability even though this justification does not entirely rationalize the additional expenditure.

In order to balance the books on disabled students, it is necessary to make assumptions regarding what is valuable and what is not. Pragmatism cannot establish the value of anything because it assumes its value. For example, the value of a university education must first be assumed before any pragmatic action as to its organization and implementation can take place. The value of a student body which the university intends to serve must first be assumed before a university can measure the benefits and costs of serving them. If such value is not assumed, the pragmatist would fall into the never-ending question "Well, what's the benefit of doing that?"[6]

The doing of "little things" for disabled persons reflects their assumed value—their value is so minimal that "little things" are all that is required to be done. This "minimalist" version of disability ensures that there is minimal expense and minimal reorganization to the university, especially to the sense of its intentionality. At best, disabled persons raise the issue of the intentions of an environment. But the environment responds to the raising of the question of its intention by pointing to the intention itself as a justification for minimal acts of minimal inclusion, i.e., for the doing of little things. Disabled students are costly participants insofar as disability represents what is not intended by an environment. This version of pragmatism produces disabled persons as an unintended minority. This production of the unintended lies at the heart of the social significance of disability and severely restricts the horizon of interpretive possibilities in relation to disability as a form of life.

The interpretation of disabled persons as "unintended" is not idiosyncratic in character. For example, the institutionalized accommodation mechanisms at Harry's university are also grounded in this understanding. Individual disabled students are expected to file a request with the Senate Committee contact person, who will "communicate with students with disabilities" and who "will make arrangements with the appropriate administrative office for assistance" which "might respond to their [disabled students'] special needs." The students are expected to inform the contact person of their "personal" accommodation needs. Consider, for example, that the university environment is often not accessible to persons who use wheelchairs. Thus, these individuals must request that space be organized to accommodate their wheelchairs in the particular classrooms, and only those classrooms, in which they will be attending classes. This is why there are only a few classrooms that are wheelchair accessible at Harry's university. An assumption guiding the functionality of this system of personal requests is that disabled students will conceive of themselves as unintended participants and request only those types of accommodation that will not radically influence the environment's intentions to conceive of them as such. Despite this piecemeal accommodation policy, it is not idiosyncratic. This policy represents the dominant standpoint which articulates disabled students as unintended. Harry represents this standpoint, he did not invent it on his own, and therefore his concept of disabled students cannot be interpreted simply as an idiosyncratic point of view.

The environment reaffirms its intention by continually raising the unintended character of disability and, thus, the environment is committed to the doing of "little things," since any "big thing" would mean a radical change to the intention of the environment. Even though disabled persons exist "in the environment," there are few signs of full integration of disabled persons with the environment.[7] Disabled persons remain the unintended and unexpected minority even though this minority may not be so minor.[8] Anyone at anytime and anywhere may become disabled. As Gadacz says, disability is "a social category whose membership is always open" (xi). Given the age of tenured professors and staying within the language of "probability," these professors, including Harry, have a good chance of joining the ranks of the disabled population.

Pragmatism as a Relation Between Disability and the Environment

Even though a pragmatic point of view has much to say about disability, it does not typically understand itself as a relationship between disability and the environment. There is no doubt that pragmatism sees a difference between disabled people and those who are not and even sees that the two hold different environmental requirements. But pragmatism frames these differences as a "gap" between that which is intended and that which is not. This gap, moreover, is only to be filled with practical action or justifications for inaction. This understanding can lead ironically to both the segregation of disabled persons (a university "all set up for them") and the beginnings of integration (the doing of "little things"). This gap between environment and disability is a specter which haunts both exclusionary and inclusionary discursive practices based on pragmatism as a taken-for-granted good. But until pragmatism is understood as a relationship between disabled persons and the environment, segregation and integration will be orientations that have equal justification in an environment understood as intended strictly for those who are able-bodied.

Disability, like able-bodiedness, is never only a pragmatic matter. Disability is always lived within an environment, and the relation between the two is always-already a matter of development. I end with some thoughts on the development of such a relation.

The relatively new, but rapidly growing, field of disability studies[9] often turns its analytic gaze to the environment within which disabled persons move and live. Recall, Gadacz's formulation: "Disability can be viewed as a relationship between a person with a physical or mental impairment and the social and physical environment around him or her" (5). Disabled and able-bodied persons alike find themselves in the midst of a social and physical environment. The difference between disability and able-bodiedness springs from the imputed intention of an environment. For whom is the environment intended? For whom is it constructed? It is only when the answer to these questions is "able-bodiedness" that the difference between persons who are disabled and those who are not emerges. The relation between disability and the environment is, therefore, framed by the problem of living in an environment which neither intends nor expects disability.

The relation between a person and the social and physical environment is not only one way that disability "can be viewed"; it is often the only way. Disability often comes into view as a confrontation with a social and physical environment. Pragmatism frames relations with disability within the intended/unintended dichotomy understood as confrontation. This standpoint reveals pragmatism as a dominant value that organizes both theoretic and practical approaches to disability.

Pragmatism encourages us to read the interaction between people and their environment as if it were only a text of institutionalized intentionality. This intentionality appears remarkably clear when I observe a person in a wheelchair confronted by a flight of stairs. Regardless of the standpoint from which disability is viewed—whether from rehabilitation (e.g., Harrison and Crow), from university administration (e.g., accommodation policy), from consumerism (e.g., Gadacz, Shapiro), or from disability itself (e.g., Murphy, Zola)—the text of the intention of the physical and social environment is inscribed, to borrow from Foucault, upon the lives of disabled persons as they move through it.

Theorizing forms of exclusion, Dorothy Smith reminds us that "Texts are the primary medium (though not the substance) of power" ("Peculiar Eclipsing" 374). The text of an environment's intentions is mediated through the interaction between the physical and social environment and the lives of disabled and able-bodied persons. But this mediation, says Smith, is not the substance of power. The substance of power lies elsewhere; it lies in the discursive practices of people who have chosen to read the interaction between disabled persons and the environment in a pragmatic way. The power of pragmatism lies in its exclusion of any imaginative relation to disability other than that of practicality.

Theorizing the relation between reading and power can assist in developing the relation between disability and the environment. Despite the fact that the discipline of cultural studies generally occludes the identity category of disability,[10] it has spent much energy theorizing the relation between reading and power. Atkinson and Middlehurst, for example, say

> Questions regarding the manufacture and institutional legitimation of social inequality, together with how counter-power challenges these forces, are axiomatic as prioritized concerns in the critical theorization of culture. . . ; however, even here scant regard has been given to the fact that texts are multiply read and their meanings negotiated, even resisted. (113)

The interaction between rival interpretations (e.g., institutionalized inequality and counter-power challenges) stands as "axiomatic" for the critical theorization of cultural organization and the possibility of "resistance." The crossroads of rival interpretations present us with the possibility of alternative readings or, at least, with readings which can attend to the standpoints that ground them. Perhaps this is why Goffman refers to interactions between the "normals" and the "stigmatized" as "one of the primal scenes of sociology" (*Stigma* 13), and why Ricoeur claims that it is only in the conflict of rival interpretations that we are able to glean the meaning of anything.

That there are multiple ways to read the way in which the environment inscribes its intentions onto the lives of disabled persons is thus highly significant. Focusing our reading on the interactional accomplishment of an environment's supposed intentionality allows for a reading that goes beyond pragmatic interests such as assessing the cost of accommodation or measuring the extent to which disabled persons have been excluded from the environment. If the text of disability is understood so as to reveal the interpretive axes of able-bodiedness/disability and structure/agency, then not only will rival interpretations come into focus but readers can also begin to ask, along with Zola, "Why [has] a society been created and perpetuated which has excluded so many of its members?" (244).

The confrontation between disability and an environment often seduces members of a community (able-bodied and disabled alike) into conceiving of pragmatism as the only way of reading the interactions that occur between an environment and its people. This is not to say that pragmatically oriented readings of the environment, which serve to endow the environment with intentionality, are not decisive acts, for they certainly are. However, they are not acts that must remain steeped in mystification. It is, after all, people who produce such intentionality and reproduce it through pragmatic justifications and practices.

Finally, the sensibility of pragmatically justified exclusion does not lie in the cost that disabled persons represent. The radical exclusion of the pragmatically organized environment does not exist only in an abundance of stairs, poor lighting, missing hand rails, doors that can be opened only by a "strong man," or elevators without braille markings. Instead, it exists through a reading of disability and the environment that maintains the rational and reasonable character of exclusion itself.

Notes

1. For excellent examples of relationships between disability and the able-bodied public, see Cahill and Eggleston 140–50; Davis; Gadacz; Zola.

2. Even though race and gender are distinguishable from disability within the concepts of "belonging," it is important to note that race and gender are social constructions and any "natural" appearance of these categories are such only when constructed to appear as "natural."

3. Canadian as well as American legislation have "accommodation within reason" provisions. For a review of such legislation, see Driedger; Gadacz; Jones; Shapiro.

4. Many established members of the university, including faculty and administrators, have told me about this "totally accessible" university. "That university, twenty years ago, decided to become accessible," or "that university receives all the funding for disability issues." (But many students have insisted such total funding is a myth.) As true as these comments may be, it is also true that moving, living, and working with disabled persons on this university campus inevitably leads to stories about "that university." The story of the "totally accessible" university is the story of a "little utopia" that does not intend to exclude disabled persons. At the same time, these stories function as a morality tale for disabled persons and not for the able-bodied members of Harry's university. The moral of the story is that all reasonable and rational disabled persons ought to go to the "totally accessible" university.

5. That disabled students represent an additional expense to a university is only so when such students are not understood as essential to the university. Whether or not the day will come when our society understands accommodations to disabled persons as a routine part of organizational life and thus not as an additional expense is difficult to say, since disability may always be viewed as an "unfortunate" aspect of human life.

6. Taylor puts the issue this way: "The utilitarian lives within a moral horizon which cannot be explicated by his own moral theory. This is one of the great

weaknesses of utilitarianism" (31–32). The pragmatist bases his/her decisions on their eventual utility and thus never addresses the "moral theory" that generates these decisions.

7. For an excellent review of the exclusion of disabled persons from aspects of Canadian life such as employment, recreation, education, etc., see Gadacz (esp. chs. 2 and 3).

8. Statistics Canada (1991) documents the disability rate of the working-age population at 17.7 percent. Zola, working with United States data, says that illness may be a "statistical norm" and that any American "is at best momentarily able-bodied [and] . . . will at some point suffer from one or more chronic diseases and be disabled, temporarily or permanently, for a significant portion of their lives" (242–43). Gadacz, working with Canadian data, comes close to the same conclusion.

9. In one of the first disability studies readers, editor Lennard Davis says, "So, this reader appears at the moment that disability, always an actively repressed *momento mori* for the fate of the normal body, gains a new, non-medicalized, and positive legitimacy both as an academic discipline and as an area of political struggle" (1). Like any new area of study, attaining legitimacy is a difficult political struggle. This struggle has been particularly difficult for disability studies insofar as the study of disabled people has been dominated by research produced from an ableist perspective such as the medico-rehabilitative model. For the genesis of disability studies, see Oliver. Other excellent examples of work in this new field can be found in Ingstad and Whyte and in Mitchell and Snyder.

10. For example, see Ferguson et al., *Out There: Marginalization and Contemporary Culture,* in which disability is never imagined as an identity category even when long lists of marginal people are generated. This occlusion leads to the cultural reproduction of disability as simply a metaphor for lack. For example, West describes the "New World *bricoleurs*" of the Cultural Politics of Difference as "persons from all countries, cultures, genders, sexual orientations, ages and regions with protean identities who avoid ethnic chauvinism and faceless universalisms" (25–26). These are the "flexible" people who avoided the "silences and blindnesses" (26, 35) of male WASP hegemony. For an analysis of this occlusion, see Michalko, *The Two-in-One;* Titchkosky, "Disability Studies: The Old and the New."

Works Cited

Adam, Barbara, and Stuart Allan, eds. *Theorizing Culture: An Interdisciplinary Critique After Postmodernism.* New York: New York UP, 1995.

Arendt, Hannah. "Action and the Pursuit of Happiness," paper delivered at the meeting of the American Science Association, Sept. 1960.

———. *The Human Condition.* Chicago: U of Chicago P, 1958.

———. *Men in Dark Times.* New York: Harcourt Brace, 1955.

Atkinson, Karen, and Rob Middlehurst. "Representing AIDS: The Textual Politics of Health Discourse." Adam and Allan 113–28.

Bailey, Gordon, and Noga Gayle, eds. *Sociology: An Introduction from the Classics to Contemporary Feminists.* Toronto: Oxford UP, 1993.

Bauman, Zygmunt. *Thinking Sociologically.* Oxford: Basil Blackwell, 1990.

Bordo, Susan. *Unbearable Weight: Feminism, Western Culture, and the Body.* Berkeley: U of California P, 1993.

Cahill, Spencer E., ed. *Inside Social Life: Readings in Sociological Psychology and Microsociology.* Los Angeles: Roxbury, 1998.

Cahill, Spencer E., and Robin Eggleston. "Wheelchair Users' Interpersonal Management of Emotions." Cahill 140–50.

Cormack, Patricia. "The Paradox of Durkheim's Manifesto: Reconsidering *The Rules of Sociological Method.*" *Theory and Society* 25 (1996): 85–104.

Davis, Lennard J. *The Disability Studies Reader.* New York: Routledge, 1997.

Driedger, Diane. *The Last Civil Rights Movement: Disabled People's International.* New York: St. Martin's, 1989.

Ferguson, Russel, Martha Gever, Trinh T. Minh-ha, and Cornel West, eds. *Out There: Marginalization and Contemporary Cultures.* Cambridge: MIT Press, 1990.

Foucault, Michel. *The History of Sexuality.* New York: Vintage Books, 1980.

Fries, Kenny, ed. *Staring Back: The Disability Experience from the Inside Out.* New York: Plume, 1997.

Gadacz, Rene. *Re-Thinking Dis-Ability: New Structures, New Relationships.* Edmonton: U of Alberta P, 1994.

Gliedman, John, and William Roth. *The Unexpected Minority: Handicapped Children in America.* New York: Harcourt Brace Jovanovich, 1980.

Goffman, Erving. *Behaviour in Public Places: Notes on the Social Organization of Gatherings.* New York: Free Press, 1963.

———. *The Presentation of Self in Everyday Life.* New York: Doubleday-Anchor, 1959.

———. *Stigma: Notes on the Management of Spoiled Identity.* Englewood Cliffs, NJ: Prentice-Hall, 1963.

Harrison, Felicity, and Mary Crow. *Living and Learning with Blind Children: A Guide for Parents and Teachers of Visually Impaired Children.* Toronto: U of Toronto P, 1993.

Higgins, Paul C. "Outsiders in a Hearing World." Rubington and Weinberg 335–44.

Ingstad, Benedicte, and Susan Reynolds Whyte, eds. *Disability and Culture.* Berkeley: U of California P, 1995.

Jenks, Chris, ed. *Visual Culture.* London: Routledge, 1995.

Jones, Ruth J. E. *Their Rightful Place: Society and Disability.* Toronto: Canadian Academy of the Arts, 1994.

Liggett, Helen. "Stars Are Not Born: An Interpretive Approach to the Politics of Disability." *Disability, Handicap, and Society* 3.3 (1988): 263–75.

Michalko, Rod. "Accomplishing a Sighted World." *Reflections: Canadian Journal of Visual Impairment* 1 (1982): 9–30.

———. *The Mystery of the Eye and the Shadow of Blindness.* Toronto: U of Toronto P, 1998.

―――. *The Two-in-One: Walking with Smokie, Walking with Blindness*. Philadelphia: Temple UP, 1999.

Mitchell, David T., and Sharon L. Snyder, eds. *The Body and Physical Difference: Discourses of Disability*. Ann Arbor: U of Michigan P, 1997.

Murphy, Robert F. *The Body Silent*. New York: W. W. Norton, 1987.

Murphy, R., J. Scheer, Y. Murphy, and R. Mack. "Physical Disability and Social Liminality: A Study in the Rituals of Adversity." *Social Science and Medicine*. 26.2 (1988): 235–42.

Oliver, Michael. *The Politics of Disablement*. Basingstoke, UK: Macmillan, 1990.

―――. *Understanding Disability: From Theory to Practice*. New York: St. Martin's P, 1996.

Rajchman, John, ed. *The Identity in Question*. New York: Routledge, 1995.

Razack, Sherene H. *Looking White People in the Eye: Gender, Race, and Culture in Courtrooms and Classrooms*. Toronto: U of Toronto P, 1998.

Ricoeur, Paul. *The Conflict of Interpretations: Essays in Hermeneutics*. Ed. Don Ihde. Evanston: Northwestern UP, 1974.

Rubington, Earl, and Martin S. Weinberg, eds. *Deviance: The Interactionist Perspective*. 6th ed. Boston: Allyn and Bacon, 1996.

Scott, Robert A. *The Making of Blind Men: A Study of Adult Socialization*. New Brunswick, NJ: Transaction Books, 1981.

Shapiro, Joseph P. *No Pity: People with Disabilities Forging a New Civil Rights Movement*. New York: Times Books, 1993.

Shklar, Judith N. *The Faces of Injustice*. New Haven: Yale UP, 1990.

Smith, E. Dorothy. *The Everyday World as Problematic: A Feminist Sociology*. Toronto: U of Toronto P, 1987.

―――. "A Peculiar Eclipsing: Women's Exclusion from Man's Culture." Bailey and Gayle 347–70.

Statistic Canada. "Health and Activity Limitation Survey." 1991. <www.statcan.ca/english/Pgdb/People/health/health12b.htm>.

Taylor, Charles. *Sources of the Self: The Making of Modern Identity*. Cambridge: Harvard UP, 1989.

Thomson, Rosemarie Garland. *Extraordinary Bodies: Figuring Physical Disability in American Culture and Literature*. New York: Columbia UP, 1997.

Titchkosky, Tanya. "Disability Studies: The Old and the New." *Canadian Journal of Sociology* 25.2 (2000): 197–224.

―――. "Women, Anorexia, and Change." *Dharma* 23.4 (1998).

Townsend, Elizabeth. *Good Intentions Overruled: A Critique of Empowerment in the Routine Organization of Mental Health Services*. Toronto: U of Toronto P, 1998.

Turner, Stephen P, ed. *Social Theory and Sociology: The Classics and Beyond*. Cambridge, MA: Basil Blackwell, 1996.

Wendell, Susan. "Toward a Feminist Theory of Disability." *The Disability Studies Reader*. Ed. Lennard J. Davis. 260–78.

West, Cornel. "A Matter of Life and Death." Rajchman 15–32.

―――. "The New Cultural Politics of Difference." Ferguson, Gevner, Trinh, and West 19–36.

Wolfe, Alan. *The Human Difference: Animals, Computers, and the Necessity of Social Science.* Berkeley: U of California P, 1993.
Zola, Irving Kenneth. *Missing Pieces: A Chronicle of Living with a Disability.* Philadelphia: Temple UP, 1982.

12

The Rhetoric of AIDS:
A New Taxonomy

Emily F. Nye

AIDS has become commonplace in modern life. Our children learn about it in their early grades, and education continues through high school and adulthood. Most people know, or know of, someone with AIDS or HIV, and we have accepted the fact that AIDS is here to stay.

But AIDS has changed since the 1980s. An increasing number of people are able to live with HIV. In fact, with early drug treatment, thousands with HIV are living for years without contracting AIDS. Where once people died from AIDS, now people live with AIDS. In the case of HIV and AIDS, the "disability," like the disease, is acquired. Some people who test HIV positive may never choose to use the label "disabled." Perhaps it is a stretch to compare AIDS with a more "conventional" disability, but I argue that people with AIDS undergo a similar perception of being disabled—they live with a physical and emotional stigma because of their "impairment." By examining the rhetoric of AIDS, we understand the idea of "disability" from a different vantage point.

In this chapter, I argue that AIDS discourse requires a new paradigm of thought. Given the complex rhetoric of AIDS, as well as its medical description and history, an evolving framework is needed for viewing the disease/condition, and this idea applies to how we approach any disability. I compose a view in four parts: AIDS the Divider, AIDS the Reformer, AIDS the Empowerer, and AIDS the Educator. My purpose is to use the existing discourse(s) of AIDS, complete with metaphors, in a way that links constructively with Cindy Patton's conception of "new knowledge." She writes that if "interactions are prolonged and power relations reordered, this knowledge produces a new thought style which is the possession of a new community" (74). The new thought style would almost certainly be a more informed and unbiased attitude about AIDS; the new community might be a more effective alliance of the diverse people and groups working in AIDS. The framework is not meant to denote a linear process from the various categories outlined. These categories coexist, and each poses a way of making sense of AIDS. A closer look at the language we use to define AIDS—and particularly metaphorical language—follows.

AIDS and Its Metaphors

The discourse of AIDS reflects the society that constructs it. This discourse consists of certain metaphors and language that influence our understanding and experience of the disease. The structure and style of AIDS discourse—rhetoric—is of central concern. Lee Edelman suggests that AIDS is an unmanageable subject for writing. Both Edelman and Susan Sontag call AIDS a plague of discourse, while Paula Treichler says that in addition to being a lethal disease, it is also an epidemic of meaning and signification. The mention of AIDS evokes a cross between awe and horror.

Because AIDS is a complicated "disability," a solely sentimental portrayal can be misleading. Sontag asks us to examine the social and ideological implications embedded within our language regarding AIDS. This article attempts to expose AIDS discourse(s) and lead the reader through a deconstruction and reconstruction of a particular rhetoric, an approach that may be applied to examine the rhetoric of other disabilities.

An important factor in how society perceives AIDS is how we learn about it. The mass media image of AIDS (television and movies) is one influence, and the rhetoric of AIDS as transmitted through the popular press is another. This discussion of the rhetoric of AIDS begins by exploring how metaphor functions and then by exploring how language use is determined by and determines the "discourse communities" surrounding AIDS.

Metaphors in language carry value as well as meaning. People need metaphors from daily life in order to understand scientific concepts. But Patton points out that if the "right" metaphors are found, "the information given to the lay person is roughly equivalent in its practical effects to that produced by science" (72). Therefore, we must question the language used to describe AIDS and examine metaphor closely. Patton, as well as many AIDS activists and scholars, maintains a distrustful attitude toward science and the media. Sontag goes so far as to suggest that those who write about AIDS are concerned with gaining rhetorical control over the illness. She asks us to question how the disease "is possessed, assimilated in argument and in cliché" (184).

The most common metaphors used to describe AIDS include military metaphors, end-of-the-world metaphors, plague metaphors, and contamination or pollution metaphors (Neil). These metaphors perpetuate a divisive quality of strife, which I will discuss under AIDS the Divider. In general, the AIDS virus is viewed as something mysterious and deadly. It takes on its own character of being, according to Patton, as a hunk of protein that refuses to reveal its secrets (25). A peripheral metaphor of communication can be detected in AIDS discourse: Dealing with the virus requires understanding codes, transcription, messenger, RNA, and evasion. This depiction of AIDS portrays a language incomprehensible to most lay people, but penetrable by the experts. We have therefore developed a reliance on the experts to teach us about AIDS. The common person remains detached and powerless to understand the disease.

Military metaphors abound in the rhetoric of AIDS. Such metaphors borrow militaristic language and imagery. When journalists used such terms as "lost in action" to describe those who died of AIDS, victimization could be implied. A sense of tragic loss and mystery prevailed. When gay writers used similar metaphors, the effect could be interpreted differently. In *And the Band Played On*, Randy Shilts used chapter titles like "Enemy Time" and "Battle Lines" to establish the sense of a raging war. Historian Michael Sherry states that the war imagery implies enemies, allies, and battle plans. He believes that this language of war served to "galvanize collective action against AIDS" (40).

Sontag takes an opposing view as she notes the prevalence of military metaphors in the literature of AIDS. The effect of military imagery on thinking about sickness and health, she writes, overmobilizes, overdescribes, "and powerfully contributes to the excommunicating and stigmatizing of the ill" (182). Donna Haraway applies the metaphor framework to the larger picture of immunology, saying that as AIDS moves to the realm of "high" science, the World War II military metaphors (battles, struggles) have upgraded to the language of postmodern warfare (communication, coding) (cited in Treichler 59).

Sontag also cites an overall end-of-the-world metaphor concerning AIDS. She attributes this to the fact that AIDS "seems the very model of the catastrophes privileged populations feel await them" (172). Authoritarian political ideologies, according to Sontag, benefit from promoting fear and a sense of takeover by aliens. AIDS is already predisposed to be a disease of otherness because of its association with homosexuality as well as drug use. An end-of-the-world rhetoric conjures up apocalyptic scenarios. But it also suggests the chance to begin again. This, claims Sontag, is a very modern American proposition. For people dealing with AIDS on a daily basis, the apocalyptic scenario could be overwhelmingly negative. Many people with AIDS would debate the "chance to begin again" proposition as being naive and "Pollyanna-ish."

AIDS as a plague and as a contaminating agent are other common metaphors. Sander Gilman compares the depiction of people with AIDS to representations of people with syphilis. Syphilis patients were isolated and shunned in much the same way that AIDS patients are today. Gilman suggests that popular media images of people with AIDS reflect poses reminiscent of the classical iconography of melancholy (252).

The language used to describe AIDS seems understandable, but actually is complex and full of intricate meaning. We have all heard (and believe we understand) the term *safe sex*, but Patton offers a closer reading. Safe sex distinguishes itself from *natural sex*. Safe people can have sex naturally, without condoms. But everyone else "fails" and is punished with unnatural sex. She also suggests that certain terms may work together to inform people constructively about safe sex. For example, *bodily fluids* is a term criticized by some AIDS activists for being more vague than the specific terms *semen* and *blood*. Patton defends *bodily fluids*: "Such use avoids the difficulties of the heavy moral baggage carried by both semen and blood in this culture—both are already constructed as venal, fatal fluids" (45). If the basic goal is to prevent the spread of AIDS, those who construct information about the disease must acknowledge the hidden meanings, the "heavy moral baggage" that comes packed in language.

Metaphorical language represents the intellectual, cultural, and moral constitution of its speakers. This brief overview suggests some of the complexities that require a careful reading of the discourses of AIDS—including questioning the very language we may take for granted when reading about AIDS in various contexts and through various disciplinary lenses.

AIDS Discourse Communities

A school of thought in composition theory helps draw a parallel between how social historians and critics like Gilman, Patton, and Sontag approach the discourse of AIDS and how I as a composition teacher approach the examination of discourse. In composition, many teachers and scholars follow a social construction view of discourse. Language is not something we practice in isolation. Language, according to James Boyd White, reflects a social world:

> Whenever you speak, you define a character for yourself and for at least One other—your audience—and make a community at least between the two of you; and you do this in a language that is of necessity provided to you by others and modified in your use of it. (xi)

Language thus functions only in relation to others. The relationship between the individual and culture is integrally linked with the other, and language is one conduit. Language is not static; it is ever-changing and "remade by its speakers, who are themselves remade both as individuals and as communities, in what they say" (x). As a community changes, so does its discourse.

Ken Bruffee applies this social constructivist theory to writing, which he claims is "internalized social talk made public and social again" (641). Individuals think to themselves and speak out loud. Bruffee writes, "To the extent that thought is internalized conversation, then, any effort to understand how we think requires us to understand the nature of community life that generates and maintains conversation" (640). Through a social construction view of discourse, we must carefully examine "community life" in its full linguistic and contextual complexity. Who belongs to the community? How do they think? What do they believe? Bruffee writes about a "community of knowledgeable peers—people who accept, and whose work is guided by, the same paradigms and the same code of values and assumptions" (642). Those engaged in conversation constitute what James Kinneavy calls a discourse community, while Jay Robinson calls it membership in a literacy community. He states that, as language users and social beings, humans must learn to be "critical, participatory members of the literacy club [they] join" (46). Pertaining to AIDS, this "club" consists of those infected with HIV. They would constitute a community of discourse.

Readers of "human interest journalism" constitute another community of discourse. People who need to know the technical angles of safe sex constitute another discourse community. A distinction begins to emerge between public education (i.e., AIDS information conveyed in general terms for the "majority" of readers) and community education (information geared toward individuals with particular concerns and characteristics). Treichler defines this as a continuum between popular and biomedical discourse. Patton discerns three main discourse communities concerning AIDS: AIDS experts, people with AIDS, and volunteers. From the emergence of AIDS to the present, each community has developed its own parlance. Many people with AIDS have a great deal of medical knowledge and emotional experience with the disease, yet if they begin to speak out of character as "experts," they are not taken seriously.

To interact effectively with the array of people who have AIDS, it is important for all people who deal with AIDS to have an understanding of the interrelationships of discourse communities. These individuals should also be aware of their own discourse. Treichler says that AIDS is a nexus where multiple stories, meanings, and discourses overlap and intersect, reinforcing and subverting each other (31). This nexus is rich and complex, but it is a mixed blessing. It is tempting to listen only to the loudest or more prominent stories being told or to oversimplify the meanings expressed. In fact, such a nexus offers the potential to illuminate the less visible stories, and it challenges us to untangle various competing views.

Indeed, different communities may have distinct agendas. Brochures and booklets produced from government funds are mandated to use language that is accessible but not "offensive" to a range of educated adults. Clearly, what one reader finds offensive the next may find to be persuasive. For example, when the Centers for Disease Control completed their first national sweep of AIDS information in 1988, they needed to produce a range of brochures. In Latino communities, the photos featured Latinos and Spanish text; in gay communities like San Francisco, the photos were more explicitly sexual (and would probably have been considered "offensive" by other communities of readers).

An analysis of the early rhetoric of AIDS illustrates how discourse reflects the mores of the scientific community. Carol Reeves studied the rhetoric of three reports on AIDS. She contested Merton's assertion that a phenomenon should be established before it is explained. AIDS was not easy to "establish" because of the implications surrounding it and the little that was known about it in its early years. Some members of the gay community believed that measures like closing the bathhouses were illegal violations of privacy. Because of the high risk and high rate of virus transmission, the amount of suffering, and the need to define the risk groups and risks, explaining came before establishing. Early rhetoric established AIDS as a new medical mystery (in order to persuade the medical community that it was worthy of further study). This rhetoric emphasized the "tragic course" of AIDS and science's failure to treat the disease. These were strategies which appealed to medical and science communities and established a "technical" (as opposed to popular) rhetoric of AIDS.

Seidel's study of the rhetoric used in AIDS education pamphlets in Uganda reflects how discourse functions in a cultural, political, and religious context. Uganda has an official AIDS agency, the AIDS Campaign Programme. But because of historically corrupt governments and civil wars, the country relies heavily on nongovernmental agencies that are primarily run by churches. The ACP AIDS brochures maintain a western scientific approach: "What everybody needs to know about 'Slim' disease, AIDS. Love carefully: Learn the facts to protect yourself and those you love. Health Education Division/Ministry of Health" (Seidel 69) By contrast, the Christian brochures recommend compassion and appropriate Christian behavior: "Love Faithfully: Protect those you love, yourself, and society. Learn real facts. Respect God's law. Uganda Catholic Medical Bureau/Catholic Secretariat" (Seidel 68).

Each agency must carefully construct its AIDS awareness message in a way that will reach those who are at risk. But the ideology behind a particular rhetoric may exclude or oppress those who need information and resources. While most people accept "science" as a reliable source of information about AIDS, it does not have all the answers, and it can, in fact, silence or distort the speech and culture of some minority communities. Patton states, "Knowledge about surviving with a chronic illness, and about reinventing sexual pleasures in a disaster zone, about finding the courage to transcend the narrowly defined roles of the AIDS service industry—these knowledges are either pushed to the margins of scientific knowledge, or are re-written as scientific data about the odds of survival or aggregate behavior change" (53). These "knowledges" are, in fact, the more constructive dimensions of AIDS. They are often based in creative grassroots education projects that encourage speaking out— and of character. Whenever multiple discourse communities exist (or coexist), the problem emerges of how to make various voices heard and acknowledged. I agree with Treichler, who states that we must insist that many voices contribute to the construction of official definitions of AIDS (69). This insistence leads us to deal with layers of discourse, which we must patiently hear, sort out, and place in perspective.

Lee Edelman points out that politics and AIDS are inseparable: They cannot be disentangled from their linguistic and rhetorical implications. A close analysis of a single symbol in AIDS discourse reveals the many layers of meaning packed into the Silence=Death slogan. In his analysis, Edelman suggests the interaction of discourse, defense, and disease. AIDS attacks the body's defense system, and once it does, science cannot provide a defense. The West itself, says Edelman in "The Mirror and the Tank," is trying to defend itself against the intolerance of the dominant culture. And even science and political institutions are defending their prestige.

The Silence=Death slogan appeals to these defensive properties inherent in the discourse(s) of AIDS. In "The Plague of Discourse," Edelman formulates and reconfigures the equation as Discourse=Defense. Silence=Death, therefore, calls for the production of discourse, or text "as a mode of defense against the opportunism of medical and legislative responses to the epidemic. But what can be said beyond the need to speak? What discourse can this call to discourse desire? Just what is the discourse of defense that will immunize the gay body politic against the opportunistic infections of the demagogic rhetoric?" (299).

Edelman concludes by condemning any discourse on AIDS that appropriates AIDS for its own purposes. He warns that we must be wary of the "temptations of the literal for discourse, alas, is the only defense with which we can counteract discourse, and there is no available discourse on AIDS that is not itself diseased" (304).

Several years ago when I conducted a writing group for people with

HIV as part of my dissertation research, I experienced the difficulty of trying to enter the HIV community. As much as I tried to claim that I was both observing and participating in the AIDS community, I had to acknowledge the constraints of my viewpoint. As I positioned myself within the larger social framework, I took inventory of the different discourse communities to which I belong: I am female (and feminist), white, middle class, lesbian. Perhaps the most obvious fact to mention is that I did not have AIDS, yet I was proposing to conduct an ethnography of those who did. I really didn't know what it was like to have AIDS. I have never experienced night sweats, chronic diarrhea, or the plummeting of my immune system. I was not part of the "we" which constitutes an HIV/AIDS membership club. Patti Lather similarly explores her position as a researcher of women living with HIV/AIDS. She was careful not to position herself as an expert, "but rather as witness . . . giving testimony to what is happening to these women" (1). Lather points out the complexity of the inside/outside dichotomy. "But where is the outside of this pandemic?" she writes. "Who is the we/they?" (24). She cites the master's thesis of Francisco Ibanez-Carrasco: "Rather than binaries, he posits an HIV continuum where, culturally speaking, everyone is at risk and we are all involved because sexuality is a collective phenomenon" (23).

I had to adjust my position. I felt like I was a "guest" in a different landscape, and certain rules of protocol applied. Just as any guest may learn from an occasional social gaffe, I learned and gradually formulated a set of rules that allowed me to successfully traverse several discourse communities. These included communities of people with HIV/AIDS, healthcare workers, and academic "experts." My rules included being aware of the different communities being visited, the various languages spoken, and the customs respected; not assuming to speak for everyone with AIDS; presenting the people in the study with utmost care; and giving something back to the people who were the "subjects."

Therefore, I acknowledge my own appropriation of AIDS discourse. What are the symptoms of my "disabled" discourse? My discourse reflects my middle-class background and culture. I perceive a fractured view of AIDS discourse, which I attempt to "fix" or restore to wholeness. The taxonomy I propose reflects my vocation as a teacher and my belief that awareness and education lead to power and empowerment.

AIDS the Divider

The stigmatization of AIDS patients is divisive and painful. "The illness flushes out an identity that might have remained hidden from neighbor, job mates, family, and friends," Sontag states (113). According to Bertram Schaffner, writing from a clinical standpoint, diagnosis carries a disclosure of a person's lifestyle, similar to Hawthorne's scarlet letter. People with AIDS may experience feelings of guilt for their homosexuality or drug use (or other "shameful" condition). In addition to stigmatization, people with AIDS often deal with strange forms of illness. They may receive a confused diagnosis by doctors who have never treated AIDS before, and in many states people with AIDS may find it hard to obtain a hospital bed.

People with AIDS and their caretakers and support system may experience social isolation, displaced anger, denial of emotional impact, and overall helplessness. The discourse of AIDS the Divider underscores difference. While cancer victims are usually "innocent," people with AIDS are "clearly guilty" according to Michael Bronski. Sontag writes that "the unsafe behavior that produces AIDS is judged to be more than just weakness. It is indulgence, delinquency—addictions to chemicals that are illegal and to sex regarded as deviant" (113). Indeed, AIDS is a disease of the "other." "Other" now includes black foreigners, such as the influx of Haitians and Cubans across U.S. borders; patients who contracted AIDS from a mysterious Florida dentist; and Magic Johnson, the world-famous basketball player who is now also known for his sexual promiscuity and subsequent HIV-positive status.

AIDS divides people and makes the "other" visible. Elisabeth Kübler-Ross, renowned scholar on death and dying, states that AIDS is our biggest sociopolitical issue, becoming "a dividing line of religious groups, a battleground for medical researchers, and the biggest demonstration of man's inhumanity to man" (4). Sontag notes that AIDS marked a turning point in attitudes toward medicine and illness, "as well as toward sexuality and catastrophe" (160). Members of the political right wing have used AIDS to condemn homosexuality, and violence against gays has increased. Yet prejudice may affect anyone with AIDS and not just gay men.

Division also occurs within the heterosexual community. People with HIV find themselves estranged from family and friends. Insurance policies may limit or even prohibit health care. In areas with predominantly gay AIDS populations, groups may be administered by gays and geared toward the needs of the gay community. Straight people may feel their needs are not adequately addressed. Minority and female populations are the fastest growing; these groups have traditionally been marginalized. Although funding agencies are taking into consideration these demographic changes, it may take time to meet the needs of all people with AIDS.

But there may be a positive outcome to this division or at least acknowledgment of division. By becoming aware of and examining the "otherness" of AIDS, we see the parts of ourselves that we are missing.

In the context of health care for people with AIDS, support groups and friendships take the place of biological family support. A group may consist of a range of people including the parent of a child with AIDS or a spouse (either gay or straight). People may be tied to the community of drug users or the community of hemophiliacs; they may be young or old. Differences such as sexual orientation, race, and religion are ideally overlooked in the larger effort to deal with AIDS. Economic and class differences are harder to ignore; questions remain over access to medical care and privilege. Still, a greater compassion results as we become more attuned to the commonalities shared by people with AIDS.

AIDS the Reformer

Within the gay community, many changes have occurred in the past twenty years in response to the epidemic. These changes occurred at social as well as psychological levels. Initially, AIDS most seriously affected densely populated cities with large numbers of homosexual males. Studies by the Centers for Disease Control revealed that the virus was passed through sex at bathhouses in New York and San Francisco, and that multiple sexual contacts quickly spread AIDS. As gay men saw increasing numbers of deaths in their communities, they began to change their behavior, have fewer sexual partners, and partake in "safe sex." According to Shilts, a "toned-down" gay lifestyle began as early as 1983 as a vogue, and it became a trend. It eventually turned into "a full-scale sociological phenomenon" (377).

Shilts states that psychologists studying the gay community compared the feelings surrounding the epidemic to those feelings surrounding a midlife crisis. This period marks redefinition for an individual. As friends begin to die, individuals accept their own mortality. Shilts comments, "The gay community's confused response marked the start of its own collective redefinition, a process that, for all its early silliness, would become one of the more profound effects of the AIDS epidemic in the coming years" (378).

He concludes that the gay movement shifted from self-exploration (and self-alienation) to an outward and politically focused movement. In the wake of so much death and grief, the gay community responded by publicizing death. Creative production surrounding AIDS proliferated. The AIDS quilt was the first large-scale memorial to death by AIDS. Now art exhibits and productions about AIDS are widespread. Award-winning performances about AIDS include Broadway's *Angels in America* and *A Silver Lake Life,* the video account of a gay couple's deaths. Hundreds of public figures have "come out" or spoken out in support of AIDS research, protection, and legislation. In some ways, AIDS has forced communities to see their divisions and make changes.

The discourse of AIDS the Reformer is mainly accessed by those within the AIDS community. This voice urges action and change. When a call for reform comes from outside the community, one must consider the source. It may be identified as repressive, as an invasion of privacy (as in bathhouse closures), or as downright fascism (as in the case of right-wing calls to quarantine people with AIDS). Examples of effective discourse are numerous. One example is that of the late Michael Callen, a musician and writer who blended his message with rabble-rousing and wit. Sometimes these "reformers" receive criticism from within the community, as in the case of writer Larry Kramer, who was the bearer of unpopular warnings early in the epidemic.

AIDS the Empowerer

"Individual empowerment" was a term apparent in much literature about treatment of AIDS—and treatment of many chronic illnesses, for that matter. Unfortunately, the term has become something of a "buzz word." It is therefore necessary to approach the term, and the discourse surrounding it, from the purview of several fields.

People with AIDS experience loss of control: control of their bodies and often their lives. People in such situations have different ways of coping with uncertainty, ranging from constructing theories of denial to developing "normative frameworks that make their situation comprehensible" (Weitz 78). In 1979, Norman Cousins published *Anatomy of an Illness,* which documents how he took responsibility for healing himself of a serious illness. The work has parallels and implications for those involved with AIDS. Cousins states that illness is an interaction between mind and body. Everyone, according to Cousins, must accept responsibility for recovering from a disease or dealing with a disability. Similar to a cure, Cousins writes, "rehabilitation implies participation of the mind as well as of the body, integrated through volition for a creative process of adaptive change" (23). A sense of purpose, along with a will to live, are also crucial qualities for survival, as are peace of mind and acceptance.

When asked how people with AIDS could reach acceptance and peace, Kübler-Ross said that their situation was the same as that of other terminally ill people who must "receive and give themselves enough permission to express their anguish and tears, their sense of impotence against a vicious killer virus and against a society that discriminates and judges" (10). Kübler-Ross elaborated that this would entail an adequate support system, with friends who will listen. One person with AIDS told her, "My most important need right now is to communicate. Sometimes words don't really seem effective and I need not be afraid of today, or at least I need to know that I can make it through the day. Just today I need rest, peace, and quiet" (175).

When Kübler-Ross first began working with AIDS patients, she compared a collective process of acknowledgment with the process individuals undergo in grief work. These stages proceed from denial of AIDS, to anger (which may manifest as passive-aggressive hostility), bargaining (changing sexual behavior in return for another chance), depression, and acceptance. People with AIDS must confront their own mortality, often in the prime of their lives, and may go through the same life review process that senior citizens engage in, which is described by psychologist Robert Butler. Becoming involved in this process can be empowering as individuals become more aware of who they are and their strengths and weaknesses.

AIDS the Educator

Many people with AIDS reach a point where they want to speak out and educate others. This might require "coming out" for some people. Others challenge the idea that AIDS is a punishment for sin; many people want to take a public stance and teach others. Dellamora states that the way forward for people with AIDS is to "re-engage with the lives and works of others" (99).

An Ann Arbor activist, whom I will call Hank, now devotes his life to educating others about AIDS. He speaks frequently at schools, religious groups, and organizations and works with his own friends who are ill. Hank was a medical student in Iowa when he had a one-night stand twelve years ago. He went on to practice medicine until he tested positive for AIDS.

"As a doctor, I made lots of money," he said. "When I left medicine, I sold towels for a while. Then I worked as a social worker for an AIDS organization in Chicago. The pay was terrible—and I was happier than I'd ever been in my life." Like many people who face their own mortality because of a fatal illness or accident, Hank was forced to reprioritize his goals. He learned to follow only those he felt were most productive.

In John Weir's memoir about his work with a writing group for people with AIDS, he writes, "AIDS has given me what little wisdom I think I possess; it is the difference between my childhood and the rest of my life" (22). Weir was twenty-six when he facilitated the group, and he watched each of the twelve members die over the course of two years. He described each member of the group and his own observations about the cultures they came from and their style of coping (two men fell in love and got married; one man committed suicide; one man went to Italy wearing shorts, "even though he had lesions all over his legs, and educated an entire Italian town about AIDS"). "I cannot talk about myself without getting around to AIDS," Weir concludes. "It has profoundly affected my sense of New York City, of friendship, of death (which I never thought about before), of gayness, of sex; really of just about everything" (22).

Many people with AIDS have shown great heroism and have taught others about death. A participant of a writing group in Los Angeles reflected:

> This has allowed us to—or me anyway—to look at the aspects of my life. Many people go through—become 60, 70, 80 years old and they never look, don't want to look . . . God I hate people who say, AIDS has given me life you know, but it's true anyway, I mean, but just to have that—there's a sense of advantage that we do. I would not have done this. I could be 80 years old, dying of cancer or heart disease or emphysema or whatever, and I would not have traced back over my life. I would have preferred just to forget it, the way so many normal people do. (Fleming)

AIDS the Educator functions for people within the community and for people outside. People with AIDS are needed to teach others. These educators, in effect, help keep down the number of new members of the community, while trying to make others more sensitive to those who have AIDS.

Viewing AIDS from these four stances seems useful to me based on background reading and personal experience. Division, reform, empowerment, and education are emerging (and interweaving) themes in the discourse of AIDS. This framework is designed to be accessible to members of different discourse communities, including people with AIDS (or HIV), health care workers, and scholars. The Divider tears apart a community and an individual. The "reader" learns to recognize the rhetoric of division embedded in the surrounding discourse. The Reformer acts to remedy the division, but the discourse here must be carefully scrutinized in order to locate the agency of reform. The Empowerer is based in an active posture as it aims to give power back to the individual or community. The Educator is an outward-looking view of AIDS; AIDS may teach people about themselves, but also teach others about AIDS (and how to avoid it).

More than just a physical description and medical history, I have suggested a framework or taxonomy for the reader to reexamine the "disability" of AIDS. This new taxonomy is composed of the language, metaphor, social context, and politics of AIDS—components that greatly affect not only our understanding of the disease but also how we react and act in response. This construction of AIDS is based on how we use language to talk or write about AIDS. If we want to understand AIDS, we must examine this discourse before incorporating it into our own. This type of approach leads to a sensitive view of other disabilities—in their full rhetorical and contextual complexity.

Works Cited

Bronski, Michael. "War Culture: War, Language, Rape, and AIDS." Cleaver and Myers 209–217.

Bruffee, Ken. "Collaborative Learning and the 'Conversation of Mankind.'" *College English* 46 (1984): 635–52.

Butler, Robert. "The Life Review: An Interpretation of Reminiscence in the Aged." *Psychiatry* 26 (1963): 65–76.

Butters, Ronald, John Clum, and Michael Moon. *Displacing Homophobia: Gay Male Perspectives in Literature and Culture.* Durham, NC: Duke UP, 1989.

Cleaver, Richard, and Patricia Myers, eds. *A Certain Terror: Heterosexism, Militarism, Violence, and Change.* Chicago: American Friends Service Committee, 1993.

Cousins, Norman. *Anatomy of an Illness.* New York: Bantam Books, 1979.

Crimp, Douglas, and Leo Bersani, eds. *AIDS: Analysis/Cultural Activism.* Cambridge: MIT UP, 1988.

Dellamora, Richard. "Apocalyptic Utterance in Edmund White's 'An Oracle.'" Murphy and Poirier 98–116.

Edelman, Lee. "The Mirror and the Tank: 'AIDS,' Subjectivity, and the Rhetoric of Activism." Murphy and Poirier 9–38.

———. "The Plague of Discourse: Politics, Literary Theory, and AIDS." Butters, Clum, and Moon 289–306.

Fleming, Anne Taylor. "People with AIDS Who Write." Transcript of essay on *MacNeil/Lehrer Newshour.* WNET New York: 12 Oct. 1994.

Gilman, Sander, L. *Disease and Representation: Images of Illness from Madness to AIDS.* Ithaca: Cornell UP, 1988.

Haraway, Donna. "A Manifesto for Cyborgs: Science, Technology, and Socialist Feminism in the 1980s." *Socialist Review* 80 (1985): 65–108.

Ibanez-Carrasco, Francisco. "An Ethnographic Cross-Cultural Exploration of the Translations Between the Official Safe Sex Discourse and Lived Experience of Men Who Have Sex with Men." Master's thesis, Simon Frazer University, 1993.

Kinneavy, James. *A Theory of Discourse.* Englewood Cliffs, NJ: Prentice Hall, 1971.

Kir-Stimon, William, ed. *Psychotherapy and the Memorable Patient.* Los Angeles: Haworth Press, 1986.

Kübler-Ross, Elisabeth. *AIDS: The Ultimate Challenge.* New York: Collier Books, 1987.

Lather, Patti. "Validity After Poststructuralism: On (Not) Writing About the Lives of Women with HIV/AIDS." Paper delivered at AERA, New Orleans, Apr. 1994.

Murphy, Timothy. "Testimony." Murphy and Poirier 306–20.

Murphy, Timothy, and Suzanne Poirier, eds. *Writing AIDS: Gay Literature, Language, and Analysis.* New York: Columbia UP, 1993.

Neil, Ruth. "Watson's Theory of Caring in Nursing: The Rainbow of and for People Living with AIDS." Parker 277–88.

Parker, M. E. *Nursing Theories in Practice.* New York: National League for Nursing, 1990.

Patton, Cindy. *Inventing AIDS*. New York: Routledge, 1990.

Reeves, Carol. "Establishing a Phenomenon: The Rhetoric of Early Medical Reports on Aids." *Written Communication* 7.3 (1990): 393–416.

Robinson, Jay. *Conversations on the Written Word*. Portsmouth, NH: Boynton/Cook, Heinemann, 1990.

Schaffner, Bertram. "Reactions of Medical Personnel and Intimates to Persons with AIDS." Kir-Stimon 67–80.

Seidel, Gill. "'Thank God I Said No to AIDS': On the Changing Discourse of AIDS in Uganda." *Discourse and Society* 1.1 (1990): 61–84.

Sherry, Michael. "The Language of War in AIDS Discourse." Murphy and Poirier 39–53.

Shilts, Randy. *And the Band Played On: Politics, People, and the AIDS Crisis*. New York: Penguin Books, 1987.

Sontag, Susan. *AIDS and Its Metaphors*. New York: Doubleday, 1988.

Treichler, Paula A. "AIDS, Homophobia, and Biomedical Discourse: An Epidemic of Signification." Crimp and Bersani 31–70.

Weir, John. "AIDS Stories." *Harper's* 273 (1985): 22.

Weitz, Rose. *Living with AIDS*. New Brunswick: Rutgers UP, 1991.

White, James Boyd. *When Words Lose Their Meaning*. Chicago: U Chicago P, 1984.

13

Gutting the Golden Goose: Disability in Grimms' Fairy Tales
Beth Franks

"Disability imagery abounds" in the fields of "literature, linguistics, philosophy, art, aesthetics and literary criticism," and "yet because it is not analyzed, it remains as background, seemingly of little consequence" (Linton 110). Disability as background has provided a setting for the actions of others, an atmospheric backdrop, an unchanging horizon—one that can be overlooked or ignored. It has remained stable for so long that its background status is accepted as a universal truth rather than questioned as a cultural perspective. Recently, however, the Western (and predominantly medical) construction of disability has been challenged. With the advent of the Americans with Disabilities Act, the move to include all children in public education, and the creation of new fields such as disability studies, disability has destabilized. It is now fluid and mutable, no longer easily disregarded or dismissed.

As part of the reconsideration of disability, an examination of its place in folk literature is timely. Money observes, "Folk wisdom penetrates the idiom of our everyday language. We assimilate its . . . meanings, make them our own, and then, through failing to recognize what we are doing, may put them to our own use" (15). Images from the Grimms' fairy tales permeate our thinking, providing us with archetypes that augment and explain our experience. We kiss frogs, climb glass mountains, fight dragons, and, according to Thomson, attempt to conform to the accepted version of normal "in the same way that Cinderella's stepsisters attempted to squeeze their feet into her glass slipper" (*Extraordinary Bodies* 8).

Biklen and Bogdan suggest that people with disabilities are portrayed in classical literature in ten standard ways. Each of the ten themes they identify reflect highly negative and stereotyping images, ones which imply the problems attendant to disability are individual rather than cultural. Briefly, disabled people are characterized as pathetic, sinister, laughable, nonsexual, and incapable of full participation. They are burdens, victims, and their own worst enemies—or conversely they have a tendency to develop unusual compensatory talents. And they "are frequently thrown into the plot solely for the purpose of adding a little color" (Bogdan and Knoll 472). Linton identifies another stereotype, that of disabled people "as childlike, even infantlike, acting on primary drives rather than engaging in purposeful behavior" (96). Do the Grimms' household tales also stereotype disability, compromising it as lesson, metaphor, and atmosphere? Are characters with disabilities predominantly background players? If not background, are they villains whose disabled stigma add an aside on the perils of nonconformity?[1]

When I first approached the task of analyzing the presence and meaning of disability in folk and fairy tales, I found myself sympathizing with those characters who were faced with impossibly large tasks: spinning a room full of straw into gold or picking up ten sacks of millet seed that had been scattered on the ground. The body of folk literature is vast. Could an analysis be both manageable and meaningful? I needed a large enough sample to answer the above questions and a small enough number of tales to make the task possible. I chose, therefore, to limit this study to the first hundred tales in *The Complete Grimm's Fairy Tales*. I further narrowed the sample by excluding all animal tales, for example, "The Cat and the Mouse in Partnership" and "The Bremen Town Musicians." This left a total of eighty-five tales to examine.

My first question, that of the presence or absence of disability, was quickly answered. Disability was present in nearly half the tales in which human characters played major roles. (See the appendix for a list of these tales.)

Mute Maidens and Schizophrenic Stepmothers: Description or Label

Fairy tales stand in a curious position in the world of literature. Based upon an oral tradition that highlights the interaction between teller and audience, the language of the tales, the narrative sequences, even the gender of the characters is subject to change. For a five-year-old boy, Little Red Cap can be more effective as a boy than a girl. Grandmother can become grandfather, the wolf a strange man who offers Little Red Cap a ride in his car, the huntsman a helpful animal. But these tales are now read rather than told, written rather than spoken. How important, therefore, is a description of "lame" or "simple" to both the tale itself and the picture of disability that the tales convey?

On the one hand, attaching too great a weight to a description in one version distorts the analysis, since there are thousands of examples of the most popular tales. Should I use "a version written down in the 9th century" (Rooth 136) or the film *Pretty Woman?* Which particular account should be selected for analysis, and once selected, how much weight should a single descriptive adjective carry? On the other hand, the Grimms' fairy tales, the source of many of our "cultural icons," are uniquely adjective bare. There are princesses, a few beautiful and a few with skin "as white as snow," but that constitutes the whole of the descriptive variation one encounters. Dwarfs are dwarfs, and giants are giants, their presence only infrequently augmented by adjectives. Thus when the reader encounters verbal illustrations such as "withered" leg or "walked with a cane," the description takes on additional meaning. But what is that meaning? I had to try to find a path through the thorns that would present information that another scholar could build upon and that would help uncover the subtext about disability that these tales bear.

In attempting to expose the multilayered messages that disability carries, I first had to face the problem of how to work with the material. Beginning with a "head count" would establish the presence of disability for any skeptic who doubts it (and whenever I describe my work I am met with incredulity). Furthermore, as Bogdan and Knoll point out, the way disability is designated "affects the meaning, the process, and the understanding generated" (464). Although establishing categories reduces the sheer weight of information one faces, the categories themselves, with their attendant labels, are bound to influence the outcome. In fact, categorical thinking in itself is a trap. If I used categories, I was likely to find the conditions they described. Thus, although interesting patterns might emerge, I was conscious of the possibility of exacerbating the very problem I was attempting to address.

The only study examining the intersection of disability and folklore that I have been able to locate approaches the material from a medical perspective. Susan Schoon Eberly examined a large body of European stories, linking descriptions of fey beings with medical categories. If my current study was to connect to Eberly's work, then medical categories made sense, yet these categories also reflected a way of thinking that had oppressed and dominated the disabled community for years.

I chose to use a broad approach partially basing my organization on Linton's description of disability studies scholarship. According to Linton, "disability has become a more capacious category, incorporating people with a range of physical, emotional, sensory, and cognitive conditions" (12). To these four conditions I added communication difficulties and a final category in which more than one condition was present. In table 13.1, I have listed each condition and the number of times it occurs. In some tales, more than one character had a disabling condition; this brought the number of characters with disabilities to forty-five.

Table 13.1. Frequency of Six Conditions

Condition	Frequency
Cognitive	9
Communicative	3
Multiple	3
Sensory	4
Physical	22
Emotional	4

In most cases, it was a simple matter to match a description to a category. I identified the simple son (often described as foolish or even stupid) as having a cognitive condition. Maidens, communicating through silence rather than speech (and only maidens are mute), dwarfs were electively mute. The witch in "Hansel and Gretel" was both lame and short of sight. The prince, tumbling off Rapunzel's tower, blinded himself in the process. Giants, dwarfs, characters with withered limbs, or those who walked with a limp were marked by a physical difference. The ease with which the words, whether adjectives or nouns, suggested a quasi-medical or educational category was alarming.

Emotional conditions that depend primarily on behavior rather than single word descriptions were somewhat more elusive. Gambling Hansel gambles away all his possessions; today we label this kind of behavior as addictive. Clever Elsie obsessively imagines one disaster after another and, losing all sense of her own identity, disappears from her village. A stepmother ("The Juniper Tree") pushes, slaps, and cuffs her stepson around their house. Believing herself to have been entered by the Devil, she kills her stepson, makes him into a black pudding, and serves him to his father for dinner. The stepmother's beliefs and her ensuing behaviors would bring a current diagnosis of schizophrenia.

In "The Elves" a changeling is substituted for a human child. The change is abrupt, and the new child has "fixed staring eyes." Eberly suggests that the exchange of a fairy child for a normal child might be a folk interpretation of a child's failure to thrive. From this I infer that a child's strange behaviors might be explained by labeling her as a stranger (or fairy child) who had been left in the "normal" child's place. Such an interpretation lends strong support to Thomson's thesis that "the tyranny of the norm makes extraordinary bodies into freakish bodies, which both compel and repel the normate sensibility" (*Extraordinary Bodies* 130). Fairy children both attract and repel just as fairy land and its denizens attract and repel. The designation "fairy child" may have contained the emotional ambiguity that parents felt toward their different child.

Make Mine Male: Gender Distribution

Of the forty-five characters with a disability, almost 75 percent were male. This skewed distribution occurred predominately in two conditions: physical (nineteen males to three females) and cognitive (nine males to one female). The large category of physical conditions fell into two subcategories: differences in stature (dwarfs, elves, and giants) and impairments of limbs. I found the type of condition (stature or limb) to be closely related to the character's gender. In my sample, there were no female dwarfs or giants—clearly not representative of human variety.

Why is disability in fairy tales a gendered trait? There are a number of possible answers, none of them carrying a positive message. The world of the fairy tale prizes women as part of the reward (the princess—the crown—the kingdom). The lack of equal distribution of disability between men and women suggests that addition of a disability would detract from the princess's value, thus making the quest more questionable. Second, women in fairy tales are lower in status than their male counterparts. If disability also confers a low status, although such is not always the case according to Thomson *(Extraordinary Bodies)* and Hahn,[2] wedding the two would be redundant. A third possibility, at least in the case of cognitive impairment, is that the symptoms of mild impairment share a common ground with characteristics expected of normal women and thus are interpreted as normal. Women are supposed to be simple, incompetent, and helpless; actual simplicity or helplessness, therefore, might be considered role-consistent behavior. Dora, in Dickens's *David Copperfield,* provides a classic example of cognitive impairment masked as simplicity for which she is beloved.

Finally, the gendered distribution in fairy tales may be a mere consequence of the focus of the plot, which tends to be on male characters and their struggles. Winning through adversity is more admirable if the task is difficult. The presence of disability might act as an additional challenge. Just as acceptance is dependent upon initial rejection, becoming able is predicated upon initial disability.

Two Spinning Tales

I examined two tales, very similar in their plots, for the way disability was described and used. "Rumpelstiltskin" and "The Three Spinners" both feature maidens who cannot or will not perform the spinning tasks their parents expect of them. In "Rumpelstiltskin" a miller brags to the king that his daughter can spin gold from straw. In "The Three Spinners" a mother tells the queen that she has to beat her daughter to keep her from spinning. In both cases, the girls cannot or will not do the tasks their parents expect of them. To qualify for queenhood, each girl is given three rooms filled with straw/flax to be spun into gold/cloth. Each girl collapses in tears. Enter the characters with disabilities.

The well-known tale "Rumpelstiltskin" features a dwarf, who allows himself to be bested by a miller's daughter. At the end of the tale our sympathies are with the girl, though throughout the tale Rumpelstiltskin himself has acted honorably and with kindness. I wonder why we accept Rumpelstiltskin's defeat as just and proper.

Rumpelstiltskin, described as "a little man" and a "manikin," first enters, speaking kindly to the girl and willingly spins two rooms of straw into gold in exchange for a necklace and a ring. The king, clearly a greedy type, wants a third room full of gold, and the miller's daughter promises their first child to Rumpelstiltskin in exchange for more spinning. Thus far the manikin has acted benevolently and, indeed, he continues to do so. When he claims the child, the queen tries to fob him off with gold, although he can spin gold for himself. Taking pity on her, he gives her three more chances to keep her child, thus outsmarting himself. His only crime, as far as I can see, is to accept defeat with ill grace; he becomes so enraged he tears himself in two.

In the tale of "The Three Spinners," magical spinners also rescue a girl from her impossible task. Each of these spinners has been physically changed by spinning, the first sporting a "broad flat foot," the second a "great underlip," and the third a "broad thumb." The only request the spinning fairies ask in exchange for their work is to be invited to the girl's wedding as her aunts. This girl keeps her bargain and in doing so is further rewarded. When the prince sees the "aunts," he asks in horror how they became so "odious." Learning that it was brought about by spinning, he forbids his bride to ever touch a spinning wheel again.

In both stories the characters with a disability help the heroine. In one story the character with a disability is both helper and villain, in the other purely a helper. In one story the character with a disability kills himself; in the other the characters are accepted (invited to a wedding), although it is clear that their appearance is unacceptable. The difference seems to lie in Rumpelstiltskin's aspirations: to have a human child (be human himself). The three spinners know their place: they enjoy life on the fringes as aunts. As long as they remain in a marginal position, they are neither threatening nor threatened. As soon as disability presumes to normalcy, it must be ripped in two.

Not Just a Pretty Face

Fairy tales tend to be long on action and short on description. The miller's daughter is described as beautiful, but beyond this we know little of her. We know even less about the other girl. Thus, when descriptions such as "lame," "walked with a limp," and "no bigger than a thumb" appear, they carry more weight than they might in a more adjective-rich narrative. Biklen and Bogdan suggested ten stereotyping themes that disabled characters carry. Although it is tempting to use their model, it carries some of the same risks that medico-educational categories do, namely, one is bound to find what one is looking for. A cursory glance suggested that I could easily find examples of disability as laughable ("Clever Elsie"), as colorful ("Godfather Death"), and as sinister. This last category falls into a whole tradition of its own, with disability being not just descriptive but a signpost to a flawed character.

As description, disability is usually a negative marker. Phrases that use disability as metaphor do not contain positive messages (e.g., deaf to his pleas, crippled by her love, an idiotic thing to do, a withered sense of justice). Such descriptions are subtle comments on character, based upon the underlying assumption that a flawed physical appearance indicates a flawed morality. Vaudeville villains, portrayed as skulking, limping degenerates, dragged their diseased legs (and crippled morality) behind them. Mr. Hyde, Captain Hook, and Captain Ahab had moral characters that, like open wounds, stained their physical appearance. Marked by disability, hence morally flawed, hence marred by disability, they were caught in an endless loop of tautological reasoning that made perfect sense to their audiences.

The queen-turned-witch who plagues Snow White is indelibly impressed on our minds as stooped, wart-ridden, hump-backed, and dependent upon a walking stick, despite the fact that she has powers of magical transformation at her fingertips. When we picture her, she hobbles along supported by her cane, yet no cane appears in the Grimms' version of this story. Disney's visual rendition of fairy tales has fused disability and villainy (the witch) not to mention disability and mirth (the dwarfs). Although it does not excuse him, Disney was working within an accepted framework regarding disability. Broomsticks, canes, staffs, and staves can be found in some of the earliest illustrations of fairy tales.[3] And the practice of keeping dwarfs as jesters established another traditional view of disability that Disney built upon.

I wondered if the predominant message in the Grimms' tales that disability sent was a negative one. To answer this question, I examined the function that disability performs in the narrative by using an analytic model proposed by Vladimir Propp. Propp identified seven spheres of action. These correspond roughly to the roles a character plays, ranging from the familiar (hero, heroine, villain, and villainess) to those less familiar (dispatcher and donor). Propp's model was developed specifically for fairy tales and thus provided a useful vehicle for my analysis.

Characters with disabilities played all seven of Propp's roles, as can be seen in table 13.2. The most surprising outcome of the above analysis, however, was that almost three-quarters of the characters with a disability played positive roles (heroes, heroines, helpers, donors, and dispatchers).[4]

Table 13.2. Propp's Spheres of Action and Disability

Sphere	Characters
Villain/villainess	7
Donor of magical agent	2
Helper	9
Sought for person	3
Dispatcher	3
Hero/heroine	20
False hero/heroine	3

Trials, Tribulations, and Just Desserts

If the above is true, why does disability have such bad press? Is disability more than an occasionally used negative signpost? Rather than simply being attached to a good or evil character, disability itself may further the plot, punishing the evildoer, testing the hero or heroine, or taking the story in a new direction.

Disability as a test, trial, or temporary punishment occurs in five tales. In "The Six Swans," the heroine maintains complete silence for six years as she weaves six shirts from nettles. Her successful completion of the six years of silence brings about her brothers' freedom from enchantment. In the tale of Rapunzel, the prince climbs up Rapunzel's tower and is pushed by a witch into thorn bushes that blind him. Eventually Rapunzel finds him in the wilderness and restores his vision with her tears. Both the sister and the prince are restored to their original (able) state at the end of their disability sentence.

I discovered only one instance in which disability was used as a punishment. Doves blind Cinderella's selfish stepsisters[5]—a particularly horrible image, since doves are generally symbols of peace. Although both dramatic and gruesome, this act is hardly integral to the plot. (The Disney version certainly hasn't suffered financially from the omission.) The tale is easily recognized, whether or not the stepsisters are blinded. In the sample of the Grimms' tales I examined, the moral of the tale was underlined only once by punishing the villain or villainess through impairment.

Disability, functioning as trial and punishment, appears in only a fraction of the tales (see table 13.3). If quantity alone counts, fairy tales do not convey an overwhelmingly negative picture of the function of disability. In the Grimms' fairy tales, therefore, disability is neither the marker of the villain or villainess nor the moral donkey bearing the burden of retribution.

Table 13.3. Function of Disability

Function of Disability	Frequency
Punishment	1
Trial	5
Description	19
Reversal	14

Parables and Paradoxes

Although there is no question that disability may add interest, poignancy, or visual imagery, in almost half the stories, disability is primarily descriptive. Godfather Death (not a bad character) plays out his role whether his legs are withered or straight. The detail about his leg is not essential to his character or to the narrative. The size of the seven dwarfs (counted as one person) who care for Snow White is also incidental to the action of the story—except, of course, to Bruno Bettelheim, who sees everything in singularly sexual terms. Even though Hahn points out that Snow White would not have taken refuge with seven adult males unless they were small, they could, after all, have been seven friendly giants or seven furry bears without causing too great a dislocation of the battle between youth and age, gullibility and greed, simplicity and desire. In contrast, the witch in "Hansel and Gretel" walks with a limp and has poor vision. Because the witch's vision is impaired, Gretel is able to trick her into believing that Hansel is starving and, finally, to push her into the oven. The witch's poor vision aids the development of the plot; her limp does not.

In a number of the tales, the fortunes of the hero or heroine are reversed through disability. It is not the character him or herself who is responsible for the reversal but the disability itself. In each of these cases, disability is integral to the plot and provides the pivot upon which the plot turns. In "The Queen Bee" and "The Three Feathers," for example, it is the "stupidity" of the youngest son that allows him to see more clearly than others. Without simplicity of vision, the youngest son would not fulfill the tasks he sets out to accomplish, tasks that his clever and worldly wise brothers fail. Simpleton is perceptive (spotting a trapdoor where no one else had seen one), constructive, and courageous (he stands up to his brothers, not allowing them to destroy the various animals they encounter). We identify with and support Simpleton, who acts ethically and charitably. In fact, as the stories progress, Simpleton demonstrates other virtues. Persistent, he completes the requisite threefold challenge each tale presents. In contrast, his older brothers are stubborn men, nagging and "tormenting" their father. Simpleton's modesty and his eagerness to help and be helped (especially by other outcasts and animals) demonstrate his willingness to embrace variety and difference. The message his actions send is that he, and not his brothers, will make a good ruler because he recognizes the contributions everyone can make.

In the teachings of Zen, paradoxical stories or koans further the enlightenment of the student. Koans are stories in which contradiction can be resolved only through an intuitive grasp of a truth larger than the one seemingly presented. In both koan and fairy tale, the message of the tale hinges on an apparent contradiction. Most of the paradoxical Grimms' tales feature the wise fool who acts compassionately because of his simpler vision. The act of compassion, by someone who merits compassion, teaches the audience where true wisdom lies.

Filling in the Blanks

In alternate spring terms, I teach a liberal arts course entitled "Portrayal of Special Populations in Texts." As an introductory exercise, I require pairs of students to analyze ten Grimms' tales for the presence of disability. This exercise gives students the opportunity to practice content analysis on a well-defined body of work and compare their own findings with those of others. Enrollment is limited to thirty students, and the class is always full. The course is taught in a small, private liberal arts college; the students are predominantly white and middle to upper middle class. The majority of the students who enroll in the class are female; they are drawn from all academic disciplines with psychology and sociology majors dominating. Students range in age from nineteen to twenty-two.

In this course I play two roles: that of teacher and that of participant observer. Participant observation, a qualitative research method used extensively in the fields of sociology and anthropology, is a valuable tool in the study of folklore (Goldstein) as well as education. Bogdan and Biklen, educational researchers in the field of disability studies, state that "[w]hile people conducting qualitative research may develop a focus . . . they do not approach the research with specific questions to answer or hypotheses to test. They also are concerned with understanding behavior from the subject's own frame of reference" (2). Cochran-Smith and Lytle expand our understanding of qualitative research, making a distinction between research on teaching and teacher research. They argue for the practice of teacher research, or "systematic and intentional inquiry carried out by teachers" (7). Thus, the qualitative researcher or participant observer must walk a fine line, balancing between the open and the structured, allowing information to unfold naturally yet conducting her study in a way that leads to new understanding.

As a participant observer, I have become familiar with a pattern. Year after year, students express their surprise at the presence of disability in the Grimms' tales, never expecting it to be a feature, much less a focus. During the year in which I finished the study described above, I took my observation one step further and presented the analysis to students in a lecture illustrated with tables. Being interested in the effects of my presentation, I added a bonus question to a quiz I gave several weeks after the lecture. For an extra point, I asked students to describe how disability had been portrayed in the Grimms' tales. All the students responded to the question—after all, there was no penalty and there was the possibility of gaining an extra point.

Every student remembered how surprised she was to find disability present in fairy tales, but only one student remembered a positive character having a disability. One-quarter of the students remembered both positive and negative characters as having a disability, while three-quarters remembered disability being the marker of only a negative character.

How was I to understand my students' responses? In the lecture I had emphasized that disability was primarily a feature of characters who played positive roles and that it was used as a punishment in only one tale. While students had obviously remembered something from this part of the course, they did not take away the message I had expected. The following analysis is offered with the full realization that it is based on a phenomenon that was observed only once. My explanation is far from conclusive, but it does suggest a direction for further research.

Even when we note that positive characters have disabilities and that disability itself can be a positive presence, most people still remember it as acting in a negative fashion or being attached to characters who play negative roles. We remember messages that conform to our expectations and dismiss evidence to the contrary, even when that evidence is reasonably strong. Despite the association with heroes and heroines, my students remembered disability as being linked with villains and villainesses. Most students also remembered that disability functioned in a predominately negative way and cited the instance of disability punishing Cinderella's stepsisters. My students remembered the exception as the rule.

People with disabilities are rendered negatively visible (and invisible) by the very stigma that have already marginalized them. The visual cues that identify them as different also carry the cultural information that they are to be not-seen. Mothers tell children not to stare at someone with a disability. Behind a hand, an able-bodied person may whisper,

"Don't look now, but that woman only has one leg . . . or one arm . . . or a white cane." And consider the suggestion, the ultimate in invisibility, "Don't you agree they're better off dead?" In a feat worthy of a magician, the mind simultaneously erases people with disabilities from view and closes the gap that has been created.

The above study of the Grimms' tales supports Snyder's contention that disability rests on a "largely invisible legacy." Despite the obvious presence of disability in fairy tales, these stories do not immediately come to mind when we consider a literature of disability. Like the simple son, it comes in many guises. Yet almost as soon as we become aware of its presence, it eludes us. It is as if we were under a curious enchantment, recalling princes and princesses with ease, struggling to remember equally notable dwarfs, giants, simpletons, changelings, and those with limited access to voice, vision, and mobility. As Thomson points out, disabled bodies have become "enduring cultural icons that range from the cyclopic Polyphemus and the gigantic Goliath to werewolves and the seven adorable little dwarfs" (*Freakery* 1). And similar to religious icons, the presence and function of disability in fairy tales is unquestioned and unchallenged.

The Grimms' tales are not the source of the negative portrait of disability, nor can they be credited with actively perpetrating stereotypes. They are, if anything, more democratic in their handling of disability than our modern, disability-conscious society. And although characters who have a disability may be marginalized (the three spinners) or victimized (Rumpelstiltskin), these acts can stimulate concern rather than applause. The injustice of Rumpelstiltskin's fate "rattles," as Bly would say, in our unconscious, eventually forcing us to realize that it is we who have been inhuman.

The study of disability in the Grimms' fairy tales is something of an exercise in magic itself, as it seeks to make visible the invisible, give language to the unutterable, and make conscious the unconscious. The enchantment is cast by our culture, which paradoxically insists we stare with condemnation at those who do not conform and instructs us to look away from the spectacle. The clear vision of the simple son applies here as well as in the Grimms' tales, showing us that invisible attitudes limit progress as potently as visible barriers.

Appendix

Characters with Disabilities in Grimms' Fairy Tales

No.	Title	Disabling Condition	No. of Characters
3	Our Lady's Child	Communication	1
4	The Story of the Youth Who Went Forth	Cognitive	1
9	The Twelve Brothers	Communication	1
11	Brother and Sister	Sensory	1
12	Rapunzel	Sensory	1
13	The Three Little Men in the Wood	Physical	1
14	The Three Spinners	Physical	1
15	Hansel and Gretel	Multiple	1
20	The Valiant Little Tailor	Physical	1
21	Cinderella	Sensory	1
25	The Seven Ravens	Physical & Physical	2
31	The Girl Without Hands	Physical	1
32	Clever Hans	Cognitive	1
33	The Three Languages	Cognitive	1
34	Clever Elsie	Emotional	1
35	The Tailor in Heaven	Physical	1
37	Thumbling	Physical	1
39	The Elves	Physical & Emotional	2
44	Godfather Death	Physical & Sensory	2
45	Thumbling's Travels	Physical	1
47	The Juniper Tree	Emotional	1
49	The Six Swans	Communication	1
53	Little Snow-White	Physical	1
55	Rumpelstiltskin	Physical	1
57	The Golden Bird	Cognitive	1
59	Frederick and Catherine	Cognitive & Physical	2
62	The Queen Bee	Cognitive	1
63	The Three Feathers	Multiple	1
64	The Golden Goose	Cognitive	1
68	The Thief and His Master	Physical	1
78	Old Man and His Grandson	Multiple	1
82	Gambling Hansel	Emotional & Physical	2
83	Hans in Luck	Cognitive	1
90	The Young Giant	Physical	1
91	The Gnome	Physical & Cognitive	2
92	The King of the Golden Mountain	Physical	1
93	The Raven	Physical	1
97	The Water of Life	Physical	1
100	The Devil's Sooty Brother	Physical	1

In the chart above, each tale is numbered and listed as it appears in the Pantheon–Random House edition. In some cases the title has been shortened. Note that in some tales, more than one character has a disabling condition.

Notes

The pilot study for this work was published in the *Proceedings of the Society for Disability Studies* (1994) under the title "Disability and Fairy Tales: An Analysis."

1. In both her books, Thomson explores the use of the extraordinary to reinforce the normate's sense of normalcy. By displaying otherness (both in sideshows and in literature), the sense of "we" is heightened. The audience projects "cultural characteristics they themselves [disavow]" onto the person so displayed, thus furthering the distance between what was different (them) and what was the same (us) as well as sharpening the difference between what was acceptable and what was not (*Extraordinary Bodies* 55–56).

2. Hahn makes a strong case for the special status many of those with disabilities (especially court jesters) had during the Middle Ages. Thomson (*Extraordinary Bodies*) adds to this her own observations about "saints' stigmatic wounds, Oedipus's and Socrates's lameness, Tiresias's and Homer's blindness, and Philoctetes's wound [which] certainly seem[ed] to function as ennobling marks" (40).

3. Warner includes a number of illustrations from old fairy tale texts in her book, *From the Beast to the Blonde*. A notable example is a series of Mother Stork pictures dating from 1900 in which Mother Stork moves from a dependent position (pictured with a cane) to independent (standing without a cane) after she has been thrown out of her own home by her "thankless children" (232–33).

4. Since a character may operate in more than one sphere, a correspondence among character, sphere of action, and role does not always exist.

5. Cinderella's stepsisters may actually have a double disability since, as Harlan Hahn points out, they "disable themselves in order to enhance their attractiveness" (219).

Works Cited

Bettelheim, Bruno. *The Uses of Enchantment: The Meaning and Importance of Fairy Tales*. New York: Vintage, 1989.

Biklen, Douglas, and Robert Bogdan. "Media Portrayals of Disabled People: A Study in Stereotypes." *Interracial Books for Children Bulletin* 8 (1977): 4–9.

Bly, Robert. *A Little Book on the Human Shadow*. San Francisco: Harper, 1988.

Bogdan, Robert, and James Knoll. "The Sociology of Disability." *Exceptional Children and Youth: An Introduction*. 3rd ed. Ed. Thomas M. Skrtic and Edward L. Meyen. Denver: Love, 1988.

Cochran-Smith, Marilyn, and Susan L. Lytle, eds. *Inside Outside: Teacher Research and Knowledge*. New York: Teachers College P, 1993.

The Complete Grimm's Fairy Tales. New York: Random House, 1972.

Dickens, Charles. *David Copperfield*. New York: Bantam-Doubleday, 1995.

Eberly, Susan Schoon. "Fairies and the Folklore of Disability: Changelings, Hybrids, and the Solitary Fairy." *Folklore* 99 (1988): 58–77.

Goldstein, Kenneth S. *A Guide for Field Workers in Folklore*. Hatboro, PA: Folklore Associates, 1964.

Hahn, Harlan. "Can Disability Be Beautiful?" *Perspectives on Disability*. 2nd ed. Ed. Mark Nagler. Palo Alto, CA: Health Markets Research, 1993. 217–26.

Linton, Simi. *Claiming Disability: Knowledge and Identity*. New York: New York UP, 1998.

Money, John. "Paleodigms and Paleodigmatics: A New Theoretical Construct Applicable to Munchausen's Syndrome by Proxy, Child-Abuse Dwarfism, Paraphilias, Anorexia Nervosa, and Other Syndromes." *American Journal of Psychotherapy* 43.1 (1989): 15–24.

Propp, Vladimir. *Morphology of the Folktale*. 2nd ed. rev. Austin: U of Texas P, 1968.

Rooth, Anna Birgitta. "Tradition Areas in Eurasia." *Cinderella: A Casebook*. Ed. Alan Dundes. Madison: U of Wisconsin P, 1988. 129–47.

Snyder, Sharon L. "Narrative Prosthesis: Contextualizing Disability as Metaphor in the Humanities." Paper presented at the MLA's discussion group, Academics with Disabilities and Disability Studies in Literature and the Arts. San Diego, 1994.

Thomson, Rosemarie Garland. *Extraordinary Bodies: Figuring Physical Disability in American Culture and Literature*. New York: Columbia UP, 1997.

———, ed. *Freakery: Cultural Spectacles of the Extraordinary Body*. New York: New York UP, 1996.

Warner, Marina. *From the Beast to the Blonde: On Fairy Tales and Their Tellers*. 1994. New York: Noonday P, 1996.

Contributors

Index

Contributors

Ellen L. Barton is a professor in the Department of English at Wayne State University, where she teaches in the linguistics program and the composition program. "Textual Practices of Erasure: Representations of Disability and the Founding of the United Way" is drawn from a larger project, entitled "Discourses of Disability: Interactional and Textual Practices in the Social Construction of Disability." Papers from the project also have appeared in the journals *TEXT, College English, Discourse and Society, Discourse Studies, Works and Days,* and *Narrative Inquiry* and in the edited collections *Constructing Incompetence* and *Under Construction.*

Brenda Jo Brueggemann is an associate professor in the Department of English at the Ohio State University. She is a former cochair of the Modern Language Association Committee on Disability Issues in the Profession and a member of the Conference on College Composition and Communication Task Force on Disability. She is the author of *Lend Me Your Ear: Rhetorical Constructions of Deafness.* She is currently coediting the MLA Disability Studies collection expected in 2001.

G. Thomas Couser is a professor of English at Hofstra University. He has written three books on American life writing: *American Autobiography: The Prophetic Mode, Altered Egos: Authority in American Autobiography,* and *Recovering Bodies: Illness, Disability, and Life Writing.*

Nirmala Erevelles is an assistant professor in Educational Foundations, Leadership, and Technology at Auburn University. Her research interests are in disability studies, sociology of education, third world feminism, cultural studies, and qualitative research.

Beth Franks is an associate professor in the Department of Education at Hobart and William Smith Colleges, Geneva, New York. She contributes book reviews on a regular basis to the *Disability Studies Quarterly.* Her research interests include eating disorders, content analyses of texts, and the use of memoir in teaching. Her latest publication appeared in the *Wisconsin Academy Review.*

Martha Stoddard Holmes is an assistant professor of literature and writing studies at California State University–San Marcos. She moderates the DS-HUM (Disability Studies in the Humanities) listserv. She is an editor of the NYU

Medical School Literature, Arts, and Medicine database and a member of the executive committee of the MLA discussion group on disability studies. Her current book project is "Melodramatic Medicine: Dickens, Collins, and the Disability." A more extended treatment by the author of autobiographical texts of Victorians with physical disabilities appears in *Fictions of Affliction: Physical Disability in Victorian Culture,* forthcoming from the University of Michigan Press.

Hannah Joyner is an assistant professor of government and history at Gallaudet University and a Ph.D. candidate in history at the University of Pennsylvania. She is finishing her dissertation, "The 'Silent South': Growing Up Deaf in the Antebellum Southern States."

Miriamne Ara Krummel is a Ph.D candidate in the Department of English at Lehigh University and the 2000–2001 Helen Ann Mins Robbins Fellow at the University of Rochester. She is working on her dissertation, "Fables, Facts, and Fictions: Jewishness in the English Middle Ages." A commitment to cultural studies and marginalized authors informs both her scholarship and her teaching.

Cynthia Lewiecki-Wilson is a professor of English and affiliate of the women's studies program at Miami University. A member of MLA, SDS, and NCTE, she serves on the CCCC executive committee and is a former editorial board member of CCC. She has published in *CCC, TETYC,* and MLA collections. She is the author of *Writing Against the Family: Gender in Lawrence and Joyce* (Southern Illinois UP, 1994) and coauthor, with Jeff Sommers, of *From Community to College: Reading and Writing Across Diverse Contexts.* With James C. Wilson, she is the coauthor of "Constructing a Third Space: Disability Studies, the Teaching of English, and Institutional Transformation," forthcoming in *Enabling the Humanities: A Sourcebook for Disability Studies in Language and Literature.*

Deshae E. Lott is an assistant professor at the University of Illinois at Springfield, where she teaches early American literature and professional and technical writing. Her primary research interest—which has produced many conference presentations and publications in *Studia Mystica* and *Resources in American Literary Studies*—involves the intersections of literary works, social practices, and American religious cultures. She is also interested in disability studies (she has limb-girdle muscular dystrophy). She presented a version of the chapter "Going to Class with (Going to Clash with?) the Disabled Person" at the 1998 MLA conference.

Rod Michalko is an associate professor in the Department of Sociology and Anthropology at St. Francis Xavier University, Nova Scotia. He is the author of *The Mystery of the Eye and the Shadow of Blindness* and *The Two-in-One: Walking with Smokie, Walking with Blindness.*

Emily F. Nye is an associate professor of English at New Mexico Tech. She has published articles and book chapters on writing as healing, service learning, literacy, and technical communication. She has presented numerous papers at MLA, CCCC, and NCTE on rhetoric, literacy, and healing.

Catherine Prendergast is an assistant professor of English at the University of Illinois at Urbana-Champaign and editorial board member of *Written Communication*. In addition to her interests in mental disability, she is working on a book-length study of constructions of race in literary research. An article related to that study, "Race: The Absent Presence in Composition Studies," won the 1999 Richard Braddock Award for the best article on the teaching of writing to appear in CCC the previous year.

Tanya Titchkosky is an assistant professor of sociology at St. Francis Xavier University, Nova Scotia. She has written articles on disability and feminism and has recently completed a book manuscript, "Disability Stays: An Introduction to the Social Construction of Disability."

James C. Wilson, a professor in the Department of English and Comparative Literature at the University of Cincinnati, teaches professional writing and editing, medical and science writing, and American literature. He is a contributing editor to the *Heath Anthology of American Literature* (1998) and the author of *The Hawthorne and Melville Friendship: An Annotated Bibliography, Biographical and Critical Essays, and Correspondence Between the Two*. He has published articles in *ESQ*, *ATQ*, and the *Wilson Quarterly*. His work in disability studies includes "Making Disability Visible: How Disability Studies Might Transform the Medical and Science Writing Classroom" in *Technical Communication Quarterly* and, with Cynthia Lewiecki-Wilson, "Constructing a Third Space: Disability Studies, the Teaching of English, and Institutional Transformation," forthcoming in *Enabling the Humanities: A Sourcebook for Disability Studies in Language and Literature*.

Index